CANCER CARE FOR THE
WHOLE PATIENT

MEETING PSYCHOSOCIAL HEALTH NEEDS

Committee on Psychosocial Services to
Cancer Patients/Families in a Community Setting
Board on Health Care Services

Nancy E. Adler and Ann E. K. Page, *Editors*

INSTITUTE OF MEDICINE
OF THE NATIONAL ACADEMIES

THE NATIONAL ACADEMIES PRESS
Washington, D.C.
www.nap.edu

THE NATIONAL ACADEMIES PRESS   500 Fifth Street, N.W.   Washington, DC 20001

NOTICE: The project that is the subject of this report was approved by the Governing Board of the National Research Council, whose members are drawn from the councils of the National Academy of Sciences, the National Academy of Engineering, and the Institute of Medicine. The members of the committee responsible for the report were chosen for their special competences and with regard for appropriate balance.

This study was supported by Contract No. N01-OD-4-2139 between the National Academy of Sciences and the National Institutes of Health. Any opinions, findings, conclusions, or recommendations expressed in this publication are those of the author(s) and do not necessarily reflect the view of the organizations or agencies that provided support for this project.

Additional copies of this report are available from the National Academies Press, 500 Fifth Street, N.W., Lockbox 285, Washington, DC 20055; (800) 624-6242 or (202) 334-3313 (in the Washington metropolitan area); Internet, http://www.nap.edu.

Library of Congress Cataloging-in-Publication Data

Cancer care for the whole patient : meeting psychosocial health needs / Committee on Psychosocial Services to Cancer Patients / Families in a Community Setting, Board on Health Care Services ; Nancy E. Adler and Ann E.K. Page, editors.
    p. ; cm.
Includes bibliographical references and index.
ISBN 978-0-309-11107-2 (hardcover)
    1. Cancer—Patients—Care—United States. 2. Cancer—Patients—Services for—United States. 3. Cancer—Social aspects—United States. I. Adler, Nancy E. II. Page, Ann (Ann E. K.) III. National Institute of Medicine (U. S.) Committee on Psychosocial Services to Cancer Patients / Families in a Community Setting.
    [DNLM: 1. Neoplasms--psychology. 2. Neoplasms—therapy. 3. Counseling—methods. 4. Needs Assessment. 5. Psychology, Medical—methods. 6. Stress, Psychological—complications. QZ 200 C2151208 2008]
RA645.C3C332 2008
362.196'994—dc22
                                                    2008000292

For more information about the Institute of Medicine, visit the IOM home page at: www.iom.edu.

The serpent has been a symbol of long life, healing, and knowledge among almost all cultures and religions since the beginning of recorded history. The serpent adopted as a logotype by the Institute of Medicine is a relief carving from ancient Greece, now held by the Staatliche Museen in Berlin.

Suggested citation: Institute of Medicine (IOM). 2008. *Cancer care for the whole patient: Meeting psychosocial health needs.* Nancy E. Adler and Ann E. K. Page, eds. Washington, DC: The National Academies Press.

*"Knowing is not enough; we must apply.
Willing is not enough; we must do."*
—Goethe

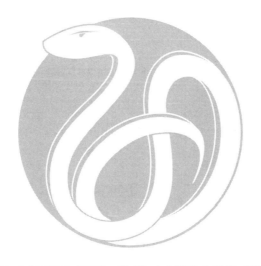

INSTITUTE OF MEDICINE
OF THE NATIONAL ACADEMIES

Advising the Nation. Improving Health.

THE NATIONAL ACADEMIES
Advisers to the Nation on Science, Engineering, and Medicine

The **National Academy of Sciences** is a private, nonprofit, self-perpetuating society of distinguished scholars engaged in scientific and engineering research, dedicated to the furtherance of science and technology and to their use for the general welfare. Upon the authority of the charter granted to it by the Congress in 1863, the Academy has a mandate that requires it to advise the federal government on scientific and technical matters. Dr. Ralph J. Cicerone is president of the National Academy of Sciences.

The **National Academy of Engineering** was established in 1964, under the charter of the National Academy of Sciences, as a parallel organization of outstanding engineers. It is autonomous in its administration and in the selection of its members, sharing with the National Academy of Sciences the responsibility for advising the federal government. The National Academy of Engineering also sponsors engineering programs aimed at meeting national needs, encourages education and research, and recognizes the superior achievements of engineers. Dr. Charles M. Vest is president of the National Academy of Engineering.

The **Institute of Medicine** was established in 1970 by the National Academy of Sciences to secure the services of eminent members of appropriate professions in the examination of policy matters pertaining to the health of the public. The Institute acts under the responsibility given to the National Academy of Sciences by its congressional charter to be an adviser to the federal government and, upon its own initiative, to identify issues of medical care, research, and education. Dr. Harvey V. Fineberg is president of the Institute of Medicine.

The **National Research Council** was organized by the National Academy of Sciences in 1916 to associate the broad community of science and technology with the Academy's purposes of furthering knowledge and advising the federal government. Functioning in accordance with general policies determined by the Academy, the Council has become the principal operating agency of both the National Academy of Sciences and the National Academy of Engineering in providing services to the government, the public, and the scientific and engineering communities. The Council is administered jointly by both Academies and the Institute of Medicine. Dr. Ralph J. Cicerone and Dr. Charles M. Vest are chair and vice chair, respectively, of the National Research Council.

www.national-academies.org

Reviewers

This report has been reviewed in draft form by individuals chosen for their diverse perspectives and technical expertise, in accordance with procedures approved by the NRC's Report Review Committee. The purpose of this independent review is to provide candid and critical comments that will assist the institution in making its published report as sound as possible and to ensure that the report meets institutional standards for objectivity, evidence, and responsiveness to the study charge. The review comments and draft manuscript remain confidential to protect the integrity of the deliberative process. We wish to thank the following individuals for their review of this report:

TERRY BADGER, College of Nursing, The University of Arizona, Tucson, Arizona

BRUCE COMPAS, Department of Psychology and Human Development, Vanderbilt University, Nashville, Tennessee

RONALD EPSTEIN, Rochester Center to Improve Communication in Health Care, University of Rochester School of Medicine and Dentistry, Rochester, New York

STEWART FLEISHMAN, Cancer Supportive Services, Continuum Cancer Centers of New York: Beth Israel and St Luke's-Roosevelt, New York

PAUL JACOBSEN, Health Outcomes and Behavior Program, Moffitt Cancer Center, and Departments of Psychology and Interdisciplinary Oncology, University of South Florida, Tampa, Florida

Although the reviewers listed above have provided many constructive comments and suggestions, they were not asked to endorse the conclusions or recommendations nor did they see the final draft of the report before its release. The review of this report was overseen by JOHANNA T. DWYER, Friedman School of Nutrition Science and Policy, Tufts University School of Medicine and Frances Stern Nutrition Center, Tufts-New England Medical Center and RICHARD G. FRANK, Department of Health Care Policy, Harvard Medical School. Appointed by the National Research Council and Institute of Medicine, they were responsible for making certain that an independent examination of this report was carried out in accordance with institutional procedures and that all review comments were carefully considered. Responsibility for the final content of this report rests entirely with the authoring committee and the institution.

Foreword

Cancer Care for the Whole Patient: Meeting Psychosocial Health Needs is an important new addition to a series of Institute of Medicine reports that prescribe actions needed to improve the quality of U.S. health care. Following in the footsteps of *Crossing the Quality Chasm: A New Health System for the 21st Century*, *Improving the Quality of Health Care for Mental and Substance Use Conditions*, and other reports in the Quality Chasm series, this report takes another step forward and attends to the psychological/behavioral and social problems that can accompany serious illness. Although the report examines psychosocial health needs from the perspective of individuals with a diagnosis of cancer, the recommendations in this report are also relevant to clinicians, other health care providers, payors, and quality oversight organizations concerned with the care of individuals with other serious and complex medical conditions.

Research has amply demonstrated the significance of psychosocial factors to health and health care. Incorporating evidence from studies of psychological and social determinants of health, clinical research on the effectiveness of psychological and behavioral services, health services research on the effective organization and delivery of health care, and biologic research in fields such as psychoneuroimmunology, this report documents the consequences of failing to meet psychosocial health needs. Importantly, it translates scientific research findings into practical applications for improving the quality of cancer care.

The result is a new standard of care for cancer care, a standard that incorporates acknowledgement, treatment, and management of psychosocial problems. While this report deals specifically with cancer patients, the lesson to improve the quality of care by focusing on the psychosocial needs of the whole patient will apply as well to many other conditions.

Harvey V. Fineberg, MD, PhD
President, Institute of Medicine

Preface

Americans place a high premium on new technologies to solve our health care needs. However, technology alone is not enough. Health is determined not just by biological processes but by people's emotions, behaviors, and social relationships. Sadly, these factors are often ignored or not defined as part of health care. Many doubt their importance and dismiss the evidence as being based on "soft science." Even when acknowledged, they are often seen as ancillary rather than central to care. High and escalating health care costs fuel the argument that addressing such concerns is a luxury rather than a necessity. These views fly in the face of evidence of the important role that psychosocial factors play in disease onset and progression, not to mention their impact on people's ability to function and maintain a positive quality of life. As this report documents, a growing body of scientific evidence demonstrates that psychological and social problems can prevent individuals from receiving needed health care, complying with treatment plans, and managing their illness and recovery. Another recent Institute of Medicine report[1] states that the purpose of health care is to "continuously reduce the impact and burden of illness, injury, and disability, and . . . improve . . . health and functioning." To accomplish this, good quality health care must attend to patients' psychosocial problems and provide services to enable them to better manage their illnesses and underlying health. To ignore these factors while pouring billions of dollars into new

---

[1]IOM. 2006. *Performance measurement: Accelerating improvement.* Washington, DC: The National Academies Press.

technologies is like spending all one's money on the latest model car and then not having the money left to buy the gas needed to make it run.

This report examines psychosocial health services from the perspective of the more than ten and a half million individuals in the United States who live with a current or past diagnosis of cancer, and who reside in 1 of every 10 U.S. households. Not only are these patients affected by their illness, but so, too, are their families. Fortunately, new advances in treatment are transforming the nature of cancer as a disease. Increasingly individuals are prevailing against acute, life-threatening diagnoses and physically demanding (and sometimes themselves life-threatening) surgical, radiation, and drug treatments. They are joining a growing segment of the U.S. population—those with chronic illnesses. This has important implications for the organization and delivery of services and for health care costs. Although the recommendations in this report address the delivery of psychosocial health services to individuals diagnosed with cancer, the committee believes the model for care delivery developed for the report and the accompanying recommendations are applicable to the health care of all with chronic illnesses. Indeed, much of the evidence of the effectiveness of individual psychosocial health services and models of care reviewed by the committee comes from services and interventions designed for individuals with other types of chronic illnesses.

The committee found evidence that was both cautionary and encouraging. Both patients and providers tell us that attention to psychosocial health needs is the exception rather than the rule in oncology practice today. We noted with dismay the many recommendations over the years calling for more attention to psychosocial concerns on which there has been no action. However, there are forces at play currently that could facilitate change as a result of this report. First, the patient care tools, approaches, and resources needed to deliver effective services for those in need are already *sufficiently* (though not *ideally*) developed. Today, every individual treated for cancer can (and should) expect to have their psychological and social needs addressed alongside their physical needs. Second, this report provides an ingredient essential to all successful change initiatives—a shared vision toward which all involved parties can direct and coordinate their efforts. This report puts forth such a vision in a standard of care articulating how psychosocial health services should be routinely incorporated into oncology care. This multidisciplinary standard can provide a common framework around which clinicians, health care organizations, patients and their advocates, payers, quality oversight organizations, and all concerned about the quality of cancer care can organize and coordinate their efforts and achieve synergy.

Finally, successful change initiatives also are characterized by their strong leadership. The United States is fortunate to have strong individual and organizational leaders who have done much to advance the quality of cancer care. This leadership is a powerful resource for change, and can do much to make the delivery of psychosocial health services a routine part of cancer care. To engage these parties in advancing the standard of care for psychosocial health services, the committee has put forth a small number of recommendations (10 in all), each targeted to key leadership—clinical leaders, advocacy organizations, health plans and purchasers, quality oversight organizations, and sponsors of research. The committee hopes that all of these leaders will join in making this new standard of care the norm—and better the health care and health of our brothers, sisters, parents, children, and ourselves—for the more than 40 percent of all Americans who will receive a diagnosis of cancer in their lifetime.

Nancy E. Adler
Chair

Acknowledgments

The Committee on Psychosocial Services to Cancer Patients/Families in a Community Setting thanks the many individuals and organizations who helped with its search for effective psychosocial health services and models for their effective delivery, and provided key information on the health care workforce and a number of policy issues. We gratefully acknowledge Carol L. Alter, MD, at the TEN Project and Georgetown University; M. Brownell Anderson, Robert Eaglen, PhD, and Robby Reynolds at the Association of American Medical Colleges; Neeraj K. Arora, PhD, at the National Cancer Institute; Terry Badger, PhD, RN, FAAN, at the University of Arizona College of Nursing; Cynthia Belar, Diane M. Pedulla, JD, Kimberley Moore, and Wendy Williams at the American Psychological Association; Thomas P. Beresford, MD, at the Department of Veterans Affairs Medical Center, University of Colorado Health Sciences Center; Joyce Bichler, ACSW, of Gilda's Club Worldwide; Elise J. Bolda, PhD, of The Robert Wood Johnson Foundation's Community Partnerships for Older Adults program at the University of Southern Maine; Cheryl Bradley, MSW, and Carson J. Pattillo, MPH, at The Leukemia & Lymphoma Society; William S. Breitbart, MD, and Andrew J. Roth, MD, at Memorial Sloan-Kettering Cancer Center; E. Dale Collins, MD, at Dartmouth Hitchcock Medical Center; Lisa Corchado and Rebecca Yowell at the American Psychiatric Association; Bridget Culhane, RN, MN, MS, CAE, and Gail A. Mallory, PhD, RN, CNAA, at the Oncology Nursing Society; Charles Darby at the Agency for Healthcare Research and Quality; Kim Day at the Board of Oncology Social Work Certification; Stephen DeMers, EdD, at the Association of State and Provincial Psychology Boards; Molla S. Donaldson, DrPH, MS, at the American Society of

Clinical Oncology; Patricia Doykos Duquette, PhD, at the Bristol-Myers Squibb Foundation; Peter D. Eisenberg, MD, at California Cancer Care; Ronit Elk, PhD, Katherine Sharpe, Nancy Single, PhD, Michael Stefanek, PhD, and Marcia W. Watts, at the American Cancer Society; Stewart Fleishman, MD, at Continuum Cancer Centers of New York: Beth Israel and St Luke's-Roosevelt; Barbara Fleming, MD, Paulette Mehta, MD, Thakor G. Patel, MD, MACP, and Shakaib Rehman, MD, FACP, at the Veterans Health Administration; Bill Given at the Charles and Barbara Given Family Care Program, Michigan State University; Mitch Golant, PhD, at The Wellness Community; Marcia Grant, RN, DNSc, FAAN, and Betty Ferrell, PhD, FAAN, at the City of Hope National Medical Center; Ethan Gray and Kathryn M. Smolinski, MSW, at the Association of Oncology Social Work; David Gustafson at the University of Wisconsin; Karmen Hanson, MA, at the National Conference of State Legislatures; John E. Hennessy, Nancy Washburn, Sandy Simmons, MSN, ARNP-C, AOCN, and Barbara Adkins, MS, ARNP-BC, AOCNP, at Kansas City Cancer Center; Joanne Hilden, MD, at St. Vincent Children's Hospital in Indianapolis, Beverly Lange, MD, at Children's Hospital of Philadelphia, and Missy Layfield, Chair of the Patient Advocacy Committee, all of the Children's Oncology Group; Caroline Huffman, LCSW, MEd, at the Lance Armstrong Foundation; Frits Huyse, MD, PhD, at the University Medical Center Groningen, The Netherlands; Paul B. Jacobsen, PhD, Nancy W. Newman, LCSW, and Donna M. Cosenzo at the H. Lee Moffitt Cancer Center and Research Institute; Barbara L. Jones, PhD, MSW, at the Association of Pediatric Oncology Social Workers; Nancy Kane, at the Payson Center for Cancer Care; Ernest Katz, Aura Kuperberg, Kathleen Meeske, PhD, Kathleen S. Ruccione, MPH, RN, FAAN, and Octavio Zavala, at the Children's Hospital Los Angeles; Anne E. Kazak, PhD, ABPP, at the University of Pennsylvania School of Medicine; Emmett B. Keeler, PhD, at the RAND Corporation; Murray Kopelow, MD, at the Accreditation Council for Continuing Medical Education; Wolfgang Linden, PhD, at the University of British Columbia, Canada; Karen Llanos at the Center for Health Care Strategies, Inc.; Kate Lorig, RN, DrPH, at Stanford University; Matthew J. Loscalzo, MSW, at the Rebecca and John Moores UCSD Cancer Center; Richard P. McQuellon, PhD, at the Wake Forest University Baptist Medical Center; Stephen Miller, MD, at the American Board of Medical Specialties; Moira A. Mulhern, PhD, at Kansas City Turning Point; Todd Peterson at the American Nurse Credentialing Center; Gail Pfeiffer, RHIA, CCS-P, at the Cleveland Clinic; William Pirl, MD, at the Massachusetts General Hospital Cancer Center; Paul A. Poniatowski at the American Board of Internal Medicine; Craig Ravesloot, PhD, at the University of Montana; Christopher J. Recklitis, PhD, MPH, at the Dana-Farber Cancer Institute; Karen Robitaille at Yale University School of Medicine; Sarah Rosenbloom, PhD, at Northwestern University Feinberg

School of Medicine; Thomas J. Smith, MD, at Virginia Commonwealth University's Massey Cancer Center; Joan Stanley at the American Association of Colleges of Nursing; Annette Stanton, PhD, at the University of California, Los Angeles; James Stockman, MD, and Jean Robillard, MD, at the American Board of Pediatrics; Ellen L. Stovall of the National Coalition for Cancer Survivorship; Bonnie Strickland at the Health Resources and Services Administration, Department of Health and Human Services; Thomas B. Strouse, MD, FAPM, DFAPA, at the Samuel Oschin Comprehensive Cancer Institute, Cedars Sinai Medical Center; Phyllis Torda at the National Committee for Quality Assurance; Douglas Tynan, PhD, at the American Board of Professional Psychology; Ginny Vaitones at the Board of Oncology Social Work Certification; Garry Welch, PhD, at Baystate Medical Center; Pamela R. West, PT, DPT, MPH, at the Centers for Medicare & Medicaid Services; Nancy Whitelaw at the National Council on Aging; Rodger Winn at the National Quality Forum; and James R. Zabora, PhD, of the National Catholic School of Social Service, Catholic University of America.

In addition, we thank M. Robin DiMatteo, Kelly B. Haskard, and Summer L. Williams, all at the University of California, Riverside, and Sheldon Cohen and Denise Janicki-Deverts, both at Carnegie Mellon University, for their papers, respectively, on "Effects of Distressed Psychological States on Adherence and Health Behavior Change: Cognitive, Motivational, and Social Factors" and "Stress and Disease." These excellent papers helped the committee think through and quickly review a growing body of evidence documenting the health effects of psychological and social stressors.

We also offer many thanks to Maria Hewitt, DrPH, formerly with the National Cancer Policy Board at the Institute of Medicine, for her generous help throughout the initial stages of this study. Rona Briere of Briere Associates, Inc., provided expert copy editing, and Alisa Decatur excellent proofreading and manuscript preparation assistance. And as always, Danitza Valdivia, administrative assistant to the Board on Health Care Services, provided ever-ready and gracious assistance regardless of the task or timeline.

Finally, we thank our project officers at the National Institutes of Health. Susan D. Solomon, PhD, senior advisor in the Office of Behavioral and Social Sciences Research, and project officer at the beginning of this study, skillfully launched the study and shaped its parameters. Julia H. Rowland, PhD, director of the National Cancer Institute's Office of Cancer Survivorship, served as project officer for the duration of the study, and provided ongoing support, thoughtful and expert guidance, and generous assistance in identifying and securing needed resources.

Contents

Tables, Figures, and Boxes

TABLES

xxi

FIGURES

BOXES

CANCER CARE FOR THE
WHOLE PATIENT

Summary

ABSTRACT

Cancer care today often provides state-of-the-science biomedical treatment, but fails to address the psychological and social (psychosocial) problems associated with the illness. This failure can compromise the effectiveness of health care and thereby adversely affect the health of cancer patients. Psychological and social problems created or exacerbated by cancer—including depression and other emotional problems; lack of information or skills needed to manage the illness; lack of transportation or other resources; and disruptions in work, school, and family life— cause additional suffering, weaken adherence to prescribed treatments, and threaten patients' return to health.

A range of services is available to help patients and their families manage the psychosocial aspects of cancer. Indeed, these services collectively have been described as constituting a "wealth of cancer-related community support services."

Today, it is not possible to deliver good-quality cancer care without using existing approaches, tools, and resources to address patients' psychosocial health needs. All patients with cancer and their families should expect and receive cancer care that ensures the provision of appropriate psychosocial health services. This report recommends ten actions that oncology providers, health policy makers, educators, health insurers, health plans, quality oversight organizations, researchers and research sponsors, and consumer advocates should undertake to ensure that this standard is met.

1

PSYCHOSOCIAL PROBLEMS AND HEALTH

The burden of illnesses and disabilities in the United States and the world is closely related to social, psychological, and behavioral aspects of the way of life of the population. (IOM, 1982:49–50)

Health and disease are determined by dynamic interactions among biological, psychological, behavioral, and social factors. (IOM, 2001:16)

Because health . . . is a function of psychological and social variables, many events or interventions traditionally considered irrelevant actually are quite important for the health status of individuals and populations. (IOM, 2001:27)

In previous reports the Institute of Medicine (IOM) has issued strong findings about the important role of psychological/behavioral and social factors in health and recommended more attention to these factors in the design and delivery of health care (IOM, 1982, 2001, 2006). In 2005, the IOM was asked once again to examine the contributions of these psychosocial factors to health and how best to address them—in this case in the context of cancer, which encompasses some of the nation's most serious and burdensome illnesses.

STUDY CONTEXT

The Reach and Influence of Cancer

One in ten American households today has a family member who has been diagnosed with or treated for cancer[1] within the past 5 years (USA Today et al., 2006), and 41 percent of Americans can expect to be diagnosed with cancer at some point in their lifetime (Ries et al., 2007). More than ten and a half million people in the United States live with a past or current diagnosis of cancer (Ries et al., 2007).

Early detection and improved treatments for many different types of cancer have changed our understanding of this group of illnesses from that of a single disease that was often uniformly fatal in a matter of weeks or months to that of a variety of diseases—some of which are curable, all of which are treatable, and for many of which long-term disease-free survival is possible. In the past two decades, the 5-year survival rate for the 15 most common cancers has increased from 43 to 64 percent for men and from 57 to 64 percent for women (Jemal et al., 2004).

Nonetheless, the diseases that make up cancer represent both acute life-threatening illnesses and serious chronic conditions. Their treatment is

---

[1]This excludes non-melanoma skin cancers.

typically very challenging physically to patients, requiring some combination of surgery, radiation, or chemotherapy for months or years. Even when treatment has been completed and no cancer remains, the frequently permanent, serious residua of cancer and/or the side effects of chemotherapy, radiation, hormone therapy, surgery, and other treatments can permanently impair cardiac, neurological, kidney, lung, and other body functioning, necessitating ongoing monitoring of cancer survivors' health and many adjustments in their daily living. Eleven percent of adults with cancer or a history of cancer (almost half of whom are age 65 or older) report having one or more limitations in their ability to perform activities of daily living such as bathing, eating, or using the bathroom, and 58 percent report other functional disabilities, such as the inability to walk a quarter of a mile, or to stand or sit for 2 hours (Hewitt et al., 2003). Long-term survivors of childhood cancer are at particularly elevated risk compared with others their age. Nearly 20 percent of those who survive 5 years or more report limitations in activities such as carrying groceries, climbing a flight of stairs, or walking a block (Ness et al., 2005). Significant numbers of individuals stop working or experience a change in employment after being diagnosed or treated for cancer (IOM and NRC, 2006).

Not surprisingly, significant mental health problems, such as depression and anxiety disorders, are common in patients with cancer (Spiegel and Giese-Davis, 2003; Carlsen et al., 2005; Hegel et al., 2006). Studies have also documented the presence of symptoms meeting the criteria for post-traumatic stress disorder (PTSD) and post-traumatic stress symptoms (PTSS) in adults and children with cancer, as well as in the parents of children diagnosed with cancer (Kangas et al., 2002; Bruce, 2006).[2] These mental health problems are additional contributors to functional impairment in carrying out family, work, and other societal roles; poor adherence to medical treatments; and adverse medical outcomes (Katon, 2003).

Patients with cancer (like those with other chronic illnesses) identify a number of other problems that adversely affect their health care and recovery, including poor communication with physicians, lack of knowledge about their illness and its management, lack of transportation to health care appointments, financial problems, and lack of health insurance (Wdowik et al., 1997; Eakin and Strycker, 2001; Riegel and Carlson, 2002; Bayliss et al., 2003; Boberg et al., 2003; Skalla et al., 2004; Jerant et al., 2005; Mallinger et al., 2005). Fifteen percent of households affected by cancer report having left a doctor's office without getting answers to important

---

[2]These mental health problems are not unique to cancer patients. Populations with other chronic illnesses, such as diabetes, heart disease, HIV-related illnesses, and neurological disorders, also have higher rates of depression, adjustment disorders, severe anxiety, PTSD or PTSS, and subclinical emotional distress (Katon, 2003).

questions about the illness (USA Today et al., 2006). The American Cancer Society and CancerCare report receiving more than 100,000 requests annually for transportation so patients can get to medical appointments, pick up medications, or receive other health services. In 2003, nearly one in five (12.3 million) people with chronic conditions[3] lived in families that had problems paying medical bills (May and Cunningham, 2004; Tu, 2004). Among uninsured cancer survivors, more than one in four delayed or decided not to get treatment because of its cost, and 41 percent were unable to pay for basic necessities, including food (USA Today et al., 2006). About 5 percent of the 1.5 million American families who filed for bankruptcy in 2001 reported that medical costs associated with cancer contributed to their financial problems (Himmelstein et al., 2005).

Although family and loved ones often provide substantial amounts of emotional and logistical support and hands-on personal and nursing care (valued at more than $1 billion annually) in an effort to address these needs (Hayman et al., 2001; Kotkamp-Mothes et al., 2005), they often do so at great personal cost, themselves experiencing depression, other adverse health effects, and an increased risk of premature death (Schultz and Beach, 1999; Kurtz et al., 2004). Caregivers providing support to a spouse who report strain from doing so are 63 percent more likely to die within 4 years than others their age (Schultz and Beach, 1999). The emotional distress of caregivers also can directly affect patients. Studies of partners of women with breast cancer (predominantly husbands, but also "significant others," daughters, friends, and others) find that partners' mental health correlates positively with the anxiety, depression, fatigue, and symptom distress of women with breast cancer and that the effects are bidirectional (Segrin et al., 2005, 2007).

Effects of Psychosocial Problems on Physical Health

The psychosocial problems described above can adversely affect health and health care in many ways. For example, a substantial literature has documented low income as a strong risk factor for disability, illness, and death (IOM, 2001; Subramanian et al., 2002). Inadequate income limits one's ability to purchase food, medications, and health care supplies necessary for health and health care, as well as to secure necessary transportation and obtain relief from other stressors that can accompany tasks of everyday life (Kelly et al., 2006). As noted above, lack of transportation to medical appointments, the pharmacy, the grocery store, health education classes, peer support meetings, and other out-of-home health resources is common,

---

[3]Asthma, arthritis, diabetes, chronic obstructive pulmonary disease, heart disease, hypertension, cancer, benign prostate enlargement, abnormal uterine bleeding, and depression.

and it can pose a barrier to health monitoring, illness management, and health promotion.

Depressed or anxious individuals have lower social functioning, more disability, and greater overall functional impairment than those without these conditions (Spitzer et al., 1995; Katon, 2003). Distressed emotional states also often generate additional somatic problems, such as sleep difficulties, fatigue, and pain (Spitzer et al., 1995; APA, 2000), which can confound the diagnosis and treatment of physical symptoms. Patients with major depression as compared with nondepressed persons also have higher rates of unhealthy behaviors such as smoking, a sedentary lifestyle, and overeating. Moreover, depression and other adverse psychological states thwart behavior change and adherence to treatment regimens by impairing cognition, weakening motivation, and decreasing coping abilities. Evidence emerging from the science of psychoneuroimmunology—the study of the interactions among behavior, the brain, and the body's immune system—is beginning to show how psychosocial stressors interfere with the working of the body's neuro-endocrine, immune, and other systems.

In sum, people diagnosed with cancer and their families must not only live with and manage the challenges and risks posed to their physical health, but also overcome psychosocial obstacles that can interfere with their health care and diminish their health and functioning. Unfortunately, the current medical system deploys its resources largely to address the former problems and often ignores the latter. As a result, patients' psychosocial needs frequently remain unacknowledged and unaddressed in cancer care.

Cancer Care Is Often Incomplete

Many people living with cancer report that their psychosocial health care needs are not well addressed in their care. At the most fundamental level, throughout diagnosis, treatment, and post-treatment, patients report dissatisfaction with the amount and type of information they are given about their diagnosis, their prognosis, available treatments, and ways to manage their illness and health. Health care providers often fail to communicate this information effectively, in ways that are understandable to and enable action by patients (Epstein and Street, 2007). Moreover, individuals diagnosed with cancer often report that their care providers do not understand their psychosocial needs; do not consider psychosocial support an integral part of their care; are unaware of psychosocial health care resources; and fail to recognize, adequately treat, or offer referral for depression or other sequelae of stress due to the illness in patients and their families (President's Cancer Panel, 2004; Maly et al., 2005; IOM, 2007). Twenty-eight percent of respondents to the National Survey of U.S. Households Affected by Cancer reported that they did not have a doctor who paid attention to factors beyond their direct medical care, such as sources of support for dealing with the illness (USA Today et al., 2006). A number of studies also have shown that physicians substantially underestimate oncology patients' psychosocial distress (Fallowfield et al., 2001; Keller et al., 2004; Merckaert et al., 2005). Indeed, oncologists themselves report frequent failure to attend to the psychosocial needs of their patients. In a national survey of members of the American Society of Clinical Oncology, a third of respondents reported that they did not routinely screen their patients for distress. Of the 65 percent that did do so, methods used were often untested or unreliable. In a survey of members of an alliance of 20 of the world's leading cancer centers, only 8 reported screening for distress in at least some of their patients, and only 3 routinely screened all of their patients for psychosocial health needs (Jacobsen and Ransom, 2007).

A number of factors can interfere with clinicians' addressing psychosocial health needs. These include the way in which clinical practices are designed, the education and training of the health care workforce, shortages and maldistribution of health personnel, and the nature of the payment and policy environment in which health care is delivered. Because of this, improving the delivery of psychosocial health services requires a multipronged approach.

STUDY SCOPE

In this context, the National Institutes of Health asked the IOM to empanel a committee to conduct a study of the delivery of the diverse psychosocial services needed by cancer patients and their families in community settings. The committee was tasked with producing a report describing barriers to access to psychosocial services and ways in which these services can best be provided, analyzing the capacity of the current mental health and cancer treatment system to deliver such care, delineating the associated resource and training requirements, and offering recommendations and an action plan for overcoming the identified barriers. The committee interpreted "community care" to refer to all sites of cancer care except inpatient settings.

This study builds on and complements several prior reports on cancer care. First, two recent reports address quality of care for cancer survivors. *From Cancer Patient to Cancer Survivor: Lost in Transition* (IOM and NRC, 2006) well articulates how high-quality care (including psychosocial health care) should be delivered after patients complete their cancer treatment. *Childhood Cancer Survivorship: Improving Care and Quality of Life* (IOM and NRC, 2003) similarly addresses survivorship for childhood cancer. The recommendations made in the present report complement and can be implemented consistent with the vision and recommendations put forth in those reports. Second, two other recent reports address palliative care:

Improving Palliative Care for Cancer (IOM and NRC, 2001) and *When Children Die: Improving Palliative and End-of-Life Care for Children and Their Families* (IOM, 2003). For this reason, the additional considerations involved in providing end-of-life care are not addressed in this report.

FINDINGS GIVE REASON FOR HOPE

In carrying out its charge, the IOM Committee on Psychosocial Services to Cancer Patients/Families in a Community Setting found multiple reasons to be optimistic that improvements in the psychosocial health care provided to oncology patients and their families can be quickly achieved. First, there is good evidence of the effectiveness of a variety of services in relieving the emotional distress—even the debilitating depression and anxiety—experienced by cancer patients. Strong evidence also supports the utility of services aimed at helping individuals adopt behaviors that can minimize disease symptoms and improve overall health. Other psychosocial services, such as transportation to health care or financial assistance to purchase medications or supplies, while not the subject of effectiveness research, have long-standing and wide acceptance as humane approaches to addressing health-related needs. Such services are available through many health and human service providers. In particular, the strong leadership of organizations in the voluntary sector has created a broad array of psychosocial support services, in some cases available at no cost to the consumer. Together, these resources have been described as constituting a "wealth of cancer-related community support services" (IOM and NRC, 2006:229).

However, it is not sufficient simply to have effective services; interventions to identify patients with psychosocial health needs and to link them to appropriate services are needed as well. Fortunately, many providers of health services—some in oncology, some delivering health care for other complex health conditions—understand that psychosocial problems can affect health adversely and have developed interventions to address these problems. Some of these interventions are derived from theoretical or conceptual frameworks, some are based on research findings, and some have undergone empirical testing on their own; the best have all three sources of support. Common components of these interventions point to a model for the effective delivery of psychosocial health services (see Figure S-1). This model includes processes that (1) identify psychosocial health needs, (2) link patients and families to needed psychosocial services, (3) support patients and families in managing the illness, (4) coordinate psychosocial and biomedical health care, and (5) follow up on care delivery to monitor the effectiveness of services and make modifications if needed—all of which are facilitated by effective patient–provider communication. Routine implementation of many of these processes is currently under way by a number of exemplary cancer care providers in a variety of settings, attest-

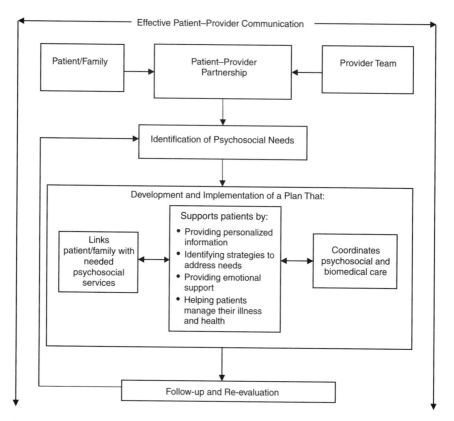

FIGURE S-1 Model for the delivery of psychosocial health services.

ing to their feasibility in settings with varying levels of resources. However, many patients do not have the benefit of these interventions, and more active steps are needed if this lack of access is to become the exception rather than the rule.

CONCLUSIONS

Based on its findings with regard to the significant impact of psychosocial problems on health and health care, the existence of effective psychosocial services to address these problems, and the development and testing of strategies for delivering these services effectively, the committee concludes that:

> *Attending to psychosocial needs should be an integral part of quality cancer care. All components of the health care system that are involved in cancer care should explicitly incorporate attention to psychosocial needs*

into their policies, practices, and standards addressing clinical health care. These policies, practices, and standards should be aimed at ensuring the provision of psychosocial health services to all patients who need them.

The committee defines psychosocial health services as follows:

Psychosocial health services are psychological and social services and interventions that enable patients, their families, and health care providers to optimize biomedical health care and to manage the psychological/behavioral and social aspects of illness and its consequences so as to promote better health.

This definition encompasses both psychosocial *services* (i.e., activities or tangible goods directly received by and benefiting the patient or family) and psychosocial *interventions* (activities that enable the provision of the service, such as needs assessment, referral, or care coordination). Examples of psychosocial needs and services that can address those needs are listed in Table S-1. Psychosocial interventions necessary for their appropriate provision are portrayed in Figure S-1. The committee offers the following recommendations for making attention to psychosocial health needs an integral part of quality cancer care.

RECOMMENDATIONS FOR ACTION

Recommendation 1: The standard of care. All parties establishing or using standards for the quality of cancer care should adopt the following as a standard:

All cancer care should ensure the provision of appropriate psychosocial health services by

- facilitating effective communication between patients and care providers;[4]
- identifying each patient's psychosocial health needs;
- designing and implementing a plan that
  - links the patient with needed psychosocial services,
  - coordinates biomedical and psychosocial care,
  - engages and supports patients in managing their illness and health; and
- systematically following up on, reevaluating, and adjusting plans.

---

[4]Although the language of this standard refers only to patients, the standard should be taken as referring to both patients and families when the patient is a child, has family members involved in providing care, or simply desires the involvement of family members.

TABLE S-1 Psychosocial Needs and Formal[a] Services to Address Them

Psychosocial Need	Health Services
Information about illness, treatments, health, and services	• Provision of information, e.g., on illness, treatments, effects on health, and psychosocial services, and help to patients/ families in understanding and using the information
Help in coping with emotions accompanying illness and treatment	• Peer support programs • Counseling/psychotherapy to individuals or groups • Pharmacological management of mental symptoms
Help in managing illness	• Comprehensive illness self-management/self-care programs

Assistance in changing behaviors to minimize impact of disease	• Behavioral/health promotion interventions, such as:
	  – provider assessment/monitoring of health behaviors (e.g., smoking, exercise)
	  – brief physician counseling
	  – patient education, e.g., in cancer-related health risks and risk reduction measures

Material and logistical resources, such as transportation	• Provision of resources
Help in managing disruptions in work, school, and family life	• Family and caregiver education • Assistance with activities of daily living (ADLs), instrumental ADLs, chores • Legal protections and services, e.g., under Americans with Disabilities Act and Family and Medical Leave Act • Cognitive testing and educational assistance
Financial advice and /or assistance	• Financial planning/counseling, including management of day-to-day activities such as bill paying • Insurance (e.g., health, disability) counseling • Eligibility assessment/counseling for other benefits (e.g., Supplemental Security Income, Social Security Disability Income) • Supplemental financial grants

[a]Family members and friends and other informal sources of support are key providers of psychosocial health services. This table includes only *formal* sources of psychosocial support— those that must be secured through the assistance of an organization or agency that in some way enables the provision of needed services (sometimes at no cost or through volunteers).

Key participants and leaders in cancer care have major roles to play in promoting and facilitating adherence to this standard of care. Their respective roles are described in the following nine recommendations.

Recommendation 2: Health care providers. **All cancer care providers should ensure that every cancer patient within their practice receives** care that meets the standard for psychosocial health care. The National Cancer Institute should help cancer care providers implement the standard of care by maintaining an up-to-date directory of psychosocial services available at no cost to individuals/families with cancer.

The committee believes that *all* providers can and should implement the above recommendation. Individual clinical practices vary by their patient population, their setting, and available resources in their clinical practice and community. Because of this, *how* individual health care practices implement the standard of care and the level at which it is done may vary. Nevertheless, as this report describes, the committee believes that it is possible for all providers to meet this standard in some way. This report identifies tools and techniques already in use by leading oncology providers to do so. There are many actions that can be taken *now* to identify and deliver needed psychosocial health services, even as the health care system works to improve their quantity and effectiveness. The committee believes that the inability to solve all psychosocial problems permanently should not preclude attempts to remedy as many as possible—a stance akin to oncologists' commitment to treating cancer even when the successful outcome of every treatment is not assured. Patient education and advocacy organizations can play a key role in bringing this about.

Recommendation 3: Patient and family education. Patient education and advocacy organizations should educate patients with cancer and their family caregivers to expect, and request when necessary, cancer care that meets the standard for psychosocial care. These organizations should also continue their work on strengthening the patient side of the patient–provider partnership. The goals should be to enable patients to participate actively in their care by providing tools and training in how to obtain information, make decisions, solve problems, and communicate more effectively with their health care providers.

A large-scale demonstration of the implementation of the standard of care at various sites would provide useful information about how to achieve its implementation more efficiently; reveal approaches to implementation in both resource-rich and non-resource-rich environments; document approaches for successful implementation among vulnerable groups, such as those with low socioeconomic status, ethnic minorities, those with low health literacy, and the socially isolated; and identify different models for reimbursement. A demonstration could also be used to examine how various types of personnel can be used to perform specific interventions encompassed by the standard and how those personnel can best be trained.

Recommendation 4: Support for dissemination and uptake. The National Cancer Institute, the Centers for Medicare & Medicaid Services (CMS), and the Agency for Healthcare Research and Quality (AHRQ) should, individually or collectively, conduct a large-scale demonstration and evaluation of various approaches to the efficient provision of psychosocial health care in accordance with the standard of care. This program should demonstrate how the standard can be implemented in different settings, with different populations, and with varying personnel and organizational arrangements.

Because policies set by public and private purchasers, oversight bodies, and other health care leaders shape how health care is accessed, what services are delivered, and the manner in which they are delivered, group purchasers of health care coverage and health plans should take a number of actions to support the interventions necessary to deliver effective psychosocial health services. The National Cancer Institute, CMS, and AHRQ also should spearhead the development and use of performance measures to improve the delivery of these services.

Recommendation 5: Support from payers. Group purchasers of health care coverage and health plans should fully support the evidence-based interventions necessary to deliver effective psychosocial health services:

- Group purchasers should include provisions in their contracts and agreements with health plans that ensure coverage and reimbursement of mechanisms for identifying the psychosocial needs of cancer patients, linking patients with appropriate providers who can meet those needs, and coordinating psychosocial services with patients' biomedical care.
- Group purchasers should review cost-sharing provisions that affect mental health services and revise those that impede cancer patients' access to such services.
- Group purchasers and health plans should ensure that their coverage policies do not impede cancer patients' access to providers with expertise in the treatment of mental health conditions in individuals undergoing complex medical regimens such as those used to treat cancer. Health plans whose networks lack this expertise should reimburse for mental health services provided by out-of-network practitioners with this expertise who meet the plan's quality and other standards (at rates paid to similar providers within the plan's network).

- Group purchasers and health plans should include incentives for the effective delivery of psychosocial care in payment reform programs—such as pay-for-performance and pay-for-reporting initiatives—in which they participate.

With respect to the above recommendation, "group purchasers" include purchasers in the public sector (e.g., Medicare and Medicaid) as well as group purchasers in the private sector (e.g., employer purchasers). Mental health care providers "with expertise in the treatment of mental health conditions in individuals undergoing complex medical regimens such as those used to treat cancer" include mental health providers who possess this expertise through formal education (such as specialists in psychosomatic medicine), as well as mental health care providers who have gained expertise though their clinical experiences, such as mental health clinicians collocated with and part of an interdisciplinary oncology practice.

Recommendation 6: Quality oversight. The National Cancer Institute, CMS, and AHRQ should fund research focused on the development of performance measures for psychosocial cancer care. Organizations setting standards for cancer care (e.g., National Comprehensive Cancer Network, American Society of Clinical Oncology, American College of Surgeons' Commission on Cancer, Oncology Nursing Society, American Psychosocial Oncology Society) and other standards-setting organizations (e.g., National Quality Forum, National Committee for Quality Assurance, URAC, Joint Commission) should

- Create oversight mechanisms that can be used to measure and report on the quality of ambulatory oncology care (including psychosocial health care).
- Incorporate requirements for identifying and responding to psychosocial health care needs into their protocols, policies, and standards.
- Develop and use performance measures for psychosocial health care in their quality oversight activities.

Ultimately, the delivery of cancer care that addresses psychosocial needs depends on having a health care workforce with the attitudes, knowledge, and skills needed to deliver such care. Thus, professional education and training should not be ignored as a factor influencing health practitioners' practices. The committee further recommends

Recommendation 7: Workforce competencies.

  a. Educational accrediting organizations, licensing bodies, and professional societies should examine their standards and licensing and certification criteria with an eye to identifying competencies in delivering psychosocial health care and developing them as fully as possible in accordance with a model that integrates biomedical and psychosocial care.
  b. Congress and federal agencies should support and fund the establishment of a Workforce Development Collaborative on Psychosocial Care during Chronic Medical Illness. This cross-specialty, multidisciplinary group should comprise educators, consumer and family advocates, and providers of psychosocial and biomedical health services and be charged with
    – identifying, refining, and broadly disseminating to health care educators information about workforce competencies, models, and preservice curricula relevant to providing psychosocial services to persons with chronic medical illnesses and their families;
    – adapting curricula for continuing education of the existing workforce using efficient workplace-based learning approaches;
    – drafting and implementing a plan for developing the skills of faculty and other trainers in teaching psychosocial health care using evidence-based teaching strategies; and
    – strengthening the emphasis on psychosocial health care in educational accreditation standards and professional licensing and certification exams by recommending revisions to the relevant oversight organizations.
  c. Organizations providing research funding should support assessment of the implementation in education, training, and clinical practice of the workforce competencies necessary to provide psychosocial care and their impact on achieving the standard for such care set forth in recommendation 1.

In addition, improving the delivery of psychosocial health services requires targeted research. This research should aim to clarify the efficacy and effectiveness of new and existing services and to identify ways of improving the delivery of these services to various populations in different geographic locations and with varying levels of resources. Doing so would be facilitated by clarifying and standardizing the often unclear and inconsistent language used to refer to psychosocial services.

Recommendation 8: Standardized nomenclature. To facilitate research on and quality measurement of psychosocial interventions, the

National Institutes of Health (NIH) and AHRQ should create and lead an initiative to develop a standardized, transdisciplinary taxonomy and nomenclature for psychosocial health services. This initiative should aim to incorporate this taxonomy and nomenclature into such databases as the National Library of Medicine's Medical Subject Headings (MeSH), PsycINFO, CINAHL (Cumulative Index to Nursing and Allied Health Literature), and EMBASE.

Recommendation 9: Research priorities. Organizations sponsoring research in oncology care should include the following areas among their funding priorities:

- Further development of reliable, valid, and efficient tools and strategies for use by clinical practices to ensure that all patients with cancer receive care that meets the standard of psychosocial care set forth in recommendation 1. These tools and strategies should include
  - approaches for improving patient–provider communication and providing decision support to cancer patients;
  - screening instruments that can be used to identify individuals with any of a comprehensive array of psychosocial health problems;
  - needs assessment instruments to assist in planning psychosocial services;
  - illness and wellness management interventions; and
  - approaches for effectively linking patients with services and coordinating care.
- Identification of more effective psychosocial services to treat mental health problems and to assist patients in adopting and maintaining healthy behaviors, such as smoking cessation, exercise, and dietary change. This effort should include
  - identifying populations for whom specific psychosocial services are most effective, and psychosocial services most effective for specific populations; and
  - development of standard outcome measures for assessing the effectiveness of these services.
- Creation and testing of reimbursement arrangements that will promote psychosocial care and reward its best performance.

Research on the use of these tools, strategies, and services should also focus on how best to ensure delivery of appropriate psychosocial services to vulnerable populations, such as those with low literacy, older adults, the socially isolated, and members of cultural minorities.

Finally, the scope of work for this study included making recommendations for how to evaluate the impact of this report. The committee believes evaluation activities would be useful in promoting action on the preceding recommendations, and makes the following recommendation to that end.

> *Recommendation 10. Promoting uptake and monitoring progress.* The National Cancer Institute/NIH should monitor progress toward improved delivery of psychosocial services in cancer care and report its findings on at least a biannual basis to oncology providers, consumer organizations, group purchasers and health plans, quality oversight organizations, and other stakeholders. These findings could be used to inform an evaluation of the impact of this report and each of its recommendations. Monitoring activities should make maximal use of existing data collection tools and activities.

Following are examples of the approaches that could be used for these monitoring efforts.

To determine the extent to which patients with cancer receive psychosocial services consistent with the standard of care and its implementation as set forth in recommendations 1 and 2, the Department of Health and Human Services (DHHS) could

- Conduct an annual, patient-level, process-of-care evaluation using a national sample and validated, reliable instruments, such as the Consumer Assessment of Healthcare Providers and Systems (CAHPS) instruments.
- Add measures of the quality of psychosocial health care for patients (and families as feasible) to existing surveys, such as the Centers for Disease Control and Prevention's Behavioral Risk Factor Surveillance System (BRFSS) and CAHPS.
- Conduct annual practice surveys to determine compliance with the standard of care.
- Monitor and document the emergence of performance reward initiatives (e.g., content on psychosocial care in requests for proposals [RFPs] and pay-for-performance initiatives that specifically include incentives for psychosocial care).

For recommendation 3 on patient and family education, DHHS could

- Routinely query patient education and advocacy organizations about their efforts to educate patients with cancer and their family caregivers about what to expect from, and how to request when necessary, oncology care that meets the standard of care set forth in recommendation 1.

- In surveys conducted to assess the extent to which oncology care meets the standard of care, include questions to patients and care-givers about their knowledge of how oncology providers should address their psychosocial needs (the standard of care) and their actual experiences with receiving such care.
- Use an annual patient-level process-of-care evaluation (such as CAHPS) to identify patient education experiences.

For recommendation 4 on dissemination and uptake of the standard of care, DHHS could report on the extent to which the National Cancer Institute/CMS/AHRQ had conducted demonstration projects and how they had disseminated the findings from those demonstrations.

For recommendation 5 on support from payers, DHHS/NCI and/or advocacy, provider, or other interest groups could

- Survey national organizations (e.g., America's Health Insurance Plans, the National Business Group on Health) about their aware-ness of and/or advocacy activities related to the recommendations in this report and the initiation of appropriate reimbursement strategies/activities.
- Monitor and document the emergence of performance reward ini-tiatives (e.g., RFP content on psychosocial care, pay for perfor-mance that specifically includes incentives for psychosocial care).
- Evaluate health plan contracts and state insurance policies for cov-erage, copayments, and carve-outs for psychosocial services.
- Assess coverage for psychosocial services for Medicare beneficiaries.

For recommendation 6 on quality oversight, DHHS could

- Examine the funding portfolios of NIH, CMS, AHRQ, and other public and private sponsors of quality-of-care research to evaluate the funding of quality measurement for psychosocial health care as part of cancer care.
- Query organizations that set standards for cancer care (e.g., the National Comprehensive Cancer Network, the American Society of Clinical Oncology [ASCO], the American College of Surgeons Commission on Cancer, the Oncology Nursing Society, the Ameri-can Psychosocial Oncology Society) and other standards-setting organizations (e.g., the National Quality Forum, the National

Committee for Quality Assurance, the URAC, the Joint Commission) to determine the extent to which they have

– created oversight mechanisms used to measure and report on the quality of ambulatory cancer care (including psychosocial care);
– incorporated requirements for identifying and responding to psychosocial health care needs into their protocols, policies, and standards in accordance with the standard of care put forth in this report; and
– used performance measures of psychosocial health care in their quality oversight activities.

For recommendation 7 on workforce competencies, DHHS could

- Monitor and report on actions taken by Congress and federal agencies to support and fund the establishment of a Workforce Development Collaborative on Psychosocial Care during Chronic Medical Illness.
- Review board exams for oncologists and primary care providers to identify questions relevant to psychosocial care.
- Review accreditation standards for educational programs used to train health care personnel to identify content requirements relevant to psychosocial care.
- Review certification requirements for clinicians to identify those requirements relevant to psychosocial care.
- Examine the funding portfolios of the NIH, CMS, AHRQ, and other public and private sponsors of quality-of-care research to quantify the funding of initiatives aimed at assessing the incorporation of workforce competencies in education, training, and clinical practice and their impact on achieving the standard for psychosocial care.

For recommendation 8 on standardized nomenclature and recommendation 9 on research priorities, DHHS could

- Report on NIH/AHRQ actions to develop a taxonomy and nomenclature for psychosocial health services.
- Examine the funding portfolios of public and private research sponsors to assess whether funding priorities included the recommended areas.

REFERENCES

APA (American Psychiatric Association). 2000. *Diagnostic and statistical manual of mental disorders, text revision (DSM-IV-TR)*. 4th ed. Washington, DC: APA.

Bayliss, E. A., J. F. Steiner, D. H. Fernald, L. A. Crane, and D. S. Main. 2003. Description of barriers to self-care by persons with comorbid chronic diseases. *Annals of Family Medicine* 1(1):15–21.

Boberg, E. W., D. H. Gustafson, R. P. Hawkins, K. P. Offord, C. Koch, K.-Y. Wen, K. Kreutz, and A. Salner. 2003. Assessing the unmet information, support and care delivery needs of men with prostate cancer. *Patient Education and Counseling* 49(3):233–242.

Bruce, M. 2006. A systematic and conceptual review of posttraumatic stress in childhood cancer survivors and their parents. *Clinical Psychology Review* 26(3):233–256.

Carlsen, K., A. B. Jensen, E. Jacobsen, M. Krasnik, and C. Johansen. 2005. Psychosocial aspects of lung cancer. *Lung Cancer* 47(3):293–300.

Eakin, E. G., and L. A. Strycker. 2001. Awareness and barriers to use of cancer support and information resources by HMO patients with breast, prostate, or colon cancer: Patient and provider perspectives. *Psycho-Oncology* 10(2):103–113.

Epstein, R. M., and R. L. Street. 2007. Patient-centered communication in cancer care: Promoting healing and reducing suffering. NIH Publication No. 07-6225. Bethesda, MD: National Cancer Institute.

Fallowfield, L., D. Ratcliffe, V. Jenkins, and J. Saul. 2001. Psychiatric morbidity and its recognition by doctors in patients with cancer. *British Journal of Cancer* 84(8):1011–1015.

Hayman, J. A., K. M. Langa, M. U. Kabeto, S. J. Katz, S. M. DeMonner, M. E. Chernew, M. B. Slavin, and A. M. Fendrick. 2001. Estimating the cost of informal caregiving for elderly patients with cancer. *Journal of Clinical Oncology* 19(13):3219–3225.

Hegel, M. T., C. P. Moore, E. D. Collins, S. Kearing, K. L. Gillock, R. L. Riggs, K. F. Clay, and T. A. Ahles. 2006. Distress, psychiatric syndromes, and impairment of function in women with newly diagnosed breast cancer. *Cancer* 107(12):2924–2931.

Hewitt, M., J. H. Rowland, and R. Yancik. 2003. Cancer survivors in the United States: Age, health, and disability. *Journal of Gerontology* 58(1):82–91.

Himmelstein, D. U., E. Warren, D. Thorne, and S. Woolhandler. 2005. Market watch: Illness and injury as contributors to bankruptcy. *Health Affairs* Web Exclusive: DOI 10.1377/hlthaff.W5.63.

IOM (Institute of Medicine). 1982. *Health and behavior: Frontiers of research in the biobehavioral sciences*. D. A. Hamburg, G. R. Elliot, and D. L. Parron, eds. Washington, DC: National Academy Press.

IOM. 2001. *Health and behavior: The interplay of biological, behavioral, and societal influences*. Washington, DC: National Academy Press.

IOM. 2003. *When children die: Improving palliative and end-of-life care for children and their families*. M. J. Field and R. E. Behrman, eds. Washington, DC: The National Academies Press.

IOM. 2006. *Improving the quality of health care for mental and substance-use conditions*. Washington, DC: The National Academies Press.

IOM. 2007. *Implementing cancer survivorship care planning*. Washington, DC: The National Academies Press.

IOM and NRC (National Research Council). 2001. *Improving palliative care for cancer*. K. M. Foley and H. Gelband, eds. Washington, DC: National Academy Press.

IOM and NRC. 2003. *Childhood cancer survivorship: Improving care and quality of life*. M. Hewitt, S. L. Weiner, and J. V. Simone, eds. Washington, DC: The National Academies Press.

IOM and NRC. 2006. *From cancer patient to cancer survivor: Lost in transition.* M. Hewitt, S. Greenfield, and E. Stovall, eds. Washington, DC: The National Academies Press.

Jacobsen, P. B., and S. Ransom. 2007. Implementation of NCCN distress management guidelines by member institutions. *Journal of the National Comprehensive Cancer Network* 5(1):93–103.

Jemal, A., L. Clegg, E. Ward, L. Ries, X. Wu, P. Jamison, P. A. Wingo, H. L. Howe, R. N. Anderson, and B. K. Edwards. 2004. Annual report to the nation on the status of cancer, 1975–2001, with a special feature regarding survival. *Cancer* 101(1):3–27.

Jerant, A. F., M. M. von Friederichs-Fitzwater, and M. Moore. 2005. Patients' perceived barriers to active self-management of chronic conditions. *Patient Education and Counseling* 57(3):300–307.

Kangas, M., J. Henry, and R. Bryant. 2002. Posttraumatic stress disorder following cancer. A conceptual and empirical review. *Clinical Psychology Review* 22(4):499–524.

Katon, W. J. 2003. Clinical and health services relationships between major depression, depressive symptoms, and general medical illness. *Biological Psychiatry* 54(3):216–226.

Keller, M., S. Sommerfeldt, C. Fischer, L. Knight, M. Riesbeck, B. Löwe, C. Herfarth, and T. Lehnert. 2004. Recognition of distress and psychiatric morbidity in cancer patients: A multi-method approach. *European Society for Medical Oncology* 15(8):1243–1249.

Kelly, M. P., J. Bonnefoy, A. Morgan, and F. Florenza. 2006. *The development of the evidence base about the social determinants of health.* World Health Organization Commission on Social Determinants of Health Measurement and Evidence Knowledge Network. http://www.who.int/social_determinants/resources/mekn_paper.pdf (accessed September 26, 2006).

Kotkamp-Mothes, N., D. Slawinsky, S. Hindermann, and B. Strauss. 2005. Coping and psychological well being in families of elderly cancer patients. *Critical Reviews in Oncology-Hematology* 55(3):213–229.

Kurtz, M. E., J. C. Kurtz, C. W. Given, and B. A. Given. 2004. Depression and physical health among family caregivers of geriatric patients with cancer—a longitudinal view. *Medical Science Monitor* 10(8):CR447–CR456.

Mallinger, J. B., J. J. Griggs, C. G. Shields. 2005. Patient-centered care and breast cancer survivors' satisfaction with information. *Patient Education and Counseling* 57(3):342–349.

Maly, R. C., Y. Umezawa, B. Leake, and R. A. Silliman. 2005. Mental health outcomes in older women with breast cancer: Impact of perceived family support and adjustment. *Psycho-Oncology* 14(7):535–545.

May, J. H., and P. J. Cunningham. 2004. *Tough trade-offs: Medical bills, family finances and access to care.* Washington, DC: Center for Studying Health System Change.

Merckaert, I., Y. Libert, N. Delvaux, S. Marchal, J. Boniver, A.-M. Etienne, J. Klastersky, C. Reynaert, P. Scalliet, J.-L. Slachmuylder, and D. Razavi. 2005. Factors that influence physicians' detection of distress in patients with cancer. Can a communication skills training program improve physicians' detection? *Cancer* 104(2):411–421.

Ness, K. K., A. C. Mertens, M. M. Hudson, M. M. Wall, W. M. Leisenring, K. C. Oeffinger, C. A. Sklar, L. L. Robison, and J. G. Gurney. 2005. Limitations on physical performance and daily activities among long-term survivors of childhood cancer. *Annals of Internal Medicine* 143(9):639–647.

President's Cancer Panel. 2004. *Living beyond cancer: Finding a new balance. President's Cancer Panel 2003–2004 annual report.* Bethesda, MD: National Cancer Institute, National Institutes of Health, Department of Health and Human Services.

Riegel, B., and B. Carlson. 2002. Facilitators and barriers to heart failure self-care. *Patient Education and Counseling* 46(4):287–295.

Ries, L., D. Melbert, M. Krapcho, A. Mariotto, B. Miller, E. Feuer, L. Clegg, M. Horner, N. Howlader, M. Eisner, M. Reichman, and B. E. Edwards. 2007. *SEER cancer statistics review, 1975–2004.* Bethesda, MD: National Cancer Institute.

Schultz, R., and S. R. Beach. 1999. Caregiving as a risk factor for mortality: The caregiver health effects study. *Journal of the American Medical Association* 282(23):2215–2219.

Segrin, C., T. A. Badger, P. Meek, A. M. Lopez, E. Bonham, and A. Sieger. 2005. Dyadic interdependence on affect and quality-of-life trajectories among women with breast cancer and their partners. *Journal of Social and Personal Relationships* 22(5):673–689.

Segrin, C., T. Badger, S. M. Dorros, P. Meek, and A. M. Lopez. 2007. Interdependent anxiety and psychological distress in women with breast cancer and their partners. *Psycho-Oncology* 16(7):634–643.

Skalla, K. A., M. Bakitas, C. T. Furstenberg, T. Ahles, and J. V. Henderson. 2004. Patients' need for information about cancer therapy. *Oncology Nursing Forum* 31(2):313–319.

Spiegel, D., and J. Giese-Davis. 2003. Depression and cancer: Mechanism and disease progression. *Biological Psychiatry* 54(3):269–282.

Spitzer, R. L., K. Kroenke, M. Linzer, S. R. Hahn, J. B. Williams, F. V. deGruy, D. Brody, and M. Davies. 1995. Health-related quality of life in primary care patients with mental disorders. Results from the PRIME-MD 1000 study. *Journal of the American Medical Association* 274(19):1511–1517.

Subramanian, S., P. Belli, and I. Kawachi. 2002. The macroeconomic determinants of health. *Annual Review of Public Health* 23:287–302.

Tu, H. T. 2004. *Rising health costs, medical debt and chronic conditions.* Issue Brief No. 88. Washington, DC: Center for Studying Health System Change.

USA Today, Kaiser Family Foundation, and Harvard School of Public Health. 2006. *National survey of households affected by cancer: Summary and chartpack.* Menlo Park, CA, and Washington, DC: USA Today, Kaiser Family Foundation, and Harvard School of Public Health. http://www.kff.org/Kaiserpolls/upload/7591.pdf (accessed April 24, 2007).

Wdowik, M. J., P. A. Kendall, and M. A. Harris. 1997. College students with diabetes: Using focus groups and interviews to determine psychosocial issues and barriers to control. *The Diabetes Educator* 23(5):558–562.

1

The Psychosocial Needs
of Cancer Patients

CHAPTER SUMMARY

Fully 41 percent of all Americans can expect to be diagnosed with cancer at some point in their life. They and their loved ones can take some comfort from the fact that over the past two decades, substantial progress in the early detection and treatment of multiple types of cancer has significantly extended the life expectancy of patients to the point that many people diagnosed with cancer can be cured, and the illness of many others can be managed as a chronic disease. Even so, people with cancer face the risk of substantial and permanent physical impairment, disability, and inability to perform routine activities of daily living, as well as the psychological and social problems that can result from the diagnosis and its sequelae.

Additionally worrisome, the remarkable advances in biomedical care for cancer have not been matched by achievements in providing high-quality care for the psychological and social effects of cancer. Numerous cancer survivors and their caregivers report that cancer care providers did not understand their psychosocial needs, failed to recognize and adequately address depression and other symptoms of stress, were unaware of or did not refer them to available resources, and generally did not consider psychosocial support to be an integral part of quality cancer care.

In response to a request from the National Institutes of Health, this report puts forth a plan delineating actions that cancer care providers, health policy makers, educators, health insurers, health plans, researchers and research sponsors, and consumer advocates should take to better respond to the psychological and social stresses faced by people with cancer, and thereby maximize their health and health care.

THE REACH OF CANCER

More than ten and a half million people in the United States live with a past or current diagnosis of some type of cancer (Ries et al., 2007); 1.4 million[1] Americans are projected to receive a new diagnosis of cancer in 2007 alone (Jemal et al., 2007). Reflecting cancer's reach, 1 in 10 American households now includes a family member who has been diagnosed or treated for cancer within the past 5 years (USA Today et al., 2006), and 41 percent of Americans can expect to be diagnosed with cancer at some point in their life (Ries et al., 2007).

While more than half a million Americans will likely die from cancer in 2007[2] (Jemal et al., 2007), numerous others are being effectively treated and will survive cancer-free for many years. Still others will have a type of cancer that is chronic and that will need to be controlled by intermittent or continuous treatment, not unlike patients with heart disease or diabetes.

Although cancers historically have not been thought of as such, they increasingly meet the definition of chronic diseases: "They are permanent, leave residual disability, are caused by nonreversible pathological alteration, require special training of the patient for rehabilitation, or may be expected to require a long period of supervision, observation, or care" (Timmreck, 1987:100).[3] As described in the next section, many of the more than 100 specific types of cancer frequently leave patients with residual disability and/or nonreversible pathological alteration, and require long periods of supervision, observation, or care. Treatment protocols by themselves for some cancers—such as breast, prostate, and colon cancer (among the most common types of cancers)—can last months; individuals on certain oral chemotherapeutic regimens for breast cancer or some forms of leukemia sometimes remain on chemotherapy for years. Even after completing treatment, cancer survivors (particularly survivors of pediatric cancers) often require care from multiple specialists and primary care providers to manage the long-term sequelae of the illness and its treatment. Thus the trajectories of various cancers vary according to the type of cancer, stage at diagnosis, and other factors (see Figure 1-1).

In addition to coping with the worry and stress brought about by their diagnosis, patients with cancer and their families must cope with the stresses induced by physically demanding (and also often life-threatening) treatments for the illness and the permanent health impairment and

---

[1]This figure excludes non-melanoma skin cancers and in situ carcinomas except in the urinary bladder.

[2]One in four deaths in the United States is due to cancer—the leading cause of death for those under age 85 (Jemal et al., 2007).

[3]The definition of chronic disease used in the National Library of Medicine's Medical Subject Headings (MeSH).

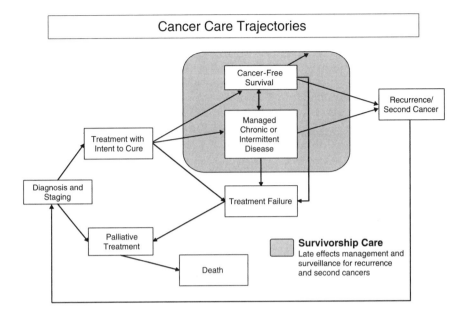

FIGURE 1-1 Cancer care trajectories.
SOURCE: Adapted from IOM and NRC, 2006.

disability, fatigue, and pain that can result, even when there are no longer any signs of the disease. These effects contribute to emotional distress and mental health problems among cancer patients, and together can lead to substantial social problems, such as the inability to work and reduced income. These effects are magnified in the presence of any psychological and social stressors that predate the onset of cancer, such as low income, lack of health insurance, and weak or absent social supports. Indeed, physical, psychological, and social stressors are often intertwined, both resulting from and contributing to each other.

These effects of cancer and its treatment are also influenced by the physical and developmental age of patients and their caregivers. More than half (approximately 60 percent) of individuals who have ever been diagnosed with cancer are age 65 or older; 39 percent are young and middle-aged adults aged 20–64; and 1 percent are age 19 or younger (NCI, undated). Among the large portion of older adults within the population living with cancer, experts in cancer care and aging note that there is great heterogeneity. Although "health and well-being, social circumstances, living arrangements, and age-related changes resulting in diminished psychologic and physical functioning vary by individual and not by chronological age" (Yancik and Ries, 2000:17), older adults with cancer are more likely to present with a preexisting chronic disease and increased functional impairment and disability, which can compound the stresses imposed by cancer (Hewitt et al., 2003). Evidence also indicates that older adults are at greater risk than younger adults for difficulties with health-related decision making (Finucane et al., 2002). Taken together, older adults may have greater need for psychosocial services. At the other end of the age continuum, the great cognitive, emotional, and developmental (as well as physical) variations among children affect the extent to which they can fully understand the implications of their disease and be involved in treatment decision making, how they cope with the physical pain and distress accompanying cancer and its treatment, and the resources available to help them cope (Patenaude and Kupst, 2005).

CANCER-INDUCED PHYSICAL STRESSORS

Health Impairment, Disability, Fatigue, and Pain

As a result of advances in early detection and treatment, in the past two decades the 5-year survival rate for the 15 most common cancers has increased for all ages—from 43 to 64 percent for men and from 57 to 64 percent for women (Jemal et al., 2004). However, these improvements in survival are sometimes accompanied by permanent damage to patients' physical health. In addition to the damage caused by the cancer itself, the side effects of chemotherapy, radiation, hormone therapy, surgery, and other cancer treatments often lead to substantial permanent impairment of several organ systems, with resultant disability (Aziz and Rowland, 2003; Oeffinger and Hudson, 2004).

Impairment and Disability

Compared with people without a history of cancer, adults with cancer (or with a history of cancer) more frequently report having fair or poor health (30 percent), other chronic medical conditions (42 percent), one or more limitations in the ability to perform activities of daily living (11 percent), other functional disabilities (58 percent), and (among those under age 65) an inability to work because of a health condition (17 percent) (Hewitt et al., 2003). These numbers may reflect in part the older age of individuals with a diagnosis of cancer; 61 percent of those with a history of cancer are more than 65 years of age (IOM and NRC, 2006). Yet one-third of those with a history of cancer who report limitations in activities of daily living or other functional areas identify cancer as the cause of their limitation, and cancer survivors in all age groups report higher rates of chronic illness compared with their counterparts with no history of the illness. National Health Interview Survey (NHIS) data from 1998, 1999, and 2000 indicate that a medical history of cancer at least doubles an individual's likelihood of poor health and disability. Individuals with a history of cancer also have significantly higher rates of other chronic illnesses, such as cardiovascular disease. When cancer and another chronic illness co-occur, poor health and disability rates are 5 to 10 times higher than otherwise expected (Hewitt et al., 2003).

Survivors of childhood cancer similarly have much higher than average rates of chronic illness beginning in their early or middle adult years. A retrospective study of more than 10,000 adults who had been diagnosed with certain cancers[4] before age 21 and who survived at least 5 years after diagnosis found that 62 percent of those between the ages of 18 and 48 (mean age 26.6 years) had at least one chronic health condition; 27 percent had a condition that was severe, life-threatening (e.g., kidney failure or need for dialysis, seizure disorder, congestive heart failure), or disabling. This was on average 17.5 years after diagnosis (range 6–31 years). Even 30 years after diagnosis, almost three-fourths had a chronic health condition; more than 40 percent had a condition that was severe, life-threatening, disabling, or fatal; and 39 percent had multiple conditions. None of these estimates include mental health problems (Oeffinger et al., 2006).

Cognitive impairment also is found in some children and adults treated for cancer. Studies of children treated for acute lymphoblastic leukemia and brain tumors (the two most common childhood cancers), for example, indicate that impairment of cognitive abilities (e.g., attention and concentration, working memory, information processing speed, sequencing ability, and visual–motor integration) is common (IOM and NRC, 2003; Butler and Mulhern, 2005). These late effects of cancer and treatment can contribute to problems in reading, language development, and ability to perform complex mathematics. Children can have difficulties doing work in the classroom and require more time to complete homework. They can also have problems in such areas as handwriting, organizing material on a page, lining up columns for arithmetic problems, and being able to complete computer-readable standardized testing forms—all of which can affect school performance and learning. Even if cancer survivors are initially asymptomatic at reentry to school, neurocognitive deficits may develop years later (IOM and NRC, 2003).

Cognitive impairment has also been documented in adults. Although the cause of such impairment (dubbed "chemobrain" by some cancer survivors)

---

[4]Leukemia, central nervous system tumor, Hodgkins disease, non-Hodgkins lymphoma, Wilms' tumor, neuroblastoma, sarcoma, or bone tumor.

is not yet clear, women treated with chemotherapy for breast cancer, for example, show subtle declines in global cognitive functioning, most particularly in language skills (e.g., word-finding ability), short-term memory, and spatial abilities; lesser impairment is found in their working and long-term memory and their speed of information processing (Stewart et al., 2006). Similar impairment of verbal memory and other executive cognitive functions has been found in adults treated for lung, colorectal, lymphoma, and other types of cancer; however, different types of cancer and their treatment vary in their cognitive effects (Anderson-Hanley et al., 2003).

Fatigue

Fatigue is the most frequently reported symptom of cancer and is identified as causing the greatest interference with patients' daily activities, although estimates of rates of fatigue among individuals with cancer vary greatly (ranging, for example, from 4 percent in breast cancer patients prior to the start of chemotherapy to 91 percent in breast cancer patients after surgery and chemotherapy and before bone marrow transplantation). Prevalence rates are difficult to interpret, however, because there is no consensus on a standard definition of fatigue, and studies use different criteria for defining its presence and severity. Fatigue is theorized to arise from a complex combination of poorly understood physical and psychological effects of illness that may be different in each patient (Carr et al., 2002). Nonetheless, it is widely recognized as a frequent side effect of both cancer and its treatment. It is different from the fatigue experienced by healthy individuals in that it persists even after rest and sleep. A 2002 review of the evidence by the Agency for Healthcare Research and Quality (AHRQ) found that mechanisms of cancer-related fatigue have been poorly explored, and current treatment options for fatigue are limited[5] (Carr et al., 2002). Fatigue among non-ill individuals generally is manifested by compromised problem solving, decreased motivation and vigor in the completion of required tasks, and overall diminished capacity for work (IOM, 2004). These effects are reported by patients with cancer as well, who also report that fatigue interferes with their physical and mental functioning (Carr et al., 2002).

---

[5]The report did identify Epoetin alfa as effective in treating chemotherapy-induced anemia and resultant fatigue, and noted that there is some evidence that exercise can reduce fatigue in women with breast cancer (Carr et al., 2002).

Pain

An estimated one-third to one-half of patients undergoing active treatment for cancer experience pain resulting from the illness, its treatment, or co-occurring illnesses. This pain often is not fully eliminated despite the administration of analgesics and other therapies, in part because it is often undertreated. Moreover, pain may continue to be a problem even when there is no longer any sign of cancer. AHRQ's 2002 evidence review documented the contribution of cancer-related pain to fatigue, impaired function, and a range of other psychosocial dimensions of health (Carr et al., 2002).

Limitations in Activities of Daily Living

The physical impairments and disabilities, as well as fatigue and pain, experienced by patients with cancer often lead to an inability to perform the routine activities of daily living that most people take for granted. Activities of daily living are defined as those age-appropriate physical and cognitive activities that individuals generally perform for themselves as part of their daily self-care. For adults, these include such activities as bathing, using the toilet, dressing, preparing meals, and feeding oneself. Instrumental activities of daily living include such tasks as using a telephone, shopping, paying bills, and using transportation. In the United States, adults with a prior diagnosis of cancer[6] are more likely than those of similar age, sex, and educational level without such a diagnosis to report needing help with activities of daily living (Yabroff et al., 2004). NHIS data for 1998–2000 show that cancer survivors without any other chronic illnesses were more than twice as likely as individuals without a history of cancer or other chronic illness to report limitations in their ability to perform activities of daily living and significantly more likely to have other functional limitations (Hewitt et al., 2003). Long-term survivors of childhood cancer are at particular risk. Nearly 20 percent of more than 11,000 such individuals (median age 26, range 5–56) diagnosed between 1970 and 1986 who survived 5 years or more reported limitations in activities such as lifting heavy objects; running or participating in strenuous sports; carrying groceries; walking uphill or climbing a flight of stairs; walking a block; or eating, dressing, bathing, or using the toilet. These limitations occurred at nearly twice the rate found in their siblings without cancer. Fewer (3, 7, and 8 percent, respectively) reported limitations in ability to eat, bathe, dress, or get around their home by themselves; perform everyday household chores; or hold a job or attend school. However, these rates were five to six times higher than those seen in their siblings without cancer (Ness et al., 2005).

---

[6]Not including non-melanoma skin cancers.

PSYCHOSOCIAL PROBLEMS

The emotional stress of living with a diagnosis of cancer and its treatment, fear of recurrence, and the distress imposed by living with the day-to-day physical problems described above can create new or worsen preexisting psychological distress for people living with cancer, their families, and other informal caregivers. Physical and psychological impairments can also lead to substantial social problems, such as the inability to work or fulfill other normative social roles.

Emotional, Mental Health, and Developmental Problems

Emotional and Mental Health Problems

Although the majority of cancer patients and their families have normal psychological functioning (Kornblith, 1998), distressed psychological states are common in individuals with cancer. The prevalence of psychological distress varies by type of cancer, time since diagnosis, degree of physical and role impairment, amount of pain, prognosis, and other variables. In one U.S. comprehensive cancer center's study of nearly 4,500 patients aged 19 and older, the prevalence of significant psychological distress ranged from 29 to 43 percent for patients with the 14 most common types of cancer[7] (Zabora et al., 2001). These rates are consistent with those found in subsequent studies of diverse populations with cancer that have reported high rates of psychological symptoms meeting criteria for such clinical diagnoses as depression, adjustment disorders, and anxiety (Spiegel and Giese-Davis, 2003; Carlsen et al., 2005; Hegel et al., 2006). Studies have also documented the presence of symptoms meeting the criteria for post-traumatic stress disorder (PTSD) and post-traumatic stress symptoms (PTSS) in adults and children with cancer, as well as in the parents of children diagnosed with the illness (Kangas et al., 2002; Bruce, 2006). Indeed, experiencing a life-threatening medical illness or observing it in another to whom one is close can be a qualifying event for PTSD according to the American Psychiatric Association's *Diagnostic and Statistical Manual of Mental Disorders (DSM-IV-TR)* (APA, 2000).

Even patients who do not develop clinical syndromes may experience worries, fears, and other forms of psychological stress that cause them significant distress. Chronic illness can bring about guilt, feelings of loss of control, anger, sadness, confusion, and fear (Charmaz, 2000; Stanton et al., 2001). Anxiety, mood disturbance, fear of recurrence, concerns about body

---

[7]Lung, brain, Hodgkin's, pancreas, lymphoma, liver, head and neck, adenocarcinoma, breast, leukemia, melanoma, colon, prostate, and gynecological.

image, and communication and other problems with family members are common in cancer patients as well (Kornblith, 1998). Patients may also experience more generalized worry; fear for the future; inability to make plans; uncertainty and a heightened sense of vulnerability; and other worries, such as about the possible development of a second cancer, changes in sexual function and reproductive ability, and changes in one's role within the family and other relationships (IOM and NRC, 2006). Moreover, cancer patients can face spiritual and existential issues involving their faith, their perceived relationship with God, and the possibility and meaning of death. Some cancer survivors report feelings of anger, isolation, and diminished self-esteem in response to such stress (NCI, 2004).

Family members also have psychological needs (Lederberg, 1998). The diagnosis of a life-threatening illness for a family member creates fear of losing the loved one and concern about the suffering he or she will endure. Family members' psychological distress can be as severe as that of the patient. A meta-analysis of studies of psychological distress in both patients and their informal caregivers (predominantly spouses or partners) found that the psychological distress of patients and their informal caregivers generally was parallel over time, although when the patient received treatment, caregivers experienced more distress than the patient (Hodges et al., 2005). Studies of partners of women with breast cancer (predominantly husbands, but also "significant others," daughters, friends, and others) find that partners' mental health correlates positively with the anxiety, depression, fatigue, and symptom distress of women with breast cancer and that the effects are bidirectional (Segrin et al., 2005, 2007). Thus, helping family members to manage their distress may have a beneficial effect on the distress level of patients.

Stress is particularly great for parents of children with cancer. Studies consistently have shown that parents have higher rates of PTSD and PTSS than either their children or adult cancer survivors, suggesting that the experience of parenting a child with cancer may be more traumatic than actually having the illness (Bruce, 2006). Children of cancer patients also are a vulnerable group, with frequent psychological problems, acting-out behaviors, and problems in school (Lederberg, 1998). Moreover, siblings of pediatric cancer patients may experience their own fears and anxieties, and may receive less attention from parents while their brother or sister is in treatment.

Family members (predominantly) and friends of individuals with cancer often provide substantial amounts of emotional and logistical support and hands-on personal and nursing care to their loved ones (Kotkamp-Mothes et al., 2005; Maly et al., 2005). The estimated value of their nonreimbursed care and support exceeds $1 billion annually (Hayman et al., 2001). Further, when their loved ones experience acute or long-term inability to care for themselves or to carry out their roles in the family, family members often step in to take up these roles. Taking on these responsibilities requires considerable adaptation (and readaptation as the course of the disease changes) on the part of family members. These experiences can add to the stress resulting from concern about the ill family member. Indeed, this stress, especially in caregivers compromised by morbidity accompanying their own aging, can be so substantial that caregivers are afflicted more by depression, other adverse health effects, and death than are patients themselves (Schultz and Beach, 1999; Kurtz et al., 2004). Caregivers who provide support to their spouse and report caregiving strain are 63 percent more likely to die within 4 years than those who do not provide care to their spouse or who provide care but report no strain (Schultz and Beach, 1999).

High stress levels in family caregivers also can interfere with their ability to provide the emotional or logistical support patients need. This can exacerbate the patient's stress and lead to the cascading consequences of elevated stress described above. Because of the changes and necessary adaptation in the family brought about by the caregiving needs of the patient, family members are sometimes considered "second-order patients" (Lederberg, 1998).

Developmental Problems

As individuals mature, they typically master and apply certain behavioral skills in their daily life. These skills include, for example, achieving self-sufficiency and physical, emotional, financial, and social independence from parents; engaging in satisfying personal relationships of varying intimacy and in meaningful work; and performing other normative social roles. The effects of cancer and its treatment can interrupt and delay the activities in which individuals typically engage to develop these skills, or can require temporarily or permanently giving up the skills and activities. As a result, individuals can experience a range of problems manifested as developmental delays, regression, or inability to perform social roles. Cancer-induced inability to perform normative activities can occur at any age. Older adults, for example, can face unplanned retirement, limitations in grandparenting abilities, inability to act as caregiver to others in their family, or limitations in their ability to work.

Children who experience numerous and prolonged hospitalizations at critical developmental periods are at particular risk for developmental problems (IOM and NRC, 2003). Adolescents can face a significant loss of independence and disruption of their social relationships at a time when they should be developing social and relationship skills critical to successful functioning in adulthood (NCI, 2004). Physical changes resulting from cancer and its treatment—such as hearing loss and vision problems; endocrine disturbances resulting in short stature, delayed puberty, and reproductive problems; and impaired sexual functioning—also can occur at any age and interfere with successful development. Adolescents and adult cancer survivors report difficulties in knowing how to plan for the future, for example, in establishing educational and career aspirations (NCI, 2004). Adolescents and young adults may have less work experience because of their illness and be at a competitive disadvantage in the labor market. This situation can be compounded if their illness or treatment causes disfigurement or requires some accommodation in the workplace. Revealing a history of cancer to a prospective employer may result in discrimination. Research has also identified some limitations in the social functioning of school-age cancer survivors (IOM and NRC, 2003). Children may return to their social network at school and beyond without hair, with amputations, or with weight gain or other physical changes resulting from their disease or its treatment. They also may have developmental problems that require attention and need help in reentering social relationships.

Social Problems

The physical and psychological problems described above can be exacerbated by or produce significant new social problems. Financial stress resulting from low income, the cost of health care, or a lack of health insurance, as well as reduced employment and income, can result in substantial stress. While the fundamental resolution of such social problems is beyond the abilities of health care providers,[8] evidence described below and in the next chapters shows why attention to these problems is an integral part of good-quality health care and how they can be addressed within the constraints of clinical practices.

Financial Stress

In 2003, nearly one in five (12.3 million) people with chronic conditions[9] lived in families that had problems paying medical bills (Tu, 2004); 63 percent of these individuals also reported problems in paying for rent, their mortgage, transportation, and food as a result of medical debt (May and Cunningham, 2004). Consistent with these findings, CancerCare, a nonprofit agency supporting individuals with cancer, reports that of those to whom it provides financial grants to pay for transportation, 18 and 11

---

[8]And beyond the scope of this report.
[9]Cancer, as well as asthma, arthritis, diabetes, chronic obstructive pulmonary disease, heart disease, hypertension, benign prostate enlargement, abnormal uterine bleeding, and depression.

percent, respectively, cited skipping medications or canceling a medical appointment in the past 3 months because of financial problems. The 2006 National Survey of U.S. Households Affected by Cancer also found that one in four families in which a member of the household had cancer in the past 5 years said the experience led the patient to use up all or most of his or her savings; 13 percent had to borrow money from their relatives to pay bills; and 10 percent were unable to pay for basic necessities such as food, heat, or housing. Seven percent took out another mortgage on their home or borrowed money, and 3 percent declared bankruptcy. Eight percent delayed or did not receive care because of the cost. As would be expected, the financial consequences were worse for those without health insurance: more than one in four delayed or decided not to get treatment because of its cost; 46 percent used all or most of their savings to pay for treatment; 41 percent were unable to pay for basic necessities; and 6 percent filed for bankruptcy (USA Today et al., 2006). About 5 percent of the 1.5 million American families who filed for bankruptcy in 2001 reported that medical costs associated with cancer contributed to their financial problems (Himmelstein et al., 2005).

Not surprisingly, members of the American Society of Clinical Oncology (ASCO), the Oncology Nursing Society (ONS), and the Association of Oncology Social Work (AOSW) report financial needs as a frequent subject of patient inquiries (Matthews et al., 2004). The American Cancer Society (ACS) and CancerCare both receive and respond to a large number of patient requests for financial assistance. In fiscal year 2006, 3,482 patients contacting CancerCare received $1,812,206 for unmet financial needs such as child care, home care, and living expenses. In the first 8 months of fiscal year 2007, 2,069 received $727,745 in such financial assistance. In fiscal year 2006, the ACS responded to 41,378 requests for financial assistance to help patients manage the costs of durable medical equipment (3,713), medications (13,013), prosthetics (128), rent (459), scholarships (2,141), utilities (657), wigs (1,674), other medical expenses (1,763), and other needs (17,830). Both agencies report that requests for financial assistance are one of the most common reasons people contact them, and often there are not enough resources to meet these needs.[10,11]

Financial needs can arise from the high costs of medical treatment, drugs, and other health support needs, such as medical supplies that are not covered by insurance and/or are beyond an individual's income level. This financial stress is compounded when a patient suffers a job loss, is not working during periods of treatment, or lacks health insurance.

[10]Personal communication, Diane Blum, Executive Director, CancerCare, June 8, 2007.
[11]Personal communication, Katherine Sharpe, American Cancer Society, June 8, 2007.

Lack of or Inadequate Health Insurance

An estimated 44.8 million Americans (15.3 percent of the population) were without health insurance in 2005 (U.S. Census Bureau, 2007), and many more have only modest insurance coverage coupled with an income level that limits their ability to pay out-of-pocket health care costs (May and Cunningham, 2004; Tu, 2004). The rate of uninsurance among cancer survivors is no higher than that among the general population (and is in fact a bit lower—11.3 percent among the nonelderly),[12] and among nonaged cancer survivors also is comparable to that observed in populations with other chronic illnesses, such as cardiovascular disease (12.1) and diabetes (12.6) (IOM and NRC, 2006). However, these figures offer little comfort. The adverse effects of no or inadequate insurance are well documented and include poorer health prior to receipt of care, delayed or no treatment, failure to get needed prescription medications, and worse outcomes of medical treatment for people with cancer as well as other diseases (IOM, 2002; Tu, 2004; IOM and NRC, 2006).

Further, analysis of the 2003 national Community Tracking Study Household Survey found that a majority of chronically ill working-age adults who reported health care cost and access problems had private health insurance. Thirteen percent of those with private insurance had out-of-pocket health care costs (not including costs for insurance premiums) that exceeded 5 percent of their income, and 16 percent lived in families that had problems paying their medical bills. Among those who were privately insured but had low income, more than one-third had problems paying their medical bills. Among the privately insured with such problems, 10 percent went without needed medical care, 30 percent delayed care, and 43 percent failed to fill needed prescriptions because of cost concerns (Tu, 2004). The National Survey of U.S. Households Affected by Cancer found that 10 percent of individuals with health insurance reached the limit of their insurance coverage, and 6 percent lost their coverage as a result of having cancer (USA Today et al., 2006).

Because health insurance in the United States for those under age 65 is most often obtained through employers, problems with health insurance are affected by problems with employment (Himmelstein et al., 2005). If an individual loses his or her job because of cancer, he or she also runs the risk of losing health insurance coverage—and income.

---

[12]And nearly all (99 percent) of patients over age 65 have health insurance through the Medicare program.

Reduced Employment and Income

In its review of studies of cancer and employment, the 2006 Institute of Medicine (IOM) report *From Cancer Patient to Cancer Survivor: Lost in Transition* found that the effect of having cancer on employment has not been well studied across all types of cancer. Nevertheless, studies across different types of cancers and populations have consistently shown that significant portions of individuals (7 to 70 percent across studies [Spelten et al., 2002]) stop working or experience a change in employment (reduction in work hours, interruption of work, change in place of employment) after being diagnosed or treated for cancer (IOM and NRC, 2006), with implications for their income. Data from the 2000 NHIS reveal that in the United States, adults aged 18 and older with a prior diagnosis of cancer[13] were less likely than individuals of similar age, sex, and educational levels to have had a job in the past month, were more likely to have limitations in the amount or type of work they could do because of health problems, and (among those with jobs) had fewer days of work in the past year (Yabroff et al., 2004). In another analysis of NHIS data from 1998–2000, 17 percent of individuals with a history of cancer reported being unable to work, compared with 5 percent of those without such a history (Hewitt et al., 2003). A retrospective cohort study carried out in five medical centers in Pennsylvania and Maryland with 1,435 cancer survivors aged 25–62 who were working at the time of their diagnosis in 1997–1999 found 41 and 39 percent of males and females, respectively, stopped working during cancer treatment. Although most (84 percent) returned to work within the 4 years after diagnosis (73 percent within the first 12 month after diagnosis), a significant minority (16 percent) did not do so. Of those who returned to work in the first year, 11 percent quit for cancer-related reasons within the next 3 years. Overall, 13 percent quit working for cancer-related reasons within 4 years of diagnosis (Short et al., 2005). Individuals whose jobs require manual labor or make other physical demands and those with head and neck cancers, cancers of the central nervous system, and stage IV blood and lymphatic cancers appear to be especially at risk for reductions in employment (Spelten et al., 2002; Short et al., 2005). The late effects of the illness or its treatment in survivors of childhood cancer can also prevent many from working (Ness et al., 2005; de Boer et al., 2006).

These changes in employment patterns can be a function of shifting priorities and values after diagnosis, a desire for retirement (consistent with the older age of most cancer patients), or changes in one's employer having nothing to do with the employee (IOM and NRC, 2006). However, many individuals with cancer report that changes in their employment or their

---

[13]Not including non-melanoma skin cancers.

ability to work are a function of changes in their health resulting from their cancer diagnosis (IOM and NRC, 2006).

OBSTACLES TO MANAGING PSYCHOSOCIAL STRESSORS

In multiple focus groups and interviews, patients with a wide variety of chronic illnesses, such as diabetes, arthritis, heart disease, chronic obstructive lung disease, depression, and asthma, have identified pain, fatigue, problems with mobility, poor communication with physicians (with resultant poor understanding of their illness and how to manage it), depression and other negative emotions, stress, lack of family support, financial problems, loss of a job, and lack of health insurance as obstacles to managing their illness and health (Wdowik et al., 1997; Riegel and Carlson, 2002; Bayliss et al., 2003; Jerant et al., 2005). Patients were often unaware of resources available to help them overcome these problems, but when they were aware, limitations in mobility, fatigue, pain, transportation problems, cost issues, and lack of insurance prevented them from taking advantage of these resources (Jerant et al., 2005). Cancer patients and their health care providers offer similar reports of these social and psychological obstacles (IOM and NRC, 2003, 2004; NCI, 2004), which add to the suffering created by the illness, prevent adherence to prescribed treatments, and interfere with patients' ability to manage their illness and their health. These problems and the effects of failing to address them are magnified in especially vulnerable and disadvantaged populations, such as those living in poverty; those with low literacy; members of cultural minorities; and those over age 65, who are more likely than younger individuals to experience the compounding effects of other chronic conditions that occur with aging.

Some of these stressors (described in the preceding sections) can come about as a consequence of cancer, others can predate the illness, while still others are imposed by the health care system itself. Although not all individuals treated for cancer face these problems, individuals who do so need the knowledge, skills, and abilities to manage them and function at their highest possible level. When these resources are not available, the ability to manage one's illness and health is decreased.

Lack of Information, Knowledge, and Skills Needed to Manage the Illness

Members of ASCO, ONS, and AOSW report that information and education about cancer are the support services most frequently requested by their patients (Matthews et al., 2004). Patients similarly rate information needs pertaining to their illness and treatments as very important (Boberg et al., 2003). Yet over the past three decades research has consistently documented many patients' and family members' dissatisfaction with the information and education they receive (Chapman and Rush, 2003) and how their health care providers communicate with them (Epstein and Street, 2007). While research has not yet yielded a comprehensive road map for how best to provide the full array of information needed at various times during and after cancer treatment, it has illuminated several characteristics of the effective provision of information. For example, information should be tailored to each patient's expectations and preferences (e.g., much detailed information in advance versus less information provided on an as-needed basis), as well as to the patient's individual diagnosis and clinical situation. Evidence also indicates that patients' wide range of information needs (e.g., information specific to their type and stage of cancer, treatment, prognosis, rehabilitation, achievement and maintenance of maximal health, coping, and financial/legal concerns) change over time, for example, during and after treatment (Rutten et al., 2005; Epstein and Street, 2007). Further, anxiety decreases satisfaction with information provided. Anxiety and other side effects of the illness and its treatment, such as pain, need to be controlled if information is to be useful (Chapman and Rush, 2003). However, evidence indicates that measures to control such side effects, as well as more basic practices to meet patients' information needs effectively, are not employed; many patients continue to have insufficient information to help them manage their illness and health (Eakin and Strycker, 2001; Boberg et al., 2003; Skalla et al., 2004; Mallinger et al., 2005). Fifteen percent of respondents to the 2006 National Survey of U.S. Households Affected by Cancer said they had had the experience of leaving a doctor's office without getting answers to important questions about their illness (USA Today et al., 2006).

Related to these findings, members of ASCO, ONS, and AOSW reported that support groups were the second most frequent subject of patient inquiries about support services (Matthews et al., 2004). Peer support programs in which people communicate and share experiences with others having a common personal experience are strong mechanisms for building one's "self-efficacy"—the belief that one is capable of carrying out a course of action to reach a desired goal (Bandura, 1997). Self-efficacy is a critical determinant of how well knowledge and skills are obtained and is an excellent predictor of behavior. There is also evidence that self-efficacy is key to individuals' successful self-management of a range of chronic illnesses, resulting in improved health outcomes (Lorig et al., 2001; Lorig and Holman, 2003). However, although peer support programs are widespread, providers are not always aware of these resources and often do not refer patients to them (IOM, 2007). Failure to refer patients to these services is associated with their low use (Eakin and Strycker, 2001).

Insufficient Logistical Resources

Even when patients have the information, knowledge, and skills to cope with their illness, a lack of logistical and material resources, such as transportation, medical equipment, and supplies, can prevent their use. As described above, the high costs of medical care (for those with and without health insurance), together with work reductions and job loss with a concomitant decrease in income, can make obtaining the needed resources difficult if not impossible. Families, friends, and other informal sources of support can provide or help secure many of these resources (Eakin and Strycker, 2001), but sometimes such sources are unavailable or overwhelmed by patients' needs. Oncology physicians, nurses, and social workers report that transportation in particular is a "paramount concern" of patients (Matthews et al., 2004:735).

Lack of Transportation

In a 2005 survey, members of AOSW identified transportation as the third greatest barrier[14] to patients and their families receiving good-quality cancer care (AOSW, 2006). The inability to get to medical appointments, the pharmacy, the grocery store, health education classes, peer support meetings, and other out-of-home resources can hinder health care, illness management, and health promotion. Indicative of this problem, ACS reports receiving more than 90,000 requests for transportation services in 2006.[15] CancerCare reports that 14,919 patients requested and were provided $3,005,679 in financial grants in fiscal year 2006 to pay for transportation. These grants (typically $100–200) were used for transportation to cancer-related medical appointments (47 percent), pharmacies or other places to pick up medications (27 percent), other medical or mental health appointments or an emergency room (8 percent), case management/client advocacy appointments (1 percent), and other destinations (17 percent). In the first 8 months of fiscal year 2007, 10,102 patients received $1,621,282 to help pay for transportation.[16]

Weak Social Support

Also, as described above, patients' informal social supports (family members and friends) provide substantial emotional, informational, and logistical support. When an individual has sufficient family members or other informal supports, such as neighbors, friends, or church groups,

---

[14]Behind inadequate health insurance and inability to pay for treatment-related expenses.
[15]Personal communication, Katherine Sharpe, American Cancer Society, March 20, 2007.
[16]Personal communication, Diane Blum, Executive Director, CancerCare, March 8, 2007.

they can perform or assist the patient in performing necessary tasks. When these informal supports are lacking, the effects of psychosocial problems are compounded.

Inattention and Lack of Support from the Health Care System

Despite the adverse effects of the psychosocial problems described above, patients report that these problems are not well addressed as part of their oncology care. At multiple meetings held across the nation with the President's Cancer Panel in 2003 and 2004, cancer survivors of all ages reported that many health care providers "still do not consider psychosocial support an integral component of quality cancer care and may fail to recognize, adequately treat, or refer for depression, anger and stress in cancer survivors, family members or other caregivers" (NCI, 2004:27). Numerous survivors and caregivers also testified that many cancer care providers did not understand their psychosocial needs, often were unaware of available resources, and/or did not provide referrals to those resources. Consistent with these reports, 28 percent of respondents to the National Survey of U.S. Households Affected by Cancer reported that they did not have a doctor who paid attention to factors beyond their direct medical care, such as a need for support in dealing with the illness (USA Today et al., 2006). A number of studies have shown that physicians substantially underestimate oncology patients' psychosocial distress (Fallowfield et al., 2001; Keller et al., 2004; Merckaert et al., 2005). Inattention to psychosocial problems on the part of oncology providers has also been reported by cancer survivors in focus groups (IOM, 2007) and other studies (Maly et al., 2005).

Two prior IOM reports (IOM, 2000, 2001) underscore that the vast majority of problems in the quality of health care are not the result of poorly motivated, uncaring, or unintelligent health care personnel, but instead result from numerous barriers to high-quality health care in the systems that prepare clinicians for their work and structure their work practices. Some of these barriers occur at the level of the patient's interaction with the clinician (e.g., poor communication between the patient and his/her health care providers, multiple demands on clinicians' time[17]),

---

[17]There is little evidence on the extent to which time is/is not sufficient to address patients' psychosocial issues. Information on both sides of the issue appears to be anecdotal. For example, examples of oncology practices described in Chapter 5 suggest that psychosocial problems can be significantly addressed. Others report that time is insufficient. One qualitative study (Bodenheimer et al., 2004) of physicians organizations' use of care management processes found that in organizations with strong leadership and a quality-focused culture, the most frequently mentioned barriers to care management—inadequate finances, payers not rewarding quality, inadequate information technology, and resistance or overwork of physicians—did not prevent the adoption of care management processes. Sites mentioning physician

some at the level of interactions among different clinicians serving the same patient (e.g., poor coordination of care across providers), some within the organization in which care is delivered (e.g., inadequate work supports, such as information technology), and some in the environment external to the delivery of care (e.g., reimbursement arrangements that financially penalize the provision of good-quality care) (Berwick, 2002).[18] Barriers at all four of these levels have been identified as potentially contributing to health care providers' failure to respond appropriately to cancer patients' psychosocial needs and are addressed in succeeding chapters.

Clinicians may not inquire about psychosocial problems because of inadequate education and training (including inadequate clinical practice guidelines) in these issues (IOM and NRC, 2004), a lack of awareness of services available to address these needs (Matthews et al., 2002), or a lack of knowledge about how to integrate attention to psychosocial health needs into their practices. The 2004 IOM report *Meeting Psychosocial Needs of Women with Breast Cancer* called particular attention to the fact that much of cancer care has shifted from inpatient to ambulatory care settings. A great deal has been written about the way in which ambulatory care practices have been constructed in the past, and the fact that their structures and work design processes need to undergo fundamental change if effective care for chronic illnesses and support for individuals' management of those illnesses is to be provided (IOM, 2001; Bodenheimer et al., 2002).

Aspects of the external environment that surrounds the delivery of health care—such as reimbursement and purchasing strategies and regulatory and quality oversight structures—also have been identified as mechanisms that as yet do not support the delivery of psychosocial health care (NCI, 2004; IOM, 2006; NCCN, 2006). Moreover, even when psychosocial problems are identified and services sought, shortages and maldistribution of health care professionals with needed expertise can be a barrier to care. In rural and other geographically remote areas, for example, there is limited availability of mental health care practitioners (IOM, 2006).

---

overwork also tended to be sites that well adopted care management processes. This study also noted how little is known about physician overwork. Because of the weakness of evidence in this area, the extent to which time allows practitioners to attend to psychosocial issues is unknown, but it is reasonable to believe it may vary according to how work is designed at each practice site.

[18] *Crossing the Quality Chasm: A New Health System for the 21st Century* identifies four different levels for intervening in the delivery of health care: (1) the experience of patients; (2) the functioning of small units of care delivery ("microsystems"), such as surgical teams or nursing units; (3) the functioning of organizations that house the microsystems; and (4) the environment of policy, payment, regulation, accreditation, and similar external factors that shape the context in which health care organizations deliver care.

The role of cancer patients and their caregivers in securing and using appropriate psychosocial health services also may need attention.

PURPOSE, SCOPE, AND ORGANIZATION OF THIS REPORT

Recognizing the impact on cancer patients and their families of unaddressed psychosocial problems, the National Institutes of Health's (NIH) Office of Behavioral and Social Sciences Research asked the IOM to empanel a committee to conduct a study of the delivery of the diverse psychosocial services needed by these patients and their families in community settings. The committee was tasked with producing a report that would

- Describe how the broad array of psychosocial services needed by cancer patients is provided and what barriers exist to accessing such care.
- Analyze the capacity of the current mental health and cancer treatment system to deliver psychosocial care, delineate the resources needed to deliver this care nationwide, and examine available training programs for professionals providing psychosocial and mental health services.
- Recommend ways to address these issues and an action plan for overcoming the identified barriers to cancer patients' receiving the psychosocial services they need.

A more detailed description of the tasks to be carried out by the committee and the methods used for the study is provided in Appendix B. Of note, this study builds on several prior IOM reports on cancer care, as well as those of other authoritative bodies (see Appendix C). This report is unique, however, in that it focuses exclusively on the delivery of psychosocial health services, and does so across all types of cancer. In shaping its scope of work, the committee took into particular consideration two recent IOM reports addressing the quality of care for cancer survivors. First, the report of the Committee on Cancer Survivorship: Improving Care and Quality of Life entitled *From Cancer Patient to Cancer Survivor: Lost in Transition* (IOM and NRC, 2006) well articulated how high-quality care (including psychosocial health care) should be delivered after patients complete their cancer treatment. The IOM report *Childhood Cancer Survivorship: Improving Care and Quality of Life* similarly addressed survivorship for childhood cancer (IOM and NRC, 2003). For this reason, the committee that conducted the present study chose to focus on how psychosocial services should be delivered during active treatment of cancer. The recommendations made in this report complement those of the two prior reports on cancer survivorship, and can be implemented for cancer survivors who have completed treatment in a manner consistent with the vision articulated in those reports. Second, two recent reports addressed palliative care: *Improving Palliative Care for Cancer* (IOM and NRC, 2001) and *When Children Die: Improving Palliative and End-of-Life Care for Children and Their Families* (IOM, 2003b). For this reason, the additional considerations involved in providing end-of-life care are not addressed in this report.

Finally, NIH directed the committee to give higher priority to in-depth as opposed to a broader array of less detailed analyses and recommendations, and noted that, given the complexity of this study, it might not be possible to thoroughly explore diversity and health disparity issues. Especially in the identification of successful models for the delivery of psychosocial services, NIH asked that the committee focus on generic models that should be promoted, with the understanding that some of these models might need to be modified to reach underserved communities. Thus, although the committee considered differences in the impact of cancer and the attendant needs of those who are socially disadvantaged, issues pertaining to health disparities (also addressed comprehensively in the recent IOM report *Unequal Treatment: Confronting the Racial and Ethnic Disparities in Health Care* [IOM, 2003a]) are not specifically addressed in this report.

With respect to the committee's charge to address "psychosocial services to cancer . . . *families* . . ." (emphasis added), the committee notes that the word "family" can mean many different things to different people; can be shaped by personal beliefs and personal, ethical, and religious values; and can have legal and political implications. The committee did not attempt to define "family" but aimed to describe what is known about cancer's effects on families as the term is variously used in qualitative and quantitative research. Most of this research has focused on the effects of cancer on spouses, parents, siblings, and children of individuals with cancer. Another large body of research focuses on "caregivers" of individuals with cancer or other illnesses. This research documents that while most caregivers are spouses and adult children of ill individuals, many other individuals, such as close friends, neighbors, and individuals from places of worship, also act as caregivers. Thus, this report incorporates research findings about "families" and "caregivers." When these words are used, we provide information on how the words are used in the research reviewed. Because of the size of this literature, and consistent with the committee's desire to address a subset of critical issues in depth, while family distress is addressed in this report, it was not possible to fully examine all of the issues families/caregivers face when a loved one is diagnosed with cancer.

The unique contributions of this report are that it

- provides an explicit definition of psychosocial health services. Although the term "psychosocial services" is frequently used, the committee found that it is used inconsistently and sometimes not at all. This inconsistency has confounded the conduct and interpretation of research on psychological and social problems that seriously interfere with patients' health care, as well as efforts to address those problems. The definition formulated by the committee and its conceptual and empirical underpinnings are presented in Chapter 2.

- identifies discrete services that are encompassed by the term psychosocial health care, evidence that supports their effectiveness, and issues needing additional research (discussed in Chapters 3 and 8).

- identifies a generic, conceptually and evidence-based model for ensuring the delivery of psychosocial health services (Chapter 4) and strategies for implementing this model in community settings with varying levels of resources (Chapter 5). In its work, the committee interpreted "community care" to mean care delivered in settings other than in-patient care sites.[19]

- identifies the support needed from policy makers in the purchasing, oversight, and regulatory arenas to facilitate routine attention to psychosocial health needs in cancer care and the delivery of psychosocial health services when needed (Chapter 6).

- identifies the knowledge, skills, and abilities needed by the workforce to implement the model for psychosocial health care, and examines how the education and training of the workforce can be improved to provide them (Chapter 7).

- identifies a research agenda to help improve psychosocial health care (Chapter 8).

Together, the recommendations presented in this report and proposed means of evaluating their successful implementation (also in Chapter 8) constitute an action plan for overcoming the identified barriers to cancer patients' receipt of the psychosocial health services they need in community settings.

---

[19]Individuals receive care for their cancer in a variety of settings, including inpatient facilities, outpatient departments attached to medical centers and hospitals, freestanding ambulatory oncology practices, and ambulatory practices of primary care physicians and other specialists. In order to address the care of as many cancer patients as possible, and recognizing that the processes and intensity of inpatient care and the needs of acutely ill inpatients differ from those associated with ambulatory care, the committee interpreted "community care" to refer to all sites of cancer care except inpatient settings.

REFERENCES

Anderson-Hanley, C., M. L. Sherman, R. Riggs, V. B. Agocha, and B. E. Compas. 2003. Neuropsychological effects of treatments for adults with cancer: A meta-analysis and review of the literature. *Journal of the International Neuropsychological Society* 9(7):967–982.

AOSW (Association of Oncology Social Work). 2006. *Member survey report*. The Association of Oncology Social Work. http://www.aosw.org/docs/MemberSurvey.pdf (accessed August 17, 2007).

APA (American Psychiatric Association). 2000. *Diagnostic and statistical manual of mental disorders, text revision (DSM-IV-TR)*. 4th ed. Washington, DC: APA.

Aziz, N. M., and J. H. Rowland. 2003. Trends and advances in cancer survivorship research: Challenge and opportunity. *Seminars in Radiation Oncology* 13(3):248–266.

Bandura, A. 1997. *Self-efficacy: The exercise of control*. New York: W.H. Freeman.

Bayliss, E. A., J. F. Steiner, D. H. Fernald, L. A. Crane, and D. S. Main. 2003. Description of barriers to self-care by persons with comorbid chronic diseases. *Annals of Family Medicine* 1(1):15–21.

Berwick, D. M. 2002. A user's manual for the IOM's quality chasm report. *Health Affairs* 21(3):80–90.

Boberg, E. W., D. H. Gustafson, R. P. Hawkins, K. P. Offord, C. Koch, K.-Y. Wen, K. Kreutz, and A. Salner. 2003. Assessing the unmet information, support and care delivery needs of men with prostate cancer. *Patient Education and Counseling* 49(3):233–242.

Bodenheimer, T., E. H. Wagner, and K. Grumbach. 2002. Improving primary care for patients with chronic illness: The chronic care model, part 2. *Journal of the American Medical Association* 288(15):1909–1914.

Bodenheimer, T., M. C. Wang, T. Rundall, S. M. Shortell, R. R. Gillies, N. Oswald, L. Casalino, and J. C. Robinson. 2004. What are the facilitators and barriers in physician organizations' use of care management processes? *Joint Commission Journal on Quality and Safety* 30(9):505–514.

Bruce, M. 2006. A systematic and conceptual review of posttraumatic stress in childhood cancer survivors and their parents. *Clinical Psychology Review* 26(3):233–256.

Butler, R. W., and R. K. Mulhern. 2005. Neurocognitive interventions for children and adolescents surviving cancer. *Journal of Pediatric Psychology* 30(1):65–78.

Carlsen, K., A. B. Jensen, E. Jacobsen, M. Krasnik, and C. Johansen. 2005. Psychosocial aspects of lung cancer. *Lung Cancer* 47(3):293–300.

Carr, D., L. Goudas, D. Lawrence, W. Pirl, J. Lau, D. DeVine, B. Kupelnick, and K. Miller. 2002. *Management of cancer symptoms: Pain, depression, and fatigue*. AHRQ Publication No. 02-E032. Rockville, MD: Agency for Healthcare Research and Quality. http://www.ahrq.gov/downloads/pub/evidence/pdf/cansymp/cansymp.pdf (accessed November 2, 2006).

Chapman, K., and K. Rush. 2003. Patient and family satisfaction with cancer-related information: A review of the literature. *Canadian Oncology Nursing Journal* 13(2):107–116.

Charmaz, K. 2000. Experiencing chronic illness. In *Handbook of social studies in health and medicine*. Edited by G. L. Albrecht, R. Fitzpatrick, and S. C. Scrimshaw. Thousand Oaks, CA: Sage Publications.

de Boer, A. G., J. H. Verbeek, and F. J. van Dijk. 2006. Adult survivors of childhood cancer and unemployment: A metaanalysis. *Cancer* 107(1):1–11.

Eakin, E. G., and L. A. Strycker. 2001. Awareness and barriers to use of cancer support and information resources by HMO patients with breast, prostate, or colon cancer: Patient and provider perspectives. *Psycho-Oncology* 10(2):103–113.

Epstein, R. M., and R. L. Street. 2007. *Patient-centered communication in cancer care: Promoting healing and reducing suffering*. NIH Publication No. 07-6225. Bethesda, MD: National Cancer Institute.

Fallowfield, L., D. Ratcliffe, V. Jenkins, and J. Saul. 2001. Psychiatric morbidity and its recognition by doctors in patients with cancer. *British Journal of Cancer* 84(8):1011–1015.

Finucane, M. L., P. Slovic, J. H. Hibbard, E. Peters, C. K. Mertz, and D. G. MacGregor. 2002. Aging and decision-making competence: An analysis of comprehension and consistency skills in older versus younger adults considering health-plan options. *Journal of Behavioral Decision Making* 15(2):141–164.

Hayman, J. A., K. M. Langa, M. U. Kabeto, S. J. Katz, S. M. DeMonner, M. E. Chernew, M. B. Slavin, and A. M. Fendrick. 2001. Estimating the cost of informal caregiving for elderly patients with cancer. *Journal of Clinical Oncology* 19(13):3219–3225.

Hegel, M. T., C. P. Moore, E. D. Collins, S. Kearing, K. L. Gillock, R. L. Riggs, K. F. Clay, and T. A. Ahles. 2006. Distress, psychiatric syndromes, and impairment of function in women with newly diagnosed breast cancer. *Cancer* 107(12):2924–2931.

Hewitt, M., J. H. Rowland, and R. Yancik. 2003. Cancer survivors in the United States: Age, health, and disability. *Journal of Gerontology* 58(1):82–91.

Himmelstein, D. U., E. Warren, D. Thorne, and S. Woolhandler. 2005. Market watch: Illness and injury as contributors to bankruptcy. *Health Affairs* Web Exclusive: DOI 10.1377/hlthaff.W5.63.

Hodges, L. J., G. M. Humphris, and G. Macfarlane. 2005. A meta-analytic investigation of the relationship between the psychological distress of cancer patients and their carers. *Social Science and Medicine* 60(1):1–12.

IOM (Institute of Medicine). 2000. *To err is human: Building a safer health system.* L. T. Kohn, J. M. Corrigan, and M. S. Donaldson, eds. Washington, DC: National Academy Press.

IOM. 2001. *Crossing the quality chasm: A new health system for the 21st century.* Washington, DC: National Academy Press.

IOM. 2002. *Care without coverage: Too little, too late.* Washington, DC: National Academy Press.

IOM. 2003a. *Unequal treatment: Confronting the racial and ethnic disparities in health care.* B. D. Smedley, A. Y. Stith, and A. R. Nelson, eds. Washington, DC: The National Academies Press.

IOM. 2003b. *When children die: Improving palliative and end-of-life care for children and their families.* M. J. Field and R. E. Behrman, eds. Washington, DC: The National Academies Press.

IOM. 2004. *Keeping patients safe: Transforming the work environment of nurses.* A. E. K. Page, ed. Washington, DC: The National Academies Press.

IOM. 2006. *Improving the quality of health care for mental and substance-use conditions.* Washington, DC: The National Academies Press.

IOM. 2007. *Implementing cancer survivorship care planning.* Washington, DC: The National Academies Press.

IOM and NRC (National Research Council). 2001. *Improving palliative care for cancer.* Edited by K. M. Foley and H. Gelband. Washington, DC: National Academy Press.

IOM and NRC. 2003. *Childhood cancer survivorship: Improving care and quality of life.* M. Hewitt, S. L. Weiner, and J. V. Simone, eds. Washington, DC: The National Academies Press.

IOM and NRC. 2004. *Meeting psychosocial needs of women with breast cancer.* Edited by M. Hewitt, R. Herdman, and J. Holland. Washington, DC: The National Academies Press.

IOM and NRC. 2006. *From cancer patient to cancer survivor: Lost in transition.* M. Hewitt, S. Greenfield, and E. Stovall, eds. Washington, DC: The National Academies Press.

Jemal, A., L. X. Clegg, E. Ward, L. A. G. Ries, X. Wu, P. M. Jamison, P. A. Wingo, H. L. Howe, R. N. Anderson, and B. K. Edwards. 2004. Annual report to the nation on the status of cancer, 1975–2001, with a special feature regarding survival. *Cancer* 101(1):3–27.

Jemal, A., R. Siegel, E. Ward, T. Murray, J. Xu, and M. J. Thun. 2007. Cancer statistics, 2007. *CA: A Cancer Journal for Clinicians* 57(1):43–66.

Jerant, A. F., M. M. von Friederichs-Fitzwater, and M. Moore. 2005. Patients' perceived barriers to active self-management of chronic conditions. *Patient Education and Counseling* 57(3):300–307.

Kangas, M., J. Henry, and R. Bryant. 2002. Posttraumatic stress disorder following cancer. A conceptual and empirical review. *Clinical Psychology Review* 22(4):499–524.

Keller, M., S. Sommerfeldt, C. Fischer, L. Knight, M. Riesbeck, B. Löwe, C. Herfarth, and T. Lehnert. 2004. Recognition of distress and psychiatric morbidity in cancer patients: A multi-method approach. *European Society for Medical Oncology* 15(8):1243–1249.

Kornblith, A. B. 1998. Psychosocial adaptation of cancer survivors. In *Psycho-oncology*. Edited by J. C. Holland. New York and Oxford: Oxford University Press.

Kotkamp-Mothes, N., D. Slawinsky, S. Hindermann, and B. Strauss. 2005. Coping and psychological well being in families of elderly cancer patients. *Critical Reviews in Oncology-Hematology* 55(3):213–229.

Kurtz, M. E., J. C. Kurtz, C. W. Given, and B. A. Given. 2004. Depression and physical health among family caregivers of geriatric patients with cancer—a longitudinal view. *Medical Science Monitor* 10(8):CR447–CR456.

Lederberg, M. S. 1998. The family of the cancer patient. In *Psycho-oncology*. Edited by J. C. Holland. New York and Oxford: Oxford University Press. Pp. 981–993.

Lorig, K., and H. Holman. 2003. Self-management education: History, definition, outcomes, and mechanisms. *Annals of Behavioral Medicine* 26(1):1–7.

Lorig, K. R., P. Ritter, A. L. Stewart, D. S. Sobel, B. W. Brown, A. Bandura, V. M. Gonzalez, D. D. Laurent, and H. R. Holman. 2001. Chronic disease self-management program—2-year health status and health care utilization outcomes. *Medical Care* 39(11):1217–1223.

Mallinger, J. B., J. J. Griggs, C. G. Shields. 2005. Patient-centered care and breast cancer survivors' satisfaction with information. *Patient Education and Counseling* 57(3):342–349.

Maly, R. C., Y. Umezawa, B. Leake, and R. A. Silliman. 2005. Mental health outcomes in older women with breast cancer: Impact of perceived family support and adjustment. *Psycho-Oncology* 14(7):535–545.

Matthews, B. A., F. Baker, and R. L. Spillers. 2002. Health care professionals' awareness of cancer support services. *Cancer Practice* 10(1):36–44.

Matthews, B. A., F. Baker, and R. L. Spillers. 2004. Oncology professionals and patient requests for cancer support services. *Supportive Care in Cancer* 12(10):731–738.

May, J. H., and P. J. Cunningham. 2004. *Tough trade-offs: Medical bills, family finances and access to care.* Washington, DC: Center for Studying Health System Change.

Merckaert, I., Y. Libert, N. Delvaux, S. Marchal, J. Boniver, A.-M. Etienne, J. Klastersky, C. Reynaert, P. Scalliet, J.-L. Slachmuylder, and D. Razavi. 2005. Factors that influence physicians' detection of distress in patients with cancer. Can a communication skills training program improve physicians' detection? *Cancer* 104(2):411–421.

NCCN (National Comprehensive Cancer Network). 2006. *Distress management. NCCN clinical practice guidelines in oncology V.I.2007.* http://www.nccn.org/professional/physicians_gls/PDF/distress.pdf (accessed January 17, 2007).

NCI (National Cancer Institute). 2004. *Living beyond cancer: Finding a new balance. President's cancer panel 2003–2004 annual report.* Bethesda, MD: Department of Health and Human Services, National Institutes of Health. http://deainfo.nci.nih.gov/ADVISORY/pcp/pcp03-04/Survivorship.pdf (accessed May 4, 2006).

NCI. undated. *Estimated U.S. cancer prevalence.* http://cancercontrol.cancer.gov/ocs/prevalence/prevalence.html#age (accessed August 14, 2007).

Ness, K. K., A. C. Mertens, M. M. Hudson, M. M. Wall, W. M. Leisenring, K. C. Oeffinger, C. A. Sklar, L. L. Robison, and J. G. Gurney. 2005. Limitations on physical performance and daily activities among long-term survivors of childhood cancer. *Annals of Internal Medicine* 143(9):639–647.

Oeffinger, K. C., and M. M. Hudson. 2004. Long-term complications following childhood and adolescent cancer: Foundations for providing risk-based health care for survivors. *CA: A Cancer Journal for Clinicians* 54(4):208–236.

Oeffinger, K. C., A. C. Mertens, C. A. Sklar, T. Kawashima, M. M. Hudson, A. T. Meadows, D. L. Friedman, N. Marina, W. Hobbie, N. S. Kadan-Lottick, C. L. Schwartz, W. Leisenring, L. L. Robison, for the Childhood Cancer Survivor Study. 2006. Chronic health conditions in adult survivors of childhood cancer. *New England Journal of Medicine* 355(15):1572–1582.

Patenaude, A., and M. Kupst. 2005. Psychosocial functioning in pediatric cancer. *Journal of Pediatric Psychology* 30(1):9–27.

Riegel, B., and B. Carlson. 2002. Facilitators and barriers to heart failure self-care. *Patient Education and Counseling* 46(4):287–295.

Ries, L., D. Melbert, M. Krapcho, A. Mariotto, B. Miller, E. Feuer, L. Clegg, M. Horner, N. Howlader, M. Eisner, M. Reichman, B. Edwards, eds. 2007. *SEER cancer statistics review, 1975–2004 National Cancer Institute.* http://seer.cancer.gov/csr/1975_2004/ (accessed June 6, 2007).

Rutten, L. J., N. K. Arora, A. D. Bakos, N. Aziz, and J. Rowland. 2005. Information needs and sources of information among cancer patients: A systematic review of research (1980–2003). *Patient Education and Counseling* 57(3):250–261.

Schultz, R., and S. R. Beach. 1999. Caregiving as a risk factor for mortality: The caregiver health effects study. *Journal of the American Medical Association* 282(23):2215–2219.

Segrin, C., T. A. Badger, P. Meek, A. M. Lopez, E. Bonham, and A. Sieger. 2005. Dyadic interdependence on affect and quality-of-life trajectories among women with breast cancer and their partners. *Journal of Social and Personal Relationships* 22(5):673–689.

Segrin, C., T. Badger, S. M. Dorros, P. Meek, and A. M. Lopez. 2007. Interdependent anxiety and psychological distress in women with breast cancer and their partners. *Psycho-Oncology* 16(7):634–643.

Short, P. F., J. J. Vasey, and K. Tunceli. 2005. Employment pathways in a large cohort of adult cancer survivors. *Cancer* 103(6):1292–1301.

Skalla, K. A., M. Bakitas, C. T. Furstenberg, T. Ahles, and J. V. Henderson. 2004. Patients' need for information about cancer therapy. *Oncology Nursing Forum* 31(2):313–319.

Spelten, E. R., M. A. G. Sprangers, and J. H. A. M. Verbeek. 2002. Factors reported to influence the return to work of cancer survivors: A literature review. *Psycho-Oncology* 11(2):124–131.

Spiegel, D., and J. Giese-Davis. 2003. Depression and cancer: Mechanism and disease progression. *Biological Psychiatry* 54(3):269–282.

Stanton, A. L., C. A. Collins, and L. A. Sworowski. 2001. Adjustment to chronic illness: Theory and research. In *Handbook of Health Psychology.* Mahwah, NJ: Lawrence Erlbaum Associates.

Stewart, A., C. Bielajew, B. Collins, M. Parkinson, and E. Tomiak. 2006. A meta-analysis of the neuropsychological effects of adjuvant chemotherapy treatment in women treated for breast cancer. *The Clinical Neuropsychologist* 20(1):76–89.

Timmreck, T. C. 1987. *Dictionary of health services management.* 2nd ed. Owings Mills, MD: National Health Publishing.

Tu, H. T. 2004. *Rising health costs, medical debt and chronic conditions.* Issue Brief No. 88. Washington, DC: Center for Studying Health System Change.

U.S. Census Bureau. 2007. Census Bureau revises 2004 and 2005 health insurance coverage estimates. Washington, DC: U.S. Department of Commerce.

USA Today, Kaiser Family Foundation, and Harvard School of Public Health. 2006. *National survey of households affected by cancer: Summary and chartpack.* Menlo Park, CA, and Washington, DC: USA Today, Kaiser Family Foundation, and Harvard School of Public Health. http://www.kff.org/Kaiserpolls/upload/7591.pdf (accessed April 24, 2007).

Wdowik, M. J., P. A. Kendall, and M. A. Harris. 1997. College students with diabetes: Using focus groups and interviews to determine psychosocial issues and barriers to control. *The Diabetes Educator* 23(5):558–562.

Yabroff, K. R., W. F. Lawrence, S. Clauser, W. W. Davis, and M. L. Brown. 2004. Burden of illness in cancer survivors: Findings from a population-based national sample. *Journal of the National Cancer Institute* 96(17):1322–1330.

Yancik, R., and L. A. G. Ries. 2000. Aging and cancer in America. *Hematology/Oncology Clinics in North America* 14(1):17–23.

Zabora, J., K. Brintzenhofeszoc, B. Curbow, C. Hooker, and S. Piantadosi. 2001. The prevalence of psychological distress by cancer site. *Psycho-Oncology* 10(1):19–28.

2

Consequences of Unmet
Psychosocial Needs

CHAPTER SUMMARY

Psychosocial problems can be created or exacerbated by cancer and its treatment, as well as predate the illness. The failure to address these problems results in needless patient and family suffering, obstructs quality health care, and can potentially affect the course of the disease. Social isolation and other social factors, stress, and untreated mental health problems contribute to emotional distress and the inability to fulfill valued social roles, and interfere with patients' ability to adhere to their treatment regimens and act in ways that promote their overall health. Additionally, these problems can bring about changes in the functioning of the body's endocrine, immune, and other organ systems, which in turn could have implications for the course of cancer and other conditions. Families and the larger community also can be affected when psychosocial problems are not addressed.

Although it is clear that psychosocial problems influence health, evidence is still emerging on just how they do so. Moreover, some such problems (such as poverty) obviously cannot be resolved by the health care system. Nevertheless, evidence clearly supports the need for attention to psychosocial problems as an integral part of good-quality health care. Psychosocial health services can enable patients with cancer, their families, and health care providers to optimize biomedical health care, manage the psychological/behavioral and social aspects of the disease, and thereby promote better health.

A significant body of research shows that the psychological and social stressors reviewed in Chapter 1—such as depression and other mental health problems, limited financial and other material resources, and inadequate social support—are associated with increased morbidity and mortality and decreased functional status. These effects have been documented both for health generally (House et al., 1988; Kiecolt-Glaser et al., 2002) and for a variety of individual health conditions and illnesses, including heart disease (Hemingway and Marmot, 1999), HIV/AIDS (Leserman et al., 2002), pregnancy (Wills and Fegan, 2001; ACOG Committee on Health Care for Underserved Women, 2006), and cancer (Kroenke et al., 2006; Antoni and Lutgendorf, 2007).

Psychosocial stressors are theorized to affect health adversely in a number of ways. First, emotional distress and mental illness can themselves be the source of suffering, diminished health, and poorer functioning through their symptoms and their adverse effects on role performance. Second, psychosocial problems can adversely affect patients' abilities to cope with and manage their illness by limiting their ability to access and receive appropriate health care resources; adhere to prescribed treatment regimens; and engage in behaviors necessary to manage illness and promote health, such as maintaining a healthy diet, exercising, and monitoring symptoms and adverse responses to treatment (Yarcheski et al., 2004; Kroenke et al., 2006). In multiple focus groups and interviews, patients with chronic illnesses such as diabetes, arthritis, heart disease, chronic obstructive lung disease, depression, and asthma have identified lack of family support, financial problems, lack of health insurance, problems with mobility, depression and other negative emotions, and stress as obstacles to dealing with their illness and health (Wdowik et al., 1997; Riegel and Carlson, 2002; Bayliss et al., 2003; Jerant et al., 2005). Moreover, a growing body of evidence is illuminating how the stress resulting from psychosocial problems can induce adverse effects within the body's cardiovascular, immune, and endocrine systems (Segerstrom and Miller, 2004; Yarcheski et al., 2004; Uchino, 2006; Miller et al., 2007). Although evidence of adverse health outcomes from these effects is strongest for cardiovascular disease, emerging evidence from animal models and some human data suggest pathways through which these effects can influence the course of other illnesses (Antoni and Lutgendorf, 2007).

A wide range of psychosocial variables may affect the course of illness. For example, several studies have found that individual psychological traits such as optimism, mastery, and self-esteem (sometimes termed psychosocial resources) protect against stress (Segerstrom and Miller, 2004). This chapter details the health effects of three psychosocial factors—social support, financial and other material resources, and emotional and mental status—for which there is strong evidence on health effects, for which there are screening and assessment tools that can be used to detect problems, and for which psychosocial health services (described in Chapter 3) exist to address identified problems. Also presented is evidence of how problems in these areas affect the way the body works and the course of certain diseases. Together, these effects reduce an individual's ability to engage in valued roles, and also have negative impacts on both families and the community.

PSYCHOSOCIAL STRESSORS AND THEIR EFFECTS ON PATIENTS

Inadequate Social Support

Humans are social animals, and inadequate social contact and support can have profound adverse consequences. It is not surprising, then, that social support plays a central role in helping cancer patients and their families manage the illness. Although there is currently no single definition of "social support" (King et al., 2006; Uchino, 2006), research reveals that it has multiple dimensions. The web of relationships that exist between a person and his or her family, friends, and other community ties and the structural and functional characteristics of that web are generally referred to as the person's "social network" (Berkman et al., 2000). The number, breadth, and depth of these relationships together make up one's degree of "social integration." Beneficial[1] social networks provide different types of support to individuals under stress, including emotional, informational, and instrumental support. Emotional support involves "the verbal and nonverbal communication of caring and concern," including "listening, 'being there,' empathizing, reassuring, and comforting" (Helgeson and Cohen, 1996:135); informational support increases knowledge and provides guidance or advice; and instrumental support involves the provision of material or logistical assistance, such as transportation, money, or assistance with personal care or household chores (Cohen, 2004). Each type of support can improve health care outcomes. For example, emotional support may help people cope more effectively with the obstacles they encounter and with their own emotional response to the challenges of illness. Insofar as knowledge may be gained from others about treatment or other aspects of care, informational support can increase the effectiveness of health care utilization. And instrumental support may help individuals act on this knowledge.

Morbidity and Mortality Effects

Epidemiological studies across a variety of illnesses have found that when individuals have low levels of social support, they experience worse outcomes, including higher mortality rates (IOM, 2001). There is strong

---

[1]Social networks can also have adverse effects, such as when they support illegal or other undesirable behaviors and attitudes.

evidence that the perception of the availability of social support protects individuals under stress from psychological distress, anxiety, and depression (Wills and Fegan, 2001; Cohen, 2004), in part by buffering them from the effects of stress (House et al., 1988; IOM, 2001). Consistent with this evidence, greater social integration has been associated with reduced mortality in multiple prospective community-based studies (Wills and Fegan, 2001). Conversely, well-designed studies have shown social isolation to be a potent risk factor for mortality across all causes of death (including cancer), as well as death due to specific conditions such as heart disease and stroke (Berkman and Glass, 2000). Indeed, the relative risk of death associated with social isolation is comparable to that associated with high cholesterol, mild hypertension, and smoking (House et al., 1988; IOM, 2001). The mechanisms by which these effects occur are not fully known, but there is evidence that social relationships that are stressful, weak, or absent can lead to decreased ability to cope with illness, negative emotions such as depression or anxiety, and immune and endocrine system dysfunction (see the discussion below) (Uchino et al., 1996; Kielcolt-Glaser et al., 2002).

Effects of social support on health outcomes have been found specifically among individuals with cancer (Patenaude and Kupst, 2005; Weihs et al., 2005). A recent study following 2,800 women with breast cancer for a median of 6 years, for example, found that women who were socially isolated before their diagnosis had a 66 percent higher risk of dying from all causes during the observation period compared with women who were socially integrated. They were also twice as likely to die from breast cancer during this period[2] (Kroenke et al., 2006).

Weakened Coping Abilities and Increased Mental Illness

Psychological adjustment to an illness involves "adaptation to disease without continued elevations of psychological distress (e.g., anxiety, depression) and loss of role function (i.e., social, sexual, vocational)" (Helgeson and Cohen, 1996:136). Positive emotional support is linked to good psychological adjustment to chronic illnesses generally and cancer specifically, and to fewer symptoms of depression and anxiety (Helgeson and Cohen, 1996; Wills and Fegan, 2001; Maly et al., 2005). Conversely, unsupportive social interactions are associated with greater psychological distress (Norton et al., 2005), decreased social role functioning (Figueiredo et al., 2004), and higher rates of post-traumatic stress disorder (PTSD) and post-traumatic stress symptoms (PTSS) in children with cancer (Bruce, 2006).

---

[2]The analysis of data adjusted for stage of cancer at diagnosis, age, and other variables that might also affect survival.

Diminished Ability to Manage Illness

The outcomes noted above are problematic in and of themselves, but they may also decrease individuals' ability to take the actions necessary to adhere to treatment, change health behaviors, and otherwise manage their illness. Individuals with greater social support are more likely to engage in health-promoting behaviors and exhibit healthy physiological functioning (IOM, 2001). In a meta-analysis of studies of predictors of positive health practices, loneliness and degree of perceived social support were found to have the largest effects (in the expected direction) on the performance of healthy behaviors (Yarcheski et al., 2004).

Insufficient Financial and Other Material Resources

Multiple studies have shown that low income is a strong risk factor for disability, illness, and death. Inadequate income limits one's ability to avoid stresses that can accompany everyday life and to purchase food, medications, transportation, and health care supplies necessary for health and health care (Kelly et al., 2006). To take just one example, lack of transportation to get to medical appointments, the pharmacy, the grocery store, health education classes, peer support meetings, and other out-of-home health resources can hinder health monitoring, illness management, and health promotion.

As discussed in Chapter 1, in 2003 nearly one in five people in the United States with chronic conditions[3] lived in families that had problems paying medical bills (Tu, 2004); 63 percent of these individuals also reported problems paying for housing, transportation, and food (May and Cunningham, 2004). Among the privately insured with problems paying medical bills, 10 percent went without needed medical care, 30 percent delayed care, and 43 percent failed to fill needed prescriptions because of cost concerns (Tu, 2004). Overall, 68 percent of families with problems paying medical bills had problems paying for other necessities, such as food and shelter (May and Cunningham, 2004). Such families may trade off medical care so they can fulfill basic needs.

The 2006 National Survey of U.S. Households Affected by Cancer similarly found that 8 percent of families having a household member with cancer delayed or did not receive care because of the cost of care. Of those without health insurance, more than one in four delayed or decided not to get treatment because of its cost, and 41 percent were unable to pay for basic necessities (USA Today et al., 2006). A longitudinal study of a cohort

---

[3]Asthma, arthritis, diabetes, chronic obstructive pulmonary disease, heart disease, hypertension, cancer, benign prostate enlargement, abnormal uterine bleeding, and depression.

of 860 men being treated for prostate cancer found that even after controlling for state of disease at the start of treatment, type of treatment, and other possible influential variables, men without health insurance achieved lower physical functioning, had more role limitations, and experienced poorer emotional well-being over time than men with health insurance. The researchers concluded that "patients undergoing aggressive treatment, which can itself have deleterious effects on quality of life, are exposed to further hardships when they do not have comprehensive health insurance upon which to support their care" (Penson et al., 2001:357). The adverse effects of no or inadequate insurance contribute to poorer health prior to the receipt of health care; undermine the effectiveness of care by increasing the chances of delayed or no treatment and the inability to obtain needed prescription medications; and contribute to worse outcomes of medical treatment for people with cancer and other diseases (IOM, 2002; Tu, 2004; IOM and NRC, 2006).

Emotional Distress and Mental Illness[4]

As discussed in Chapter 1, psychological distress is common among individuals with cancer. However, mental health problems and other types of psychological distress (which sometimes predate illness) (Hegel et al., 2006) are not unique to patients with cancer. People with chronic conditions such as diabetes, heart disease, HIV-related illnesses, and neurological disorders also are found to have high rates of depression, adjustment disorders, severe anxiety, PTSS or PTSD, and subclinical emotional distress (Katon, 2003). In a British sample of older adults living in the community, the development of serious physical illness in the respondent was frequently associated with the development of new-onset major depression (Murphy, 1982). A more recent longitudinal study in Canada found an increased risk of developing major depression to be associated with virtually any long-term medical condition (Patten, 2001). Most recently, an 8-year study followed a nationally representative sample of more than 8,000 U.S. adults aged 51–61 living in the community (and with no symptoms of depression at the start of the study) to examine the extent to which they developed symptoms of depression after a new diagnosis of several illnesses—cancer (excluding minor skin cancers), diabetes, hypertension, heart disease, arthritis, chronic lung disease (excluding asthma), or stroke. Those receiving

---

[4]Portions of this section are from a paper commissioned by the committee entitled "Effects of Distressed Psychological States on Adherence and Health Behavior Change: Cognitive, Motivational, and Social Factors" by M. Robin DiMatteo, Kelly B. Haskard, and Summer L. Williams, all of the University of California, Riverside. This paper is available from the Institute of Medicine.

a diagnosis of cancer were at the highest risk of developing symptoms of depression within 2 years (13 percent incidence), with more than triple the risk of all others combined (Polsky et al., 2005). (Those with a diagnosis of chronic lung disease, heart disease, and stroke also had higher-than-average rates of depressive symptoms.)

Depressed or anxious individuals with a variety of comorbid general medical illnesses (including cancer) report lower social functioning, more disability, and greater overall functional impairment than patients without depression or anxiety (Katon, 2003). Distressed emotional states also often generate additional somatic problems, such as sleep difficulties, fatigue, and pain (Spitzer et al., 1995; APA, 2000), which can confound the diagnosis and treatment of physical symptoms. Among patients with a variety of chronic medical conditions other than cancer, those with depressive and anxiety disorders have significantly more medically unexplained symptoms than those without depression and anxiety, even when severity of illness is controlled for. Patients with depressive and anxiety disorders also have greater difficulty learning to live with chronic symptoms such as pain or fatigue; data suggest that depression and anxiety are associated with heightened awareness of such physical symptoms. Multiple studies of patients with major depression have also found higher-than-normal rates of unhealthy behaviors such as smoking, sedentary lifestyle, and overeating (Katon, 2003). Depression is associated as well with poor adherence to prescribed treatment regimens (DiMatteo et al., 2000).

Impaired Adherence to Medical Regimens and Behavior Changes Designed to Improve Health

While serious health events can trigger health-damaging behaviors—such as use of substances and consumption of unhealthful foods—as individuals cope with the distress associated with the illness, they can also motivate people to take up a number of health-promoting behaviors (McBride et al., 2003; Demark-Wahnefried et al., 2005). One study, for example, found that 6 months after surviving a heart attack, 17 percent of patients were engaged in four health-promoting behaviors (refraining from smoking, weight reduction, sufficient physical activity, and consumption of a low-fat diet), compared with just 3 percent of patients at baseline (Salamonson et al., 2007). Another study found that following HIV diagnosis, 43 percent of individuals reported increased physical activity and 59 percent improved diet (Collins et al., 2001). In general, research indicates that following a cancer diagnosis, many patients engage in behaviors such as stress management, quitting smoking, aerobic exercise, and major dietary change (Blanchard et al., 2003; Ornish et al., 2005; Andrykowski et al., 2006; Rabin and Pinto, 2006; Humpel et al., 2007). One study found that following a cancer diagnosis, as many as half of those who smoked quit (Gritz et al., 2006). The concept of "teachable moments" has been used to explain how, after experiencing health events such as serious illness, people are motivated to take up health-promoting behaviors (McBride et al., 2003; Demark-Wahnefried et al., 2005).

Over the course of many serious acute and chronic conditions, however, patients' adherence to health professionals' recommendations for improved health can be quite low. And despite motivation, changes in actual health behaviors do not always come about or persist. For example, dozens of studies have found more than 30 percent nonadherence to dialysis, dietary and fluid restrictions, and transplant management in patients with end-stage renal disease, diabetes, and lung disease. In patients with cardiovascular disease, nonadherence to lifestyle changes, cardiac rehabilitation, and medication regimens is almost 25 percent. In patients with HIV, nonadherence to highly active antiretroviral treatment regimens and behavior change is 11.7 percent (DiMatteo, 2004). Similar rates of nonadherence have been observed in cancer patients despite the importance to survival and better health care outcomes of adhering to a treatment regimen. More than 20 percent of cancer patients have been found to be nonadherent to a variety of treatments, including oral ambulatory chemotherapy, radiation treatment, and adjuvant therapy with tamoxifen (Partridge et al., 2003; DiMatteo, 2004). For adjuvant tamoxifen, for example, adherence can be as low as 50 percent after 4 years of treatment (Partridge et al., 2003). One study of the natural progression of exercise participation after a diagnosis of breast cancer found that women did not significantly increase their levels of exercise over time and were in fact exercising below recommended levels despite their expressed intentions otherwise (Pinto et al., 2002). As discussed below, depression and other adverse psychological states can thwart adherence to treatment regimens and behavior change in a number of ways, for example, by impairing cognition, weakening motivation, and decreasing coping abilities.

Impaired Cognition

To achieve healthy lifestyles and manage chronic illness effectively, patients must first understand what they need to do to care for themselves. The necessary information may come from many sources, including the media, family members, and health professionals, and may include, for example, reasons for needed chemotherapy, the exact ways in which medication should be administered, and the importance of sleep and a good diet. Distressed psychological states can seriously challenge the cognitive functioning and information processing required to understand treatments and organize health behaviors. Stress, anxiety, anger, and depression can impair the ability to learn and maintain new behaviors (Spiegel, 1997) or to undertake complex tasks that require planning and behavioral execution (Wells and Burnam, 1991; Olfson et al., 1997).

For example, research on kidney transplant recipients' adherence to immunosuppressive medication has found that patients with poor adherence report higher levels of psychological distress relative to patients with good adherence (Achille et al., 2006). Patients undergoing dialysis treatment for end-stage renal disease have also been found to experience greater cognitive impairment and dysfunction due to depressive mood (Tyrrell et al., 2005). Disturbance of mood and motivation in HIV-positive individuals has been associated with decrements in several cognitive factors, such as neurocognitive performance, verbal memory, executive functioning, and motor speed (Castellon et al., 2006). Among patients with advanced cancer, depression and anxiety similarly have been found to contribute to cognitive impairments (Mystakidou et al., 2005). Even after controlling for the effects of pain and illness severity, anxiety and depression among patients with cancer have been independently associated with decreased cognitive functioning (Smith et al., 2003).

Moreover, when patients are distraught about the course of their illness, they may be more likely to forget health professionals' recommendations and less likely to ask questions about their care and participate in medical visits (Robinson and Roter, 1999; DiMatteo et al., 2000; Katon et al., 2004; Sherbourne et al., 2004). Lower levels of patient participation are associated with poorer health behaviors (Martin et al., 2001).

Weakened Motivation

Distressed psychological states can limit patients' concern about the importance of their health behaviors and contribute to their belief that the benefits of adherence are not worth the trouble (Fink et al., 2004). Distressed psychological states can also lead to diminished self-perceptions and limitations in personal self-efficacy,[5] which in turn negatively affect health behaviors and adherence. Pessimism about the future and about oneself can forestall the adoption of new health practices and interfere with health behaviors and adherence (Peterman and Cella, 1998; DiMatteo et al., 2000; Taylor et al., 2004). Limitations in personal self-efficacy that derive from both anxiety and depression can interfere with the behavioral commitment essential to the adoption and maintenance of new health practices. Distressed psychological states can also amplify somatic symptoms, causing

---

[5] As discussed in Chapter 1, self-efficacy is defined as the belief that one is capable of carrying out a course of action to reach a desired goal (Bandura, 1997).

additional functional disability and further reducing patients' motivation to change behavior.

Less Effective Coping

Self-efficacy and emotional resilience contribute to greater engagement in health-promoting behaviors, including adherence to treatment regimens. Conversely, these behaviors can be undermined by ineffective coping with psychological distress. Optimism and positive coping also have been explored as mechanisms through which ill individuals can become more emotionally resilient and better able to cope with and manage the course of their disease. Coping (which involves seeking of social support, positive reframing, information seeking, problem solving, and emotional expression) can bolster one's adjustment to chronic illness (Holahan et al., 1997), and improving patients' coping strategies can be effective in reducing symptoms of psychological distress that hinder health behaviors and the management of illness (Barton et al., 2003). For patients with cancer, optimism also predicts improved quality of life and functional status and the effective management of pain (Astin and Forys, 2004).

Finding meaning in the illness experience is another coping mechanism that can improve a patient's psychological adjustment (Folkman and Greer, 2000), contributing to a greater sense of control, improved psychological adjustment, and more positive focus (Fife, 1995). As many as 83 percent of patients with breast cancer come to realize at least one benefit following their diagnosis (Sears et al., 2003); such a realization involves positive reappraisal of their situation and results in better coping, mood, and health status. Research on patients with tuberculosis in South Africa found a significant relationship between assessment of meaning in life and adherence to treatment for the disease (Corless et al., 2006). Finding benefit also is linked to patients' adherence to antiretroviral therapy for HIV (Stanton et al., 2001; Luszczynska et al., 2006).

Conversely, coping mechanisms that are less adaptive can help in dealing with the immediate emotional distress associated with illness but create longer-term problems. Avoidant coping, which involves denial, emotional instability, avoidant thinking (avoiding thoughts about the reality of the illness), and immature defenses, is associated with less engagement in healthy behaviors (e.g., healthy diet, exercise, adherence to treatment), as well as the adoption of unhealthful behaviors (e.g., smoking, drinking alcohol to excess, abusing psychotropic medications) in an effort to cope with emotional distress (Stanton et al., 2007). Avoidant thinking about the illness is considered "harmful coping" because problems are not faced and solutions are not found, contributing to unhealthy behaviors and nonadherence (Carver et al., 1993).

ALTERATIONS IN BODY FUNCTIONING DUE TO STRESS[6]

Psychological stress arises from the interaction between the individual and the environment. It is said to occur when environmental demands (stressors) exceed the individual's capacity to deal with those demands (Lazarus and Folkman, 1984; Cohen et al., 1995). Stress is thought to exert its pathological effects on the body and increase the risk of disease in part by encouraging maladaptive behaviors as described above. People often cope with the negative emotions elicited by stress through behaviors that bring short-term relief but carry long-term risk. Under stress, people generally smoke more, drink more alcohol, eat foods with a higher fat and sugar content, and exercise less (Conway et al., 1981; Cohen and Williamson, 1988; Anderson et al., 1994). They also tend to have less and poorer-quality sleep (Akerstedt, 2006).

In addition, stress is thought to influence the pathogenesis or course of physical disease more directly by causing negative affective states, such as anxiety and depression, which in turn exert direct effects on biological processes that stimulate and dysregulate certain physiological systems in the body. The immune, cardiovascular, and neuro-endocrine systems are well-known respondents to stress (IOM, 2001). Long-term stressful circumstances that reduce perceptions of control and increase feelings of helplessness, hopelessness, and anxiety damage health and can lead to premature death, in part because of the immune, cardiac, and other physiological responses they produce (WHO, 2003). Individuals are even more vulnerable to the adverse physiological effects of stress when they are exacerbated by other psychosocial factors (e.g., a weak social network) or the individual has inadequate psychosocial assets to buffer the effects of exposure to stress.

Links Between Stress and Disease

There is strong evidence that chronic stress influences the development and/or progression of certain illnesses, including major depression, heart disease, HIV-related illnesses, and (to a lesser extent) cancer.

Depression

Substantial research links stressful life events to both diagnosed depression and depressive symptoms (Monroe and Simons, 1991; Kessler, 1997; Mazure, 1998; Hammen, 2005). One study found that during the 3–6

---

[6]Portions of this section are from a paper commissioned by the committee entitled "Stress and Disease," authored by Sheldon Cohen and Denise Janicki-Deverts, both of Carnegie Mellon University. This paper is available from the Institute of Medicine.

months preceding the onset of their depression, 50–80 percent of depressed persons had experienced a major life event, compared with only 20–30 percent of nondepressed persons evaluated during the same time period (Monroe and Simons, 1991). Approximately 20–25 percent of people who experience major stressful events develop depression (van Praag et al., 2004). Moreover, there is consistent evidence that severe events are more strongly associated with the onset of depression than are nonsevere events, and that there may be a dose-response relationship between the severity of major life events and the likelihood of depression onset (Monroe and Simons, 1991; Kessler, 1997). In general, major life events that are undesirable and uncontrollable, such as bereavement or job loss, are the most likely to be associated with depression (Mazure, 1998). Life-threatening illnesses have also been associated with an increased risk of depression (Dew, 1998). The greatest prevalence of depression in chronically ill patients is reported among those with greater pain, higher levels of physical disability, and more severe illness (Krishnan et al., 2002).

Cardiovascular Disease

Prospective research conducted among initially healthy populations provides considerable support for a link between stress and incident cardiovascular disease (CVD) (Rozanski et al., 1999; Krantz and McCeney, 2002; Belkic et al., 2004). Research examining the influence of chronic psychosocial stress on the risk of recurrent events among persons with preexisting CVD is not as extensive. However, findings from this literature further suggest that exposure to chronic or ongoing psychosocial stress may play a role in worsening disease prognosis among persons with a known history of CVD. Perceived life stress (Ruberman et al., 1984), excessive demands at work (Hoffmann et al., 1995), marital distress (Orth-Gomer et al., 2000; Coyne et al., 2001), and social isolation (Mookadam and Arthur, 2004) each have been related to poor CVD outcomes (i.e., recurrent events and/or mortality) among persons with preexisting CVD. In addition, short-term stressful events and episodes of anger have been shown to precipitate clinical manifestations of coronary artery disease such as myocardial infarction (Rozanski et al., 1999; Krantz and McCeney, 2002). Reviews of prospective studies generally conclude that depression is an important risk factor both for onset of CVD among initially healthy persons (Rugulies, 2002; Wulsin and Singal, 2003; Frasure-Smith and Lesperance, 2005) and for worsening prognosis among CVD patients (Barth et al., 2004; van Melle et al., 2004; Bush et al., 2005). Several studies have also shown that social support is associated with lower resting and ambulatory blood pressures (Uchino et al., 1999; Ong and Allaire, 2005)—a factor reducing the risk of the development of heart disease and lower atherosclerosis (Uchino, 2006) and the progression of cardiac disease once diagnosed.

HIV/AIDS

The typical clinical course of HIV infection is a gradual progression from an initial asymptomatic phase, to a symptomatic phase, to the onset of AIDS (CDC, 1992). Individuals differ with respect to the rate at which they progress through these phases. Some remain asymptomatic for extended periods of time and respond well to medical treatment, whereas others progress rapidly to the onset of AIDS, and suffer numerous complications and opportunistic infections (Kopnisky et al., 2004). It has been suggested that psychosocial factors, including stress and depression, may account for some of this variability (Kiecolt-Glaser and Glaser, 1988; Kopnisky et al., 2004; Pereira and Penedo, 2005).

Although the evidence published before 2000 for the influence of stress on progression through the clinical phases of HIV infection was inconsistent (Cohen and Herbert, 1996; Nott and Vedhara, 1999), several studies did report associations between stress due to negative life events and more rapid HIV progression (Goodkin et al., 1992; Kemeny and Dean, 1995; Evans et al., 1997). Studies published since 2000 have been more consistently supportive of such a link (Pereira and Penedo, 2005).[7] Evidence also suggests that an accumulation of negative life events over several years of follow-up predicts more rapid progression to AIDS (Leserman et al., 2002). Moreover, stress has been found to influence the course of specific conditions (especially virus-initiated illnesses), to which persons with HIV are especially susceptible (Pereira et al., 2003a,b).

Cancer

The literature is less clear with regard to the effects of stressful life events on the incidence of cancer. Studies of the effects of stress on the

---

[7]One difference between earlier and later studies that may explain the variable findings is that in the most recent studies (started in 1995 or later), some patients have been treated with highly active antiretroviral therapy, a regimen that has substantially reduced AIDS-related deaths among infected persons. Hence the association between stress and HIV progression may be attributable to stress interfering with adherence to this complex medication regimen. Variable findings also may be due to differences in how stress was measured (Cole and Kemeny, 2001). Studies published during the 1990s frequently used aggregate measures of the occurrence of negative life events; later studies tended to incorporate subjective ratings of the stressfulness of events and focus on specific events with highly personal consequences, such as bereavement and the threat of severe illness (Cohen and Janicki-Deverts, 2007).

onset of cancer are inconsistent; results range from no association to a strong association (Fox, 1989; Petticrew et al., 1999; Turner-Cobb et al., 2001; Duijts et al., 2003; Heffner et al., 2003; Walker et al., 2005). These conflicting findings are due in no small part to methodological limitations of this work. Some of these limitations have to do with the measurement of biological processes; newer studies are finding more linkages between stress and biological processes that may serve as mechanisms in tumor development and growth. Other limitations derive from problems in the measurement of exposure to stress and of disease outcomes. Because the incidence literature is based primarily on measures of stressful life events, associations could be obscured by the fact that those who can cope effectively with such events are less subject to disease (Eysenck, 1988; Giese-Davis and Spiegel, 2003). On the other hand, most cancers develop over many years and are diagnosed only after developing for 2–30 years, arguing against an association between recent stressful events and the onset of cancer (National Cancer Institute, 2007).

It is generally accepted that stress is more likely to influence the progression and recurrence of cancer than the initial onset of the disease (Thaker et al., 2007). This assumption is based largely on evidence that stress and depression can influence immunocompetence, and that the immune system plays an important role in tumor surveillance and growth (Cohen and Rabin, 1988; Anderson et al., 1994; Turner-Cobb et al., 2001). Yet even research in these areas has produced inconsistent results (Cohen and Herbert, 1996; Giese-Davis and Spiegel, 2003; Walker et al., 2005). The lack of impressive data on psychological stress and depression as risks for the onset, progression, or recurrence of cancer is at least partly attributable to the practical difficulties of designing and implementing adequate studies. For example, in the interest of maximizing power, studies frequently combine multiple types of cancers. Such an approach makes it difficult to interpret results, as it is likely that stress may influence the development of some types of tumors (e.g., those caused by viruses or subject to endocrine regulation) but not others. Despite the less clear evidence to date on the effect of stress on cancer, growing knowledge about the effects of stress on body function—in particular on the functioning of the immune system—adds to suspicions about the potential adverse effects of stress on the progression of some types of cancer.

Effects of Stress on Organ Systems

Although epidemiologic studies conducted to date are inconclusive about the effects of stress on the development and progression of cancer, evidence emerging from the science of psychoneuroimmunology—the study of the interactions among behavior, the brain, and the body's immune system—shows that psychological and social stressors can interfere with the working of the body's organ systems, in particular the neuro-endocrine and immune systems.[8] These effects are thought to mediate the influence of psychosocial stressors on health in general and could potentially play a role in the progression of cancer.

The body's sympathetic-adrenal medullary (SAM) system and the hypothalamic-pituitary-adrenocortical (HPA) axis are two neuro-endocrine systems that are highly responsive to psychological stress. The SAM system reacts to stress in part by increasing the production of certain hormones called catecholamines. In HPA stimulation, the pituitary gland secretes a hormone that activates the adrenal gland to secrete additional hormones called glucocorticoids (primarily cortisol in humans). Although the release of these hormones is a healthy response to an environmental stressor, their excessive or prolonged production under ongoing stressful conditions is associated with impaired functioning or dysregulation of various organs and organ systems (McEwen, 1998; Antoni and Lutgendorf, 2007). These effects can have a cascading effect on the immune system (Kielcolt-Glaser et al., 2002).

Immune system processes play a central role in protecting against infectious diseases, autoimmune diseases, coronary artery disease, and at least some cancers by identifying organisms and cells that are atypical, attacking them, and preventing their replication. Under chronic stress, however, key immune system functioning can be disrupted. Chronic stress, depression, inadequate social support, and other psychosocial stressors can create disequilibrium in immune system functioning by either overstimulating some immune system functions or suppressing others (Miller et al., 2007). For example, the unbalanced production of certain proteins (cytokines) that help regulate the body's immune system can create a pathological state of inflammation that has been linked to certain cancers, as well as a number of chronic conditions, such as CVD, arthritis, type 2 diabetes, and frailty and functional decline in older adults (Kielcolt-Glaser et al., 2002; Antoni et al., 2006). Prolonged exposure to cortisol and catecholamines under chronic stress also can adversely affect cellular replication and several regulators of cell growth. Some of these observed effects on cancer cells—such as accelerating tumor growth, enhancing tumor metabolism, assisting tumor cells in migrating and adhering to a distant site, increasing blood vessel growth in tumors, and helping tumors evade the immune system's natural killer

---

[8]Many of these studies are conducted using animals. While not perfectly matching the physiology and environmental features of humans, such studies greatly inform our understanding of the biological effects of psychosocial stress.

(NK) cells[9]—could help cancer to progress (Antoni and Lutgendorf, 2007; Thaker et al., 2007).

Multiple studies have shown that positive social support, in particular the provision of emotional support, is related to better immune system functioning and resistance to disease (Uchino et al., 1996; IOM, 2001; Uchino, 2006). In women with ovarian cancer, higher levels of social support predicted higher levels of NK cell activity, while patients with greater distress had more impaired NK cells (Lutgendorf et al., 2005).[10] Findings from two randomized controlled trials of psychosocial interventions in breast cancer patients also found improvements in immune system functioning using a variety of measures of immune system competency (Andersen et al., 2004; McGregor et al., 2004).

Studies with animals also have found increased stress to be associated with higher levels of stress hormones (catecholamines) and increased tumor mass and metastases (Thaker et al., 2007). For example, mice with mammary tumors randomly assigned to more stressful housing conditions showed greater tumor growth as well as shorter survival following chemotherapy (Kerr et al., 1997; Strange et al., 2000). Higher levels of certain pro-inflammatory cytokines (interleukin) also have been found in people living in high-stress situations, for example, female caregivers of relatives with Alzheimer's disease compared with community controls (Lutgendorf et al., 1999).

Although more research is needed to understand the extent to which, and how, these stress-induced physiological changes can influence cancer, it is clear that stress can induce pathology in several aspects of body function that affect health. Research findings also indicate that stress, mood, coping, social support, and psychosocial interventions affect neuro-endocrine and immune system activity and can influence the underlying cellular and molecular processes that facilitate the progression of cancer. Findings also suggest the plausibility of improving the health status of cancer patients by attending to their psychosocial distress (McEwen, 1998; Antoni and Lutgendorf, 2007; Thaker et al., 2007). For all these reasons, psychosocial stressors should not be ignored in the delivery of high-quality health care for people living with cancer.

---

[9]A type of white blood cell that attacks harmful body invaders, such as tumors or virus-infected cells.

[10]In this study, social support and distress appeared to operate independently.

ADVERSE EFFECTS ON FAMILIES AND
THE LARGER COMMUNITY

Failure to attend to patients' psychosocial needs can have ripple effects throughout the family, and may also affect the larger community. Some of these effects can rebound and create additional psychosocial problems for the patient.

Adverse Effects on Families

As described in Chapter 1, family members of patients with cancer experience higher-than-normal stress for multiple reasons, including fear of losing their loved one, concern about the suffering of their family member, and the additional demands of providing emotional and logistical support and hands-on care during times of acute illness (Hodges et al., 2005; Kotkamp-Mothes et al., 2005). Further, when loved ones experience acute or long-term inability to care for themselves or carry out their familial roles, family members often must assume these roles.

Providing this emotional, logistical, and hands-on care and assuming roles previously carried out by the patient require considerable adaptation (and readaptation as the course of the disease changes) on the part of family members. These experiences can add to the stress resulting from concern about the ill family member. This cumulative stress, especially in caregivers compromised by morbidity accompanying their own aging (Jepson et al., 1999), can be so substantial that family members acting as caregivers themselves have an increased likelihood of experiencing depression, other adverse health effects, and earlier death (Schultz and Beach, 1999; Kurtz et al., 2004).

Moreover, high stress levels in caregivers can interfere with their ability to provide the emotional or logistical support patients need. Problematic family relationships that predate the onset of cancer also can lead to inadequate support from the family (Kotkamp-Mothes et al., 2005). Both of these situations can exacerbate the patient's stress, which in turn can contribute to the patient's poorer adjustment to the illness. Thus, attending to the needs of the families of patients not only will benefit family members, but also may help patients with their own emotional responses and management of their disease.

Adverse Effects on the Larger Community

As described in Chapter 1, a significant percentage of adults stop working or experience a change in employment (reduction in work hours, interruption in work, change in place of employment) subsequent to a diagnosis of or treatment for cancer (IOM and NRC, 2006), with implications for their own lives and income. The evidence is not clear as to factors that do and do not affect survivors' return to work (Spelten et al., 2002). Nonetheless, to the extent that unaddressed mental health problems such as depression or other psychosocial problems associated with their disease affect patients' desire to continue or return to work or impair their performance on the job, they, their families, and the workplace will be adversely affected financially. Additionally, to the extent that caregivers give up work outside of the home or reduce their work hours to provide care to a loved one, workplace productivity will decrease.

Mental health problems associated with cancer may also have adverse financial effects on the larger economy and on health care providers. However, with respect to effects on the larger economy, the financial costs of failing to deliver psychosocial health services to individuals with cancer have not been studied. Studies that have attempted to quantify the impact of mental health problems on the cost of medical care have been based on the effect of depression and/or anxiety on those with medical illnesses other than cancer (Simon et al., 1995, 2002; Henk et al., 1996). Issues pertaining to reimbursement of psychosocial health services are addressed in Chapter 6.

CONCLUSIONS

Having examined the evidence presented in Chapter 1 about the prevalence of psychosocial problems among people with cancer and the extent to which those problems are unaddressed by health care providers, as well as the evidence reviewed in this chapter about how psychosocial problems can adversely affect health, the committee concludes that all cancer patients and their families are at heightened risk for emotional suffering, diminished adherence to treatment, impaired work and social functioning, and as a result, additional threats to their health beyond those directly imposed by their cancer. As many prior studies on disparities in health care have documented (IOM, 2003; Maly et al., 2006), these risks are greater in populations already experiencing such social stressors as poverty, limited education, language barriers, and/or membership in an ethnic or cultural minority.

Failing to address these risks can adversely affect individuals with many different types of illness. However, the trajectory of cancer often poses both an immediate threat to life and threats to lifelong physical, psychological, and social functioning as a result of the chronic physical and psychological impairment and disability that can result from both the illness and its treatment. Moreover, treatment for many cancers can itself be life-threatening.

These multiple threats make attention to psychosocial problems in cancer patients and their families critically important. Although reducing psychosocial stressors and improving psychosocial services may not increase cancer "cure rates," the committee concludes that

> Addressing psychosocial needs should be an integral part of quality cancer care. All components of the health care system that are involved in cancer care should explicitly incorporate attention to psychosocial needs into their policies, practices, and standards addressing clinical medical practice. These policies, practices, and standards should be aimed at ensuring the provision of psychosocial health services to all patients who need them.

Essential to this conclusion—and to this study overall—is the definition of "psychosocial health services" developed by the committee:

> Psychosocial health services are psychological and social services and interventions that enable patients, their families, and health care providers to optimize biomedical health care and to manage the psychological/behavioral and social aspects of illness and its consequences so as to promote better health.

Several aspects of this definition merit discussion. First, a wide variety of psychological and social services are delivered by providers of health and human services. The committee uses the term "psychosocial *health* services" to distinguish psychological/behavioral and social services that are delivered to improve health and health care from psychosocial services provided to achieve other goals. For example, psychosocial services are provided in the child welfare and criminal/juvenile justice systems to meet such goals as strengthening a family or preventing incarceration or reincarceration. These are psychosocial services, but generally are provided outside of the health care system, and in such settings are not thought of as *health care* services. While a particular psychosocial service, such as mental health care, can be delivered in more than one sector to help achieve multiple goals (e.g., improved health and prevention of incarceration), when psychosocial services are proposed as worthy of attention from the health care system, the intended effects on health and health care services should be clear. By adopting the terminology of psychosocial *health* services, the committee aims to define psychosocial services in a way that recognizes the legitimate and sometimes different purposes of such services across different health and human service sectors, while simultaneously establishing an expectation for efficacy and effectiveness in improving health or health care. Second, the committee's definition of psychosocial health services distinguishes between *services* directly needed by the patient (e.g., treatment for depression or financial assistance) and the *interventions* or strategies used to secure those services (e.g., screening, formal referral, or case management). This distinction is elaborated in Chapters

3 and 4. The rationale for and the significance of the committee's definition of psychosocial health services are discussed in detail in Appendix B.

Some might question whether effective psychosocial health services exist, exist in sufficient quantity, and are accessible to patients, and whether aiming to ensure the provision of psychosocial health services to all patients in need is a feasible goal for oncology providers. Moreover, some might question whether it is worthwhile to identify and attempt to address psychosocial problems through means not typically thought of as medical services, given that some psychosocial problems, such as poverty, are not resolvable. There are several reasons why the committee believes this to be a reasonable aim.

In the next chapter, the committee documents the finding of another recent IOM report on cancer—that a *"wealth"* of cancer-related community support services exists, many of which are available at no cost to patients (IOM and NRC, 2006:229). The committee also notes that tools and techniques needed to identify and address psychosocial problems already exist and are in use by leading oncology providers. Although these tools and techniques have not yet been perfected, and there is not currently as ample a supply of psychosocial services as would be necessary to meet the needs of all patients, the committee describes in the next three chapters psychosocial services, tools, and interventions that do exist and are being used to help patients manage their cancer, its consequences, and their health.

The committee urges all involved in the delivery of cancer care not to allow the perfect to be the enemy of the good. There are many actions that can be taken *now* to identify and deliver needed psychosocial health services, even as the health care system works to improve their quantity and effectiveness. The committee believes that the inability to solve all psychosocial problems permanently should not preclude attempts to remedy as many as possible—a stance akin to oncologists' commitment to treating cancer even when the successful outcome of every treatment is not assured.

REFERENCES

Achille, M., A. Ouellette, S. Fournier, M. Vachon, and M. Hebert. 2006. Impact of stress, distress and feelings of indebtedness on adherence to immunosuppressants following kidney transplantation. *Clinical Transplantation* 20(3):301–306.

ACOG Committee on Health Care for Underserved Women. 2006. Committee opinion: Psychosocial risk factors—perinatal screening and intervention. *Obstetrics and Gynecology* 108(2):469–477.

Akerstedt, T. 2006. Psychosocial stress and impaired sleep. *Scandinavian Journal of Work, Environment & Health* 32(6, special issue):493–501.

Andersen, B. L., W. B. Farrar, D. M. Golden-Kreutz, R. Glaser, C. F. Emery, T. R. Crespin, C. L. Shapiro, and W. E. Carson. 2004. Psychological, behavioral, and immune changes after a psychological intervention: A clinical trial. *Journal of Clinical Oncology* 22(17): 3570–3580.

Anderson, B., J. Kiecolt-Glaser, and R. Glaser. 1994. A biobehavioral model of cancer stress, and disease course. *American Psychologist* 49(5):389–404.

Andrykowski, M., A. Beacham, J. Schmidt, and F. Harper. 2006. Application of the theory of planned behavior to understand intentions to engage in physical and psychosocial health behaviors after cancer diagnosis. *Psycho-Oncology* 15(9):759–771.

Antoni, M. H., and S. Lutgendorf. 2007. Psychosocial factors and disease progression in cancer. *Current Directions in Psychological Science* 16(1):42–46.

Antoni, M. H., S. K. Lutgendorf, S. W. Cole, F. S. Dhabhar, S. E. Sephton, P. G. McDonald, M. Stefanek, and A. K. Sood. 2006. The influence of bio-behavioral factors on tumor biology: Pathways and mechanisms. *Nature Reviews: Cancer* 6(3):240–248.

APA (American Psychiatric Association). 2000. *Diagnostic and statistical manual of mental disorders, text revision (DSM-IV-TR)*. 4th ed. Washington DC: APA.

Astin, J. A., and K. Forys. 2004. Psychosocial determinants of health and illness: Integrating mind, body, and spirit. *Advances in Mind–Body Medicine* 20(4):14–21.

Bandura, A. 1997. *Self-efficacy: The exercise of control*. New York: W.H. Freeman.

Barth, J., M. Schumacher, and C. Herrmann-Lingen. 2004. Depression as a risk factor for mortality in patients with coronary heart disease: A meta-analysis. *Psychosomatic Medicine* 66(6):802–813.

Barton, C., D. Clarke, N. Sulaiman, and M. Abramson. 2003. Coping as a mediator of psychosocial impediments to optimal management and control of asthma. *Respiratory Medicine* 97(7):747–761.

Bayliss, E. A., J. F. Steiner, D. H. Fernald, L. A. Crane, and D. S. Main. 2003. Description of barriers to self-care by persons with comorbid chronic diseases. *Annals of Family Medicine* 1(1):15–21.

Belkic, K. L., P. A. Landsbergis, P. L. Schnall, and D. Baker. 2004. Is job strain a major source of cardiovascular disease risk? *Scandinavian Journal of Work, Environment and Health* 30(2):85–128.

Berkman, L. F., and T. Glass. 2000. Social integration, social networks, social support, and health. In *Social epidemiology*. Edited by L. F. Berkman and I. Kawachi. New York: Oxford University Press. Pp. 137–173.

Berkman, L. F., T. Glass, I. Brisette, and T. Seeman. 2000. From social integration to health: Durkheim in the new millenium. *Social Science and Medicine* 51(6):843–857.

Blanchard, C. M., M. M. Denniston, F. Baker, S. R. Ainsworth, K. S. Courneya, D. M. Hann, D. H. Gesme, D. Reding, T. Flynn, and J. S. Kennedy. 2003. Do adults change their lifestyle behaviors after a cancer diagnosis? *American Journal of Health Behavior* 27(3): 246–256.

Bruce, M. 2006. A systematic and conceptual review of posttraumatic stress in childhood cancer survivors and their parents. *Clinical Psychology Review* 26(3):233–256.

Bush, D. E., R. C. Ziegelstein, U. V. Patel, B. D. Thombs, D. E. Ford, J. A. Fauerbach, U. D. McCann, K. J. Stewart, K. K. Tsilidis, A. L. Patel, C. J. Feuerstein, and E. B. Bass. 2005. *Post-myocardial infarction depression. Summary*. Evidence Report/Technology Assessment No. 123. AHRQ Publication No. 05-E018-1. Rockville, MD: Agency for Healthcare Research and Quality.

Carver, C. S., C. Pozo, S. D. Harris, V. Noriega, M. F. Scheier, D. S. Robinson, A. S. Ketcham, F. L. Moffat, and K. C. Clark. 1993. How coping mediates the effect of optimism on distress: A study of women with early stage breast cancer. *Journal of Personality and Social Psychology* 65(2):375–390.

Castellon, S. A., D. J. Hardy, C. H. Hinkin, P. Satz, P. K. Stenquist, W. G. van Gorp, H. F. Myers, and L. Moore. 2006. Components of depression in HIV-1 infection: Their differential relationship to neurocognitive performance. *Journal of Clinical Experimental Neuropsychology* 28(3):420–437.

CDC (Centers for Disease Control and Prevention). 1992. 1993 revised classification system for HIV infection and expanded surveillance case definition for AIDS among adolescents and adults. *MMWR. Morbidity and Mortality Weekly Report* 41(RR-17):1–19.

Cohen, S. 2004. Social relationships and health. *American Psychologist* 59(8):676–684.

Cohen, S., and D. Janicki-Deverts. 2007. *Stress and disease*. Paper Commissioned by the Institute of Medicine Committee on Psychosocial Services to Cancer Patients and Families in a Community Setting.

Cohen, S., and T. B. Herbert. 1996. Health psychology: Psychological factors and physical disease from the perspective of human psychoneuroimmunology. In *Annual Review of Psychology*. Vol. 47. Edited by J. T. Spence, J. M. D., and D. J. Foss. El Camino, CA: Annual Review Inc. Pp. 113–142.

Cohen, S., and B. S. Rabin. 1998. Stress, immunity and cancer. *Journal of the National Cancer Institute* 90(1):3–4.

Cohen, S., and G. Williamson. 1988. Perceived stress in a probability sample of the United States. In *The Social Psychology of Health: Claremont Symposium on Applied Social Psychology*. Edited by S. Spacapan and S. Oskamp. Newbury Park, CA: Sage Publications.

Cohen, S., R. C. Kessler, and L. Underwood Gordon. 1995. Strategies for measuring stress in studies of psychiatric and physical disorder. In *Measuring stress: A guide for health and social scientists*. Edited by S. Cohen, R. C. Kessler, and L. U. Gordon. New York: Oxford University Press. Pp. 3–26.

Cole, S. W., and M. E. Kemeny. 2001. Psychosocial influences on the progression of HIV infection. In *Psychoneuroimmunology*. 3rd ed., Vol. 2. Edited by R. Ader, D. L. Felten, and N. Cohen. San Diego: Academic Press.

Collins, R. L., D. E. Kanouse, A. L. Gifford, J. W. Senterfitt, M. A. Schuster, D. McCaffrey, M. F. Shapiro, and N. S. Wenger. 2001. Changes in health-promoting behavior following diagnosis with HIV: Prevalence and correlates in a national probability sample. *Health Psychology* 20(5):351–360.

Conway, T. L., R. R. Vickers, H. W. Ward, and R. H. Rahe. 1981. Occupational stress and variation in cigarette, coffee, and alcohol consumption. *Journal of Health and Social Behavior* 22(2):155–165.

Corless, I. B., P. K. Nicholas, D. Wantland, P. McInerney, B. Ncama, B. Bhengu, C. McGibbon, and S. Davis. 2006. The impact of meaning in life and life goals on adherence to a tuberculosis medication regimen in South Africa. *The International Journal of Tuberculosis and Lung Disease* 10(10):1159–1165.

Coyne, J. C., M. J. Rohrbaugh, V. Shoham, J. S. Sonnega, J. M. Nicklas, and J. A. Cranford. 2001. Prognostic importance of marital quality for survival of congestive heart failure. *The American Journal of Cardiology* 88(5):526–529.

Demark-Wahnefried, W., N. M. Aziz, J. H. Rowland, B. M. Pinto. 2005. Riding the crest of the teachable moment: Promoting long-term health after the diagnosis of cancer. *Journal of Clinical Oncology* 23(24):5814–5830.

Dew, M. A. 1998. Psychiatric disorder in the context of physical illness. In *Adversity, stress, and psychopathology*. Edited by B. P. Dohrenwend. New York: Oxford University Press. Pp. 177–218.

DiMatteo, M. R. 2004. Variations in patients' adherence to medical recommendations: A quantitative review of 50 years of research. *Medical Care* 42(3):200–209.

DiMatteo, M. R., H. S. Lepper, and T. W. Croghan. 2000. Depression is a risk factor for noncompliance with medical treatment: Meta-analysis of the effects of anxiety and depression on patient adherence. *Archives of Internal Medicine* 160(14):2101–2107.

Duijts, S. F. A., M. P. A. Zeegers, and B. V. Borne. 2003. The association between stressful life events and breast cancer risk: A meta-analysis. *International Journal of Cancer* 107(6):1023–1029.

Evans, D. L., J. Leserman, D. O. Perkins, R. A. Stern, C. Murphy, B. Zheng, D. Gettes, J. A. Longmate, S. G. Silva, C. M. van der Horst, C. D. Hall, J. D. Folds, R. N. Golden, and J. M. Petitto. 1997. Severe life stress as a predictor of early disease progression. *American Journal of Psychiatry* 154(5):630–634.

Eysenck, H. J. 1988. Personality, stress and cancer: Prediction and prophylaxis. *British Journal of Medical Psychology* 61(Part 1):57–75.

Fife, B. L. 1995. The measurement of meaning in illness. *Social Science and Medicine* 40(8): 1021–1028.

Figueiredo, M. I., E. Fries, and K. M. Ingram. 2004. The role of disclosure patterns and unsupportive social interactions in the well-being of breast cancer patients. *Psycho-Oncology* 13(2):96–105.

Fink, A. K., J. Gurwitz, W. Rakowski, E. Guadagnoli, and R. A. Silliman. 2004. Patient beliefs and tamoxifen discontinuance in older women with estrogen receptor—positive breast cancer. *Journal of Clinical Oncology* 22(16):3309–3315.

Folkman, S., and S. Greer. 2000. Promoting psychological well-being in the face of serious illness: When theory, research and practice inform each other. *Psycho-Oncology* 9(1):11–19.

Fox, B. H. 1989. Depressive symptoms and risk of cancer (editorial). *Journal of the American Medical Association* 262(9):1231.

Frasure-Smith, N., and F. Lesperance. 2005. Reflections on depression as a cardiac risk factor. *Psychosomatic Medicine* 67(Supplement 1):S19–S25.

Giese-Davis, J., and D. Spiegel. 2003. Emotional expression and cancer progression. In *Handbook of affective sciences*. Edited by R. J. Davidson, K. R. Scherer, and H. H. Goldsmith. New York: Oxford University Press. Pp. 1053–1082.

Goodkin, K., I. Fuchs, D. Feaster, J. Leeka, and D. Rishel. 1992. Life stressors and coping style are associated with immune measures in HIV-1 infection: A preliminary report. *International Journal of Psychiatry in Medicine* 22(2):155–172.

Gritz, E. R., M. C. Fingeret, D. J. Vidrine, A. B. Lazev, N. V. Mehta, and G. P. Reece. 2006. Successes and failures of the teachable moment: Smoking cessation in cancer patients. *Cancer* 106(1):17–27.

Hammen, C. 2005. Stress and depression. *Annual Review of Clinical Psychology* 1:293–319.

Heffner, K. L., T. J. Loving, T. F. Robles, and J. K. Kiecolt-Glaser. 2003. Examining psychosocial factors related to cancer incidence and progression: In search of the silver lining. *Brain, Behavior and Immunity* 17(Supplement 4):S109–S111.

Hegel, M. T., C. P. Moore, E. D. Collins, S. Kearing, K. L. Gillock, R. L. Riggs, K. F. Clay, and T. A. Ahles. 2006. Distress, psychiatric syndromes, and impairment of function in women with newly diagnosed breast cancer. *Cancer* 107(12):2924–2931.

Helgeson, V. S., and S. Cohen. 1996. Social support and adjustment to cancer: Reconciling descriptive, correlational, and intervention research. *Health Psychology* 15(2):135–148.

Hemingway, H., and M. Marmot. 1999. Psychosocial factors in the aetiology and prognosis of coronary heart disease: Systematic review of prospective cohort studies. *British Medical Journal* 318(7196):1460–1467.

Henk, H., D. Katzelnick, K. Kobak, J. Greist, and J. Jefferson. 1996. Medical costs attributed to depression among patients with a history of high medical expenses in a health maintenance organization. *Archives of General Psychiatry* 53(10):899–904.

Hodges, L. J., G. M. Humphris, and G. Macfarlane. 2005. A meta-analytic investigation of the relationship between the psychological distress of cancer patients and their carers. *Social Science and Medicine* 60(1):1–12.

Hoffmann, A., D. Pfiffner, R. Hornung, H. Niederhauser. 1995. Psychosocial factors predict medical outcome following a first myocardial infarction. *Coronary Artery Disease* 6(2):147–152.

Holahan, C. J., R. H. Moos, C. K. Holahan, and P. L. Brennan. 1997. Social context, coping strategies, and depressive symptoms: An expanded model with cardiac patients. *Journal of Personality and Social Psychology* 72(4):918–928.

House, J., K. Landis, and D. Umberson. 1988. Social relationships and health. *Science* 241(4865): 540–545.

Humpel, N., C. Magee, and S. C. Jones. 2007. The impact of a cancer diagnosis on the health behaviors of cancer survivors and their family and friends. *Supportive Care Cancer* 15(6):621–630.

IOM (Institute of Medicine). 2001. *Health and behavior: The interplay of biological, behavioral, and societal influences.* Washington, DC: National Academy Press.

IOM. 2002. *Care without coverage: Too little, too late.* Washington, DC: National Academy Press.

IOM. 2003. *Unequal treatment: Confronting racial and ethnic disparities in health care.* B. D. Smedley, A. Y. Stith, and A. R. Nelson, eds. Washington, DC: The National Academies Press.

IOM and NRC (National Research Council). 2006. *From cancer patient to cancer survivor: Lost in transition.* M. Hewitt, S. Greenfield, and E. Stovall, eds. Washington, DC: The National Academies Press.

Jepson, C., R. McCorkle, D. Adler, I. Nuamah, and E. Lusk. 1999. Effects of home care on caregivers' psychosocial status. *Image: The Journal of Nursing Scholarship* 31(2):115–120.

Jerant, A. F., M. M. von Friederichs-Fitzwater, and M. Moore. 2005. Patients' perceived barriers to active self-management of chronic conditions. *Patient Education and Counseling* 57(1):300–307.

Katon, W. J. 2003. Clinical and health services relationships between major depression, depressive symptoms, and general medical illness. *Biological Psychiatry* 54(3):216–226.

Katon, W. J., J. Unutzer, and G. Simon. 2004. Treatment of depression in primary care: Where we are, where we can go. *Medical Care* 42(12):1153–1157.

Kelly, M. P., J. Bonnefoy, A. Morgan, and F. Florenza. 2006. *The development of the evidence base about the social determinants of health.* World Health Organization Commission on Social Determinants of Health–Measurement and Evidence Knowledge Network. http://www.who.int/social_determinants/resources/mekn_paper.pdf (accessed May 2006).

Kemeny, M. E., and L. Dean. 1995. Effects of AIDS-related bereavement on HIV progression among New York City gay men. *AIDS Education and Prevention* 7(5 Supplement):36–47.

Kerr, L. R., M. S. Grimm, W. A. Silva, J. Weinberg, and J. T. Emerman. 1997. Effects of social housing condition on the response of the Shionogi mouse mammary carcinoma (sc115) to chemotherapy. *Cancer Research* 57(6):1124–1128.

Kessler, R. C. 1997. The effects of stressful life events on depression. *Annual Review of Psychology* 48:191–214.

Kiecolt-Glaser, J. K., and R. Glaser. 1988. Psychological influences on immunity: Implications for AIDS. *American Psychologist* 43(11):892–898.

Kielcolt-Glaser, J. K., L. McGuire, T. F. Robles, and R. Glaser. 2002. Emotions, morbidity, and mortality: New perspectives from psychoneuroimmunnology. *Annual Review of Psychology* 53:83–107.

King, G., C. Willoughby, J. A. Specht, and E. Brown. 2006. Social support processes and the adaptation of individuals with chronic disabilities. *Qualitative Health Research* 16(7):902–925.

Kopnisky, K. L., D. M. Stoff, and D. M. Rausch. 2004. Workshop report: The effects of psychological variables on the progression of HIV-1 disease. *Brain, Behavior, and Immunity* 18(3):246–261.

Kotkamp-Mothes, N., D. Slawinsky, S. Hindermann, and B. Strauss. 2005. Coping and psychological well being in families of elderly cancer patients. *Critical Reviews in Oncology-Hematology* 55(3):213–229.

Krantz, D. S., and M. K. McCeney. 2002. Effects of psychological and social factors on organic disease: A critical assessment of research on coronary heart disease. *Annual Review of Psychology* 53:341–369.

Krishnan, K. R., M. Delong, H. Kraemer, R. Carney, D. Spiegel, C. Gordon, W. McDonald, M. A. Dew, G. Alexopoulos, K. Buckwalter, P. D. Cohen, D. Evans, P. G. Kaufmann, J. Olin, E. Otey, and C. Wainscott. 2002. Comorbidity of depression with other medical diseases in the elderly. *Biological Psychiatry* 52(6):559–588.

Kroenke, C. H., L. D. Kubzansky, E. S. Schernhammer, M. D. Holmes, and I. Kawachi. 2006. Social networks, social support, and survival after breast cancer diagnosis. *Journal of Clinical Oncology* 24(7):1105–1111.

Kurtz, M. E., J. C. Kurtz, C. W. Given, and B. A. Given. 2004. Depression and physical health among family caregivers of geriatric patients with cancer—a longitudinal view. *Medical Science Monitor* 10(8):CR447–CR456.

Lazarus, R. S., and S. Folkman. 1984. *Stress, appraisal and coping*. New York: Springer.

Leserman, J., J. M. Petitto, H. Gu, B. N. Gaynes, J. Barroso, R. N. Golden, D. O. Perkins, J. D. Folds, and D. L. Evans. 2002. Progression to AIDS, a clinical AIDS condition and mortality: Psychosocial and physiological predictors. *Psychological Medicine* 32(6):1059–1073.

Luszczynska, A., Y. Sarkar, and N. Knoll. 2006. Received social support, self-efficacy, and finding benefits in disease as predictors of physical functioning and adherence to antiretroviral therapy. *Patient Education and Counseling* 66(1):37–42.

Lutgendorf, S., L. Garand, K. Buckwalter, T. Reimer, S. Hong, and D. Lubaroff. 1999. Life stress, mood disturbance, and elevated interleukin-6 in healthy older women. *The Journals of Gerontology. Series A, Biological Sciences and Medical Sciences* 54A:M434–M439.

Lutgendorf, S. K., A. K. Sood, B. Anderson, S. McGinn, H. Maiseri, M. Dao, J. I. Sorosky, K. D. Geest, J. Ritchie, and D. M. Lubaroff. 2005. Social support, psychological distress, and natural killer cell activity in ovarian cancer. *Journal of Clinical Oncology* 23(28):7105–7113.

Maly, R. C., Y. Umezawa, B. Leake, and R. A. Silliman. 2005. Mental health outcomes in older women with breast cancer: Impact of perceived family support and adjustment. *Psycho-Oncology* 14(7):535–545.

Maly, R. C., Y. Umezawa, C. T. Ratliff, B. Leake. 2006. Racial/ethnic group differences in treatment decision-making and treatment received among older breast carcinoma patients. *Cancer* 106(4):957–965.

Martin, L. R., M. R. DiMatteo, and H. S. Lepper. 2001. Facilitation of patient involvement in care: Development and validation of a scale. *Behavioral Medicine* 27(3):111–120.

May, J. H., and P. J. Cunningham. 2004. *Tough trade-offs: Medical bills, family finances and access to care*. Washington, DC: Center for Studying Health System Change.

Mazure, C. M. 1998. Life stressors as risk factors in depression. *Clinical Psychology: Science and Practice* 5(3):291–313.

McBride, C. M., K. M. Emmons, and I. M. Lipkus. 2003. Understanding the potential of teachable moments: The case of smoking cessation. *Health Education and Research* 18(2):156–170.

McEwen, B. S. 1998. Seminars in medicine of the Beth Israel Deaconess Medical Center: Protective and damaging effects of stress mediators. *New England Journal of Medicine* 338(3):171–179.

McGregor, B. A., M. H. Antoni, A. Boyers, S. M. Alferi, B. B. Blomberg, and C. S. Carver. 2004. Cognitive-behavioral stress management increases benefit finding and immune function among women with early-stage breast cancer. *Journal of Psychosomatic Research* 56(1):1–8.

Miller, G. E., E. Chen, and E. S. Zhou. 2007. If it goes up, must it come down? Chronic stress and the hypothalamic-pituitary-adrenocortical axis in humans. *Psychological Bulletin* 133(1):25–45.

Monroe, S. M., and A. D. Simons. 1991. Diathesis-stress theories in the context of life stress research: Implications for depressive disorders. *Psychological Bulletin* 110(3):406–425.

Mookadam, F., and H. M. Arthur. 2004. Social support and its relationship to morbidity and mortality after acute myocardial infarction: Systematic overview. *Archives of Internal Medicine* 164(14):1514–1518.

Murphy, E. 1982. Social origins of depression in old age. *British Journal of Psychiatry* 141(2):135–142.

Mystakidou, K., E. Tsilika, E. Parpa, E. Katsouda, A. Galanos, and L. Vlahos. 2005. Assessment of anxiety and depression in advanced cancer patients and their relationship with quality of life. *Quality of Life Research* 14(8):1825–1833.

National Cancer Institute. 2007. *Psychological stress and cancer.* http://www.cancer.gov/cancertopics/factsheet/Risk/stress/ (accessed August 1, 2007).

Norton, T. R., S. L. Manne, S. Rubin, E. Hernandez, J. Carlson, C. Bergman, and N. Rosenblum. 2005. Ovarian cancer patients' psychological distress: The role of physical impairment, perceived unsupportive family and friend behaviors, perceived control, and self-esteem. *Health Psychology* 24(2):143–152.

Nott, K. H., and K. Vedhara. 1999. Nature and consequences of stressful life events in homosexual HIV-positive men: A review. *AIDS Care* 11(2):235–243.

Olfson, M., B. Fireman, M. M. Weissman, A. C. Leon, D. V. Sheehan, R. G. Kathol, C. Hoven, and L. Farber. 1997. Mental disorders and disability among patients in a primary care group practice. *American Journal of Psychiatry* 154(12):1734–1740.

Ong, A. D., and J. C. Allaire. 2005. Cardiovascular intraindividual variability in later life: The influence of social connectedness and positive emotions. *Psychology and Aging* 20(3):476–485.

Ornish, D., G. Weidner, W. R. Fair, R. Marlin, E. B. Pettengill, C. J. Raisin, S. Dunn-Emke, L. Crutchfield, F. N. Jacobs, R. J. Barnard, W. J. Aronson, P. McCormac, D. J. McKnight, J. D. Fein, A. M. Dnistrian, J. Weinstein, T. H. Ngo, N. R. Mendell, and P. R. Carroll. 2005. Intensive lifestyle changes may affect the progression of prostate cancer. *Journal of Urology* 174(3):1065–1069; discussion 1069–1070.

Orth-Gomer, K., S. Wamala, M. Horsten, K. Schenck-Gustafsson, N. Schneiderman, and M. A. Mittleman. 2000. Marital stress worsens prognosis in women with coronary heart disease: The Stockholm female coronary risk study. *Journal of the American Medical Association* 284(23):3008–3014.

Partridge, A., P. Wang, E. Winer, and J. Avorn. 2003. Nonadherence to adjuvant tamoxifen therapy in women with primary breast cancer. *Journal of Clinical Oncology* 21(4):602–606.

Patenaude, A. F., and M. J. Kupst. 2005. Psychosocial functioning in pediatric cancer. *Journal of Pediatric Psychology* 30(1):9–27.

Patten, S. 2001. Long-term medical conditions and major depression in a Canadian population study at waves 1 and 2. *Journal of Affective Disorders* 63(1-3):35–41.

Penson, D. F., M. L. Stoddard, D. J. Pasta, D. P. Lubeck, S. C. Flanders, and M. S. Litwin. 2001. The association between socioeconomic status, health insurance coverage, and quality of life in men with prostate cancer. *Journal of Clinical Epidemiology* 54(4):350–358.

Pereira, D. B., and F. J. Penedo. 2005. Psychoneuroimmunology and chronic viral infection: HIV infection. In *Human psychoneuroimmunology*. Edited by K. Vedhara and M. Irwin. Oxford, UK: Oxford University Press. Pp. 165–194.

Pereira, D. B., M. H. Antoni, A. Danielson, T. Simon, J. Efantis-Potter, C. S. Carver, R. E. Durán, G. Ironson, N. Klimas, M. A. Fletcher, and M. J. O'Sullivan. 2003a. Life stress and cervical squamous intraepithelial lesions in women with human papillomavirus and human immunodeficiency virus. *Psychosomatic Medicine* 6(3)5:427–434.

Pereira, D. B., M. H. Antoni, A. Danielson, T. Simon, J. Efantis-Potter, C. S. Carver, R. E. Durán, G. Ironson, N. Klimas, M. A. Fletcher, and M. J. O'Sullivan. 2003b. Stress as a predictor of symptomatic genital herpes virus recurrence in women with human immunodeficiency virus. *Journal of Psychosomatic Research* 54(3):237–244.

Peterman, A. H., and D. F. Cella. 1998. Adherence issues among cancer patients. In *The handbook of health behavior change*. 2nd ed. Edited by S. Shumaker, E. B. Schron, J. K. Ockene, and W. L. McBee. New York: Springer. Pp. 462–482.

Petticrew, A., J. Fraser, and M. Regan. 1999. Adverse life events and risk of breast cancer: A meta-analysis. *British Journal of Health and Psychology* 4(1):1–17.

Pinto, B. M., J. Trunzo, P. Reiss, and S. Y. Shiu. 2002. Exercise participation after diagnosis of breast cancer: Trends and effects on mood and quality of life. *Psycho-Oncology* 11(5):389–400.

Polsky, D., J. A. Doshi, S. Marcus, D. Oslin, A. Rothbard, N. Thomas, and C. L. Thompson. 2005. Long-term risk for depressive symptoms after a medical diagnosis. *Archives of Internal Medicine* 165(11):1260–1266.

Rabin, C., and B. Pinto. 2006. Cancer-related beliefs and health behavior change among breast cancer survivors and their first-degree relatives. *Psycho-Oncology* 15(8):701–712.

Riegel, B., and B. Carlson. 2002. Facilitators and barriers to heart failure self-care. *Patient Education and Counseling* 46(4):287–295.

Robinson, J. W., and D. L. Roter. 1999. Psychosocial problem disclosure by primary care patients. *Social Science and Medicine* 48(10):1353–1362.

Rozanski, A., J. A. Blumenthal, and J. Kaplan. 1999. Impact of psychological factors on the pathogenesis of cardiovascular disease and implications for therapy. *Circulation* 99(16):2192–2217.

Ruberman, W., E. Weinblatt, J. D. Goldberg, and B. S. Chaudhary. 1984. Psychosocial influences on mortality after myocardial infarction. *New England Journal of Medicine* 311(9):552–559.

Rugulies, R. 2002. Depression as a predictor for coronary heart disease: A review and meta-analysis. *American Journal of Preventive Medicine* 23(1):51–61.

Salamonson, Y., B. Everett, P. Davidson, and S. Andrew. 2007. Magnitude of change in cardiac health-enhancing behaviours 6 months following an acute myocardial infarction. *European Journal of Cardiovascular Nursing* 6(1):66–71.

Schultz, R., and S. R. Beach. 1999. Caregiving as a risk factor for mortality: The caregiver health effects study. *Journal of the American Medical Association* 282(23):2215–2219.

Sears, S. R., A. L. Stanton, and S. Danoff-Burg. 2003. The yellow brick road and the emerald city: Benefit finding, positive reappraisal coping and posttraumatic growth in women with early-stage breast cancer. *Health Psychology* 22(5):487–497.

Segerstrom, S. C., and G. E. Miller. 2004. Psychological stress and the human immune system: A meta-analytic study of 30 years of inquiry. *Psychological Bulletin* 130(4):601–630.

Sherbourne, C., M. Schoenbaum, K. B. Wells, and T. W. Croghan. 2004. Characteristics, treatment patterns, and outcomes of persistent depression despite treatment in primary care. *General Hospital Psychiatry* 26(2):106–114.

Simon, G., M. V. Korff, and W. Barlow. 1995. Health care costs of primary care patients with recognized depression. *Archives of General Psychiatry* 52(10):850–856.

Simon, G. E., D. Chisholm, M. Treglia, and D. Bushnell. 2002. Course of depression, health services cost, and work productivity in an international primary care study. *General Hospital Psychiatry* 24(5):328–335.

Smith, E., S. Gomm, and C. Dickens. 2003. Assessing the independent contribution to quality of life from anxiety and depression in patients with advanced cancer. *Palliative Medicine* 17(6):509–513.

Spelten, E. R., M. A. G. Sprangers, and J. H. A. M. Verbeek. 2002. Factors reported to influence the return to work of cancer survivors: A literature review. *Psycho-Oncology* 11(2):124–131.

Spiegel, D. 1997. Psychosocial aspects of breast cancer treatment. *Seminars in Oncology* 24(Supplement 1):S1-36–S1-47.

Spitzer, R. L., K. Kroenke, M. Linzer, S. R. Hahn, J. B. Williams, F. V. deGruy, D. Brody, and M. Davies. 1995. Health-related quality of life in primary care patients with mental disorders. Results from the PRIME-MD 1000 study. *Journal of the American Medical Association* 274(19):1511–1517.

Stanton, A. L., C. A. Collins, and L. Sworowski. 2001. Adjustment to chronic illness: Theory and research. In *Handbook of health psychology.* Edited by A. Baum, T. A. Revenson, and J. E. Singer. Mahwah, NJ: Lawrence Erlbaum Associates. Pp. 387–404.

Stanton, A. L., T. A. Revenson, and H. Tennen. 2007. Health psychology: Psychological adjustment to chronic disease. *Annual Review of Psychology* 58(13):13.11–13.28.

Strange, K. S., L. R. Kerr, H. N. Andrews, J. T. Emerman, and J. Weinberg. 2000. Psychosocial stressors and mammary tumor growth: An animal model. *Neurotoxicology and Teratology* 22(1):89–102.

Taylor, K. L., R. Shelby, E. Gelmann, and C. McGuire. 2004. Quality of life and trial adherence among participants in the prostate, lung, colorectal, and ovarian cancer screening trial. *Journal of the National Cancer Institute* 96(14):1083–1094.

Thaker, P. H., S. K. Lutgendorf, and A. K. Sood. 2007. The neuroendocrine impact of chronic stress on cancer. *Cell Cycle* 6(4):430–433.

Tu, H. T. 2004. *Rising health costs, medical debt and chronic conditions.* Issue Brief No. 88. Washington, DC: Center for Studying Health System Change.

Turner-Cobb, J. M., S. E. Sephton, and D. Spiegel. 2001. Psychosocial effects on immune function and disease progression in cancer: Human studies. In *Psychoneuroimmunology.* 3rd ed., Vol. 2. Edited by R. Ader, D. L. Felten, and N. Cohen. New York: Academic Press. Pp. 565–582.

Tyrrell, J., L. Paturel, B. Cadec, E. Capezzali, and G. Poussin. 2005. Older patients undergoing dialysis treatment: Cognitive functioning, depressive mood and health-related quality of life. *Aging and Mental Health* 9(4):374–379.

Uchino, B. N. 2006. Social support and health: A review of physiological processes potentially underlying links to disease outcomes. *Journal of Behavioral Medicine* 29(4):377–387.

Uchino, B. N., J. T. Cacioppo, and J. K. Kiecolt-Glaser. 1996. The relationship between social support and physiological processes: A review with emphasis on underlying mechanisms and implications for health. *Psychological Bulletin* 119(3):488–531.

Uchino, B. N., J. Holt-Lunstad, D. Uno, and R. Betancourt. 1999. Social support and age-related differences in cardiovascular function: An examination of potential mediators. *Annals of Behavioral Medicine: A Publication of the Society of Behavioral Medicine* 21(2):135–142.

USA Today, Kaiser Family Foundation, and Harvard School of Public Health. 2006. *National survey of households affected by cancer: Summary and chartpack.* Menlo Park, CA, and Washington, DC: USA Today, Kaiser Family Foundation, and Harvard School of Public Health. http://www.kff.org/Kaiserpolls/upload/7591.pdf (accessed April 24, 2007).

van Melle, J. P., P. de Jonge, T. A. Spijkerman, J. G. P. Tijssen, J. Ormel, D. J. van Veldhuisen, R. H. van den Brink, and M. P. van den Berg. 2004. Prognostic association of depression following myocardial infarction with mortality and cardiovascular events: A meta-analysis. *Psychosomatic Medicine* 66(6):814–822.

van Praag, H. M., E. R. de Kloet, and J. van Os. 2004. *Stress, the brain and depression.* Cambridge, UK: Cambridge University Press.

Walker, L. G., V. L. Green, J. Greenman, A. A. Walker, and D. M. Sharp. 2005. Psychoneuroimmunology and chronic malignant disease: Cancer. In *Human Psychoneuroimmunology*. Edited by M. Irwin and V. Vedhara. New York: Oxford University Press.

Wdowik, M. J., P. A. Kendall, and M. A. Harris. 1997. College students with diabetes: Using focus groups and interviews to determine psychosocial issues and barriers to control. *The Diabetes Educator* 23(5):558–562.

Weihs, K. L., S. J. Simmens, J. Mizrahi, T. M. Enright, M. E. Hunt, and R. S. Siegel. 2005. Dependable social relationships predict overall survival in stages II and III breast carcinoma patients. *Journal of Psychosomatic Research* 59(5):299–306.

Wells, K. B., and M. A. Burnam. 1991. Caring for depression in America: Lessons learned from early findings of the medical outcomes study. *Psychiatric Medicine* 9(4):503–519.

WHO (World Health Organization). 2003. *Social determinants of health: The solid facts.* Copenhagen, Demark: WHO.

Wills, T. A., and M. F. Fegan. 2001. Social networks and social support. In *Handbook of health psychology*. Edited by A. Baum, T. A. Revenson, and J. E. Singer. Mahwah, NJ: Lawrence Erlbaum Associates. Pp. 209–234.

Wulsin, L. R., and B. M. Singal. 2003. Do depressive symptoms increase the risk for the onset of coronary disease? A systematic quantitative review. *Psychosomatic Medicine* 65(2):201–210.

Yarcheski, A., N. E. Mahon, T. J. Yarcheski, and B. L. Cannella. 2004. A meta-analysis of predictors of positive health practices. *Journal of Nursing Scholarship* 36(2):102–108.

3

Psychosocial Health Services

CHAPTER SUMMARY

A range of services can help patients and their families manage the psychological/behavioral and social aspects of illness that can adversely affect their health care and outcomes. An individual's own psychological and informal social resources often counteract many of these stressors. However, when these resources are not available or are overwhelmed by the number, magnitude, or duration of stressors, or when a problem requires professional intervention, formal services are needed.

Evidence supports the effectiveness of services aimed at relieving the emotional distress that accompanies many chronic illnesses, including cancer, even in the case of debilitating depression and anxiety. Good evidence also underpins a number of interventions designed to help individuals adopt behaviors that can help them manage disease symptoms and improve their overall health. Other psychosocial health services, such as transportation to health care or financial assistance to purchase medications or supplies, while not the subject of effectiveness research, have wide acceptance as humane interventions to address related needs, and are long-standing components of such public programs as Medicaid and the Older Americans Act. Many health and human service providers deliver one or more of these services. In particular, strong leadership of organizations in the voluntary sector has created a broad array of psychosocial support services—sometimes available at no cost to patients. Together, these services have been described as constituting a "wealth of cancer-related community support services" (IOM and NRC, 2006:229).

A DIVERSITY OF SERVICES

An array of services exists to address the varied psychosocial problems and needs (summarized in Chapter 1) that often accompany cancer and its treatment (see Table 3-1). As defined in Chapter 2, psychosocial health services are those psychological and social services that enable patients, their families, and health care providers to optimize biomedical health

TABLE 3-1 Psychosocial Needs and Formal[a] Services to Address Them

Psychosocial Need	Health Services
Information about illness, treatments, health, and services	• Provision of information, e.g., on illness, treatments, effects on health, and psychosocial services, and help to patients/ families in understanding and using the information
Help in coping with emotions accompanying illness and treatment	• Peer support programs • Counseling/psychotherapy to individuals or groups • Pharmacological management of mental symptoms
Help in managing illness	• Comprehensive illness self-management/self-care programs
Assistance in changing behaviors to minimize impact of disease	• Behavioral/health promotion interventions, such as: – Provider assessment/monitoring of health behaviors (e.g., smoking, exercise) – Brief physician counseling – Patient education, e.g., in cancer-related health risks and risk-reduction measures
Material and logistical resources, such as transportation	• Provision of resources
Help in managing disruptions in work, school, and family life	• Family and caregiver education • Assistance with activities of daily living (ADLs), instrumental ADLs, chores • Legal protections and services, e.g., under Americans with Disabilities Act and Family and Medical Leave Act • Cognitive testing and educational assistance
Financial advice and/or assistance	• Financial planning/counseling, including management of day-to-day activities such as bill paying • Insurance (e.g., health, disability) counseling • Eligibility assessment/counseling for other benefits (e.g., Supplemental Security Income, Social Security Disability Income) • Supplement financial grants

[a]The committee notes that, as discussed in Chapters 1 and 2, family members and friends and other informal sources of support are key providers of psychosocial health services. This table includes only formal sources of psychosocial support—those that must be secured through the assistance of an organization or agency that in some way enables the provision of needed services (sometimes at no cost or through volunteers).

care and to manage the psychological/behavioral and social aspects of illness and its consequences so as to promote better health. We note that some level of psychosocial support (e.g., providing emotional support and information about one's illness) accompanies much of routine health care. Family members and other informal supports also meet many emotional and logistical needs in times of illness. However, when this level or type of support is insufficient to address a patient's needs, more formal services are needed. Definitions and descriptions of these services and the extent of evidence supporting their effectiveness in meeting identified patient needs are discussed below.

In addition to these *services* to address problems that arise at the level of the patient (the need for which will likely vary among individuals), psychosocial *interventions* are needed on a more uniform basis within clinical practices to address problems arising at the level of the health care system, such as failure to identify patients' psychosocial needs, to link patients to effective services, and to support them in managing their illness and health. These more consistently needed provider- and system-level interventions to deliver effective psychosocial services are discussed in Chapters 4 and 5.

EVIDENCE OF EFFECTIVENESS

The effectiveness of some psychosocial health services has been substantiated through research. Others (such as the provision of transportation or financial assistance to purchase medications) have such long-standing and wide acceptance that they have not been the subject of much research interest. Others addressed in more recent effectiveness research appear promising, but require further study to clarify the extent of their effectiveness. Interest remains high in still others that have not yet shown effectiveness in research studies as multiple parties seek effective ways to meet pressing needs. This variation in the extent to which psychosocial health services are evidence based is similar to the variation seen in research findings supporting the effectiveness of individual biomedical health care services (Neumann et al., 2005; IOM, 2007). The approach used by the committee to evaluate the effectiveness of individual psychosocial health services is described in Appendix B.

Limitations in Taxonomy and Nomenclature

A serious problem encountered by the committee as it sought to identify and evaluate evidence of the effectiveness of psychosocial health services is the lack of a taxonomy and nomenclature for referring to these services. This is manifest in the controlled vocabularies of major bibliographic databases and other indexing services. For example, the term "psychosocial" is not a medical subject heading (MeSH) used for indexing publications by the National Library of Medicine, and as of April 30, 2007, no conceptual definition of "psychosocial" could be found in the National Cancer Institute's *Metathesaurus* (http://ncimeta.nci.nih.gov) or *Dictionary of Cancer Terms* (http://www.cancer.gov/dictionary/). Moreover, when the terminology "psychosocial services" is used in health care, it is used inconsistently. As a result, the committee's first task was to agree upon a definition of psychosocial services to guide its work. The committee's review of different definitions in the field and its considerations in developing the definition put forth in Chapter 2 are discussed in Appendix B.

Examining the effectiveness of *individual* psychosocial services is similarly confounded by absent or imprecise terminology within and across databases such as MeSH/Medline, PsycINFO, CINAHL (Cumulative Index to Nursing and Allied Health Literature), and EMBASE. For example, "peer support" is not a MeSH heading. Moreover, even when different researchers use the same word, it may not always refer to the same intervention. For example, group psychotherapy (Goodwin, 2005), peer support delivered in a group situation (Ussher et al., 2006), group education (Weis, 2003), and varying combinations of these (Weis, 2003) (not always identified as multicomponent interventions) are all frequently labeled "support group" interventions—which unsurprisingly have been found to have inconsistent effects. Similarly, "illness self-management" or "self-management" is not a MeSH heading; it awkwardly and imprecisely maps to "self-care" in the MeSH database. In oncology, many illness self-management or self-care interventions are also referred to as psychoeducation or, more recently, cognitive-behavioral interventions.

The imprecise and unreliable vocabulary used to refer to psychosocial services is manifest in evidence reviews and analyses of the effectiveness of "psychosocial services" in toto. For example, the series of articles entitled "The Great Debate" (Relman and Angell, 2002; Williams and Schneiderman, 2002; Williams et al., 2002)—whose titles ("Resolved: Psychosocial Interventions Can Improve Clinical Outcomes in Organic Disease [Pro]" and "Resolved: Psychosocial Interventions Can Improve Clinical Outcomes in Organic Disease [Con]") and some of their content suggest the methodological soundness (and desirability) of lumping together divergent psychosocial health services and rendering an overarching judgment about their effectiveness. Reviews of the effectiveness of aggregate psychosocial services are problematic just as such reviews of the effectiveness of biomedical health care in the aggregate would be unhelpful (and unlikely)—a point made in the concluding article in the "Great Debate" series (see Lundberg, 2002). The committee determined that the absence of a controlled vocabulary impedes the identification, interpretation, and implementation of research findings on psychosocial health care, and therefore makes the following recommendation.

Recommendation: Standardized nomenclature. To facilitate research on and quality measurement of psychosocial interventions, the National Institutes of Health (NIH) and the Agency for Healthcare Research and Quality (AHRQ) should create and lead an initiative to develop a standardized, transdisciplinary taxonomy and nomenclature for psychosocial health services. This initiative should aim to incorporate this taxonomy and nomenclature into such databases as the National Library of Medicine's Medical Subject Headings (MeSH), PsycINFO, CINAHL (Cumulative Index to Nursing and Allied Health Literature), and EMBASE.

Evidence Reviews

Provision of Information

As discussed in Chapter 1, individuals who are being treated for cancer express the need for a wide range of information on their clinical condition and care. Patients need information about the onset, progression, treatment, and management of their disease and help in interpreting sometimes overwhelming quantities of complex information. They need to be able to find out about the normal course of their condition, the treatments that are available, and those treatments' expected outcomes and side effects so they can make treatment decisions that are consistent with their preferences and care for themselves on a daily basis. Continuing changes in health care delivery and financing also make it increasingly important for cancer patients to have information that will help ensure that they receive high-quality care. This means having access to information about the qualifications of physicians; the relative quality ratings for hospitals and the insurance plans in which they participate; and costs for diagnostic tests, treatments, and hospitalization. It also means being able to obtain information on such services as transportation and other logistical resources, financial assistance, and support groups in the area.

As with the array of psychosocial health services generally, the effectiveness of providing patients with these different types of information has not uniformly been the subject of research. The provision of information about insurance coverage or sources for obtaining wigs, financial support, or logistical assistance, for example, typically is not questioned as a useful service. The broad range of voluntary organizations that provide such information at no cost to consumers and the volume of patient inquiries they handle are further testimony to their usefulness. (A table listing selected nationwide sources of information on cancer and cancer-related services available at no cost to patients is presented in the next section of this chapter.)

In contrast, providing patients with information to enable them to care for themselves on a daily basis and make treatment decisions that best meet their goals and values has been the subject of much research. Indeed, the Institute of Medicine (IOM) has previously recommended that, "patients should be given the necessary information and the opportunity to exercise the degree of control they choose over health care decisions that affect them. The health system should be able to accommodate differences in patient preferences and encourage shared decision making" (IOM, 2001:8).

Although there is little evidence that providing information about the onset, progression, treatment, and management of their disease systematically affects patient behaviors that in turn influence health outcomes, a substantial literature documents the beneficial effects of interventions aimed at improving patients' participation in their care (Coulter and Ellins, 2006). While providing patients with information about their illness and potential treatments will always be only one of many factors that influence a specific behavior, it is clearly an important aspect of improving their participation in their care.

The effect of providing condition-specific information tailored to the individual patient's medical situation or condition has been the subject of many randomized controlled trials involving patients with cancer and other conditions, such as low back pain, diabetes, arthritis, and asthma. An analysis of systematic reviews of the effects of provision of health information found that, although the provision of information on the treatment and management of disease did not affect health status, written information improved knowledge and recall of health information, and the provision of verbal and written information together had a greater impact than the provision of either alone (Coulter and Ellins, 2006).

A variety of strategies for transmitting information about their disease and its treatment to cancer patients have been tested in high-quality randomized controlled trials. Such strategies include presenting information through print materials, audiotapes, CD-ROMs, computer decision aids, and videotapes. These studies have found evidence for the effectiveness of such strategies in increasing knowledge and satisfaction with decision making, as well as reducing decisional conflict (Epstein and Street, 2007).

For example, McPherson and colleagues (2001) conducted a systematic review to determine effective methods of information delivery to cancer patients. Ten studies met the inclusion criteria, covering interventions using audiovisual aids, audiotapes, interactive media, and written information. Written information was found to enhance recall and knowledge, and patients and their families valued practical information booklets. Two important findings from the review are that cancer patients are a heterogeneous population whose information needs differ according to their preferences and coping styles, and that tailoring information to the patient reduces the amount of information needed and increases the relevance and recall of the information provided (McPherson et al., 2001).

Another systematic review of cancer patients' use of the Internet and its impact on health outcomes identified 24 surveys representing a total of 8,679 patients with cancer. Four types of Internet use were identified: communication (e-mail), community (virtual support groups), content (health information), and e-commerce. While a great majority of the studies on providing information to cancer patients have evaluated print materials and computer-based personalization of information, the modest amount of research findings on Internet-based information indicates that it has positive effects on self-efficacy (a person's belief in his/her ability to carry out a course of action to reach a desired goal) and task behavior, encourages patients to make health-related decisions, and improves confidence in the doctor–patient encounter. However, patients reported feeling overwhelmed by the sheer volume of information available on line and were confused by conflicting medical information on cancer treatment (Eysenbach, 2003).

It is particularly important to provide patients with information about treatment decisions so that they can participate in choosing among available effective options. Decision-support tools array such information in a way that enables patients to compare the risks and benefits of different treatments that are suited to their situation. An analysis of systematic reviews of decision aids for patients found that, as with the provision of information on disease and its treatment generally, such aids improve knowledge and information recall and lead to increased involvement in the decision-making process, and that patients who use them experience less decisional conflict. There is limited evidence that decision aids affect health service utilization in a way that in some cases leads to reduced costs, but no effects on health outcomes have been demonstrated (Coulter and Ellins, 2006).

Multicomponent educational interventions, such as those including use of an educational audiotape, workbook, and values clarification exercise, also have been designed to provide the information patients need. One well-conducted randomized controlled trial (Goel et al., 2001) among surgical practices in Canada involving women with breast cancer who needed to decide between breast-conserving treatment and mastectomy found evidence of the effectiveness of such a multicomponent intervention, but only for women who were uncertain about what decision to make. There is some evidence that nonprint formats are of greater benefit for underserved groups and that these formats have an impact on health behavior (Coulter and Ellins, 2006). Nonprint formats are also useful in communicating with individuals with low literacy.

Services to Help Cope with Emotions

A wide variety of mental health therapies have been developed to treat emotional distress and mental health problems.[1] Although it was beyond the scope of this report to examine the evidence in support of all types of services to address all manifestations of emotional distress and mental health problems in individuals with cancer,[2] the discussion below reviews peer support programs selected because of their widespread use and availability, as well as counseling/psychotherapy and medications that address depression and anxiety—among the most common mental health conditions affecting individuals diagnosed with cancer.

Peer support programs   Peer support is defined as a relationship in which people with the same condition provide emotional support to each other and share knowledge about dealing effectively with that condition. Vicariously experiencing the successes of others similar to oneself is a primary pathway to building one's own self-efficacy (Bandura, 1997). Self-efficacy is viewed as a key predictor of how effectively individuals can motivate themselves and persevere in the face of adversity, how much effort they will make in pursuing a course of action, and what their emotional reactions to the course of events will be. Self-efficacy is also an important determinant of how extensively knowledge and skills are obtained (Pajares, 2002), and there is evidence that it is a critical factor in an individual's successful self-management of a range of chronic illnesses (Lorig et al., 2001; Lorig and Holman, 2003).

Peer support programs can provide one-on-one support (as in the American Cancer Society's Reach to Recovery program) or support from groups. Peer support groups (also called self or mutual support groups) have been studied most often. Emotional support is a primary component of peer support groups (Weis, 2003; Ussher et al., 2006). These groups also typically provide information and education, sharing of coping skills, acceptance by others in similar situations, a sense of normalcy, and diminished social isolation (Barlow et al., 2000; Campbell et al., 2004). Many of these supports are the same as those provided by beneficial informal social networks described in Chapter 2, which have been found to reduce

---

[1]In child and adolescent therapy alone, for example, it is conservatively estimated that, even if one omits various combinations of treatments and variants of treatments that are not substantially different, there are more than 550 psychotherapies in use (Kazdin, 2000).

[2]For example, this report does not address the unique clinical treatment issues of individuals with mental illnesses such as schizophrenia and psychotic disorders. However, the access to specialized mental health services described in Chapter 6 pertains to cancer patients with all types of mental health problems and illness, not just those described in this chapter. The reader is directed to a recent IOM report, *Improving the Quality of Health Care for Mental and Substance-Use Conditions* (IOM, 2006), which addresses approaches to coordinating mental health care with other medical care for all types of mental health conditions.

morbidity and mortality. Expected outcomes include increased confidence and a sense of control in relation to self, improved coping with one's illness, and more effective interactions with others, particularly medical professionals. Together, these outcomes promote a helpful sense of self-efficacy in dealing with the varied challenges of the illness and its treatment (Bandura, 1997; Thaxton et al., 2005; Ussher et al., 2006).

Peer support groups are widely used to help people with a broad range of illnesses. One of the largest and most successful is Alcoholics Anonymous. Support groups for people living with HIV or AIDS are another example (Spirig, 1998). Such groups are often developed by individuals who feel marginalized socially by their illness because of the associated stigma, disfigured appearance, embarrassment, disability, or threat to life (Davison et al., 2000). After World War II, assisted by the American Cancer Society, patients who had had a laryngectomy, colostomy, or mastectomy began to form support groups in major cities to help cope with these permanent and stigmatizing body changes. Today, support groups for cancer patients are organized through nonprofit advocacy organizations—some devoted to patients with a particular form of cancer (e.g., The Leukemia & Lymphoma Society) and others, such as Gilda's Clubs, The Wellness Community, and CancerCare, with a more general focus. These support groups are the most widely available form of free psychological assistance for patients with cancer.

Peer groups have developed to help patients of all ages cope with cancer in all of its stages: at diagnosis, during active treatment, and during advanced disease (Plante et al., 2001). They are used most widely by patients with particular forms of cancer, the most common being prostate and breast (e.g., Us Too groups for prostate cancer and breast cancer support groups) (Goodwin, 2005). Today, the support offered by such groups frequently includes services from a health or human services professional, such as a physician, nurse, psychologist, or social worker, who facilitates group meetings or provides patient education or other services to the group. In fact, many groups that are called peer groups actually have co-leaders who are professionals. This involvement from health care providers often makes a "pure" peer group difficult to define; most groups today are to some extent hybrids involving both consumer peers and professionals. Research comparing peer and professionally led support groups has found no difference as long as the sense of community and mutual respect is maintained (Barlow et al., 2000).

Research on the effectiveness of peer support groups has been difficult because such groups often arise naturally out of communities when people sense a need,[3] and therefore do not easily lend themselves to the control of variables as is required to conduct controlled clinical trials. The varied

---

[3] And not all patients want to participate in a support group.

components of support groups (e.g., group psychotherapy, informal emotional support, education and information) and the diverse participants and facilitators also confound the interpretation of research findings. According to Davison and colleagues (2000:216) in their review of the state of the art of peer support, "Support groups constitute a category with fuzzy boundaries, and as such they make scientists uneasy. In the interest of elegance and experimental control, we often prefer mutually exclusive categories and singular causal models. . . . Support groups cannot be replicated in the lab, but the tendency of some types of patients to seek each other's company . . . emerges statistically as a clear pattern replicated across cities."

Although evidence for the effectiveness of peer support interventions is less clear than desirable, overall it supports their effectiveness in bringing about a number of desirable outcomes—such as improved knowledge, coping skills, and sense of self-efficacy—across a wide range of mental and general medical conditions, including HIV/AIDS (Spirig, 1998) and cancer (Barlow et al., 2000; Dunn et al., 2003; National Breast Cancer Centre and National Cancer Control Initiative, 2003; Campbell et al., 2004; Zabalegui et al., 2005; Ussher et al., 2006). However, not all patients may need or benefit equally from participation in peer support groups (Helgeson et al., 2000); those with the lowest self-esteem and self-efficacy in coping with depressive symptoms appear to benefit most (Helgeson et al., 2006).

Better understanding of the effectiveness of peer support groups will require more randomized controlled trials in which the participants, content, and outcome variables are clearly delineated. These trials also should involve multiple centers so as to encompass populations of sufficient size to allow study of subsamples and types, duration, and content of interventions. Use of a standard set of outcome measures across studies also would allow more meaningful comparisons across studies through meta-analysis. Research is needed as well that compares group formats so as to identify the treatment and personal variables that lead to the best and poorest outcomes. Moreover, most peer support groups have developed in middle-class, Caucasian, and female populations; studies involving other ethnic and socioeconomic groups and men are needed, as are studies of one-to-one forms of peer support.

The Internet is widely used for providing "virtual" peer support groups. Although such groups are difficult to monitor with respect to their delivery and quality of services (when no facilitator modulates interactions) and will not be easy to evaluate for efficacy, their increasing use suggests that research also should be directed toward assessment of their efficacy, especially since they provide a means to reach home-bound and geographically isolated patients at minimal expense (Eysenbach et al., 2004; Hoybye et al., 2005; Lieberman and Goldstein, 2005; Winefield, 2006; Stein et al., 2007).

Counseling and psychotherapy Counseling and psychotherapy encompass "a wide range of techniques used by a designated professional that have as their common feature the attempt to influence the patient's behavior, emotions, thoughts, and attitudes through psychological techniques, most often verbal interchange, in the relationship between the psychotherapist and the patient" (Klerman, 1989:1730). Although counseling and psychotherapy have been found to be effective for a number of different mental health problems in patients with a range of general medical illnesses (Wells et al., 1988; Schulberg et al., 1998), findings on their effectiveness in helping patients with cancer and analyses of these findings in the aggregate have been mixed.

The large number of research trials of psychotherapeutic interventions with adult patients[4] (conducted at all stages of disease, though focusing mainly on newly diagnosed patients, those in active treatment, and those with metastatic disease) has enabled several meta-analyses and other systematic reviews of the evidence. These reviews also have yielded mixed results because of variations in the criteria established for inclusion as an adequately designed clinical trial; however, they generally have found that evidence supports the efficacy of psychotherapy in the treatment of anxiety and depressive symptoms in adults (Devine et al., 1995; Meyer and Mark, 1995; Sheard and Maguire, 1999; AHRQ, 2002; Barsevick et al., 2002; Rehse and Pukrop, 2003; Pirl, 2004; Jacobsen et al., 2006). In a debate in the *Annals of Behavioral Medicine*, Andrykowski and Manne (2006) reason that clinically relevant efficacy can be assumed on the basis of two or more well-conducted randomized controlled trials utilizing Consolidated Standards of Reporting Trials (CONSORT) criteria. When criteria for efficacy are highly restrictive (as in Newell et al., 2002—that is, requiring greater than half of outcome measures to be statistically significant)—evidence for efficacy appears to be weaker (Coyne et al., 2006). An additional problem contributing to the mixed results of these analyses appears to be related in part to the fact that most early studies of these psychosocial services did not require elevation of a baseline target symptom in subjects, thus diminishing the likelihood of showing a significant reduction in the identified symptom in some studies. Jacobsen and colleagues' (2006) comprehensive review found that fewer than 5 percent of studies had required a clinically significant baseline level of distress in their design, an observation made by Sheard and Maguire (1999) years earlier. Nonetheless, the norm for studies of these psychosocial interventions has been to include all patients, regardless of their level of distress.

---

[4]Less research has been conducted on psychological interventions with children with cancer, in part because of their small numbers and evidence showing low levels of psychopathology in children as a group (Patenaude and Kupst, 2005; Pai et al., 2006).

Having reviewed the various systematic reviews and individual studies, the committee concludes that there is statistically significant, clinically relevant evidence to support the effectiveness of psychotherapeutic interventions in helping to manage anxiety or depression in adults with cancer—across disease sites, treatments, and types of interventions (e.g., psychoeducation, supportive therapies, cognitive therapies, relaxation techniques), and delivered to both individuals and groups. These findings apply despite the wide range of interventions, diversity of patients, and variety of study designs. The review of 60 studies by Jacobsen and colleagues (2006), examining only well-designed controlled studies with clinically relevant outcome data, found support for incorporating tested interventions into clinical practice guidelines. The National Cancer Control Initiative in Australia similarly found strong evidence for interventions that used cognitive-behavioral, supportive, and psychoeducational approaches for the management of depression and anxiety (National Breast Cancer Centre and National Cancer Control Initiative, 2003). Evidence with respect to three key types of psychotherapies is summarized below:

- *Cognitive-behavioral therapy*—This approach has been the most widely studied in randomized controlled trials and has been shown to help reduce psychological symptoms (anxiety and depression), as well as the physical symptoms of pain, nausea/vomiting, and fatigue, most effectively during the initial and treatment phases of illness. The approach involves teaching problem solving, reframing of thoughts, and ways of constructive coping, and often includes relaxation and guided imagery. The adjuvant therapy developed by Greer and colleagues is a well-studied model based on these principles (Greer et al., 1992; Moorey et al., 1994; Moynihan et al., 1998). Two studies (Nezu et al., 2003; Boesen et al., 2005) using cognitive-behavioral skill-based interventions found they were most beneficial for those who entered the trial with highest distress.
- *Supportive psychotherapy*—This approach involves providing emotional support and encouragement, focusing on emotional responses, and encouraging adaptive coping. Randomized trials have tested manualized supportive-expressive and supportive-existential psychotherapy for patients with early and advanced disease. All of these trials have shown efficacy in reducing distress, improving quality of life, and helping patients cope with the physical aspects of illness. Overall, there is strong evidence from clinical trials that these approaches yield benefits in reducing anxiety and depressive symptoms and improving well-being (Spiegel et al., 1981; Goodwin et al., 2001; Kissane et al., 2007). Another type of supportive psychotherapy—interpersonal psychotherapy—focuses on

the role changes and the conflicts and strains related to illness. The approach has been studied for treatment of depression in patients with HIV/AIDS (Markowitz et al., 1993) with good results. Similar results were obtained in small trials in which the approach was adapted for use with cancer patients, being delivered face to face and by telephone for homebound patients by trained counselors using a manual (Alter et al., 1996; Donnelly et al., 2000). In practice, supportive psychotherapy is a flexible therapeutic approach in which a skilled therapist applies aspects of cognitive-behavioral therapy and psychodynamic concepts while providing emotional support. The emphasis varies depending on the stage of illness and the level of severity of psychosocial and physical problems (Berglund et al., 1994a; Evans and Connis, 1995; McArdle et al., 1996). It is difficult to design controlled clinical trials that take into account the need for such flexibility in therapy.

- *Family and couples therapy*—While not widely studied in controlled trials involving patients with cancer, therapies that result in increased communication and cohesion and reduction of conflicts due to the strain of illness in one member appear to be of most benefit for families with dysfunctional issues (Kissane et al., 2006). The approach taken may be largely cognitive-behavioral or supportive therapy. Couples therapy has been studied in patients with cancer and has been found to be useful in reducing illness-related conflicts, particularly when there is sexual dysfunction involved (Manne et al., 2006).

In addition to evidence on the effectiveness of specific types of counseling or psychotherapy, there is interest in the effectiveness of counseling and psychotherapy when delivered via telephone, Internet, or other electronic communication technologies (e.g., teleconferencing). Telepsychiatry and counseling via phone have been recommended as approaches for delivering mental health services to patients in remote locations or in areas with a shortage of mental health professionals (McGinty et al., 2006), and there is evidence of their effectiveness (Marcus et al., 1998; Ruskin et al., 2004). (See Chapter 5 for a discussion of the use of remote resources to meet psychosocial health needs.) A recent systematic review of telephone-based interventions for mental illness also found evidence of their effectiveness, but noted that the limited number of studies conducted, their small sample sizes, and the lack of a randomized controlled trial methodology prevent drawing firm conclusions. The authors call for large-scale, randomized controlled trials to increase understanding of the efficacy of telephone interventions (Leach and Christensen, 2006). A recent IOM report similarly noted that use of Internet-mediated and other communications technologies for the delivery of mental health services requires additional effectiveness research, as well as specialized training of clinicians, additional protection of consumer information, and mechanisms for ensuring the competencies of those who provide such forms of care (IOM, 2006).

More helpful evidence about how best to deliver psychotherapeutic services could be produced through (1) use of large randomized trials of psychotherapeutic interventions of high quality using CONSORT guidelines; (2) intervention studies of patients with particularly stigmatizing forms of cancer, such as lung cancer; (3) more studies of men with a range of cancers, particularly prostate and colon; (4) more studies with children; (5) effectiveness and dissemination studies designed to adapt, implement, and test interventions with proven efficacy in routine clinical settings (as well as adaptations for telephone or Internet application); (6) studies of psychotherapeutic interventions in ethnically diverse populations; (7) intervention trials that would identify patients with elevated levels of targeted symptoms of anxiety or depression, or both, at baseline to permit assessment of clinically relevant levels of symptom change; and (8) studies including analysis of data from clinical trial settings with respect to cost in real-world clinical settings.

Psychopharmacological services   Psychopharmacological services comprise the use of a range of medications known as psychotropic drugs to reduce anxiety, depression, and other mental health symptoms. These drugs have been well tested in clinical trials in depressed adults with cardiac disease, stroke, and diabetes, with results strongly supporting their efficacy (Jacobsen and Weinger, 1998; Lustman et al., 1992; Glassman et al., 2002; Rassmussen et al., 2003; Gill and Hatcher, 2006; Simon et al., 2007). Yet there have been few large-scale randomized controlled trials of psychotropic agents in patients with cancer, in part because of (1) high rates of attrition of study participants due to progressive illness and (2) symptoms of cancer, such as fatigue, that mimic symptoms of depression.

However, recent research and systematic reviews of research on the use of antidepressants (tricyclics, selective serotonin reuptake inhibitors [SSRIs], atypical antidepressants, a psychostimulant) and antianxiety drugs (benzodiazepines) in adult cancer patients suggest that they reduce depressive symptoms, major depression, and anxiety in these patients, though fewer of the studies focused on anxiety (National Breast Cancer Centre and National Cancer Control Initiative, 2003; Pirl, 2004; Jacobsen et al., 2006; Williams and Dale, 2006; Rodin et al., 2007). Results of several modest-sized trials also suggest the efficacy of antidepressants in the control of anxiety and depressive symptoms in adult patients with cancer (Costa et al., 1985; Holland et al., 1991, 1998; Wald et al., 1993; Heeringen and Zivkov, 1996; Razavi et al., 1996, 1999; Ly et al., 2002; Fisch et al., 2003;

Jacobsen et al., 2006). The review of Jacobsen and colleagues (2006) found that antidepressants and anxiolytics are effective in preventing and relieving depression and anxiety and may be recommended in clinical practice guidelines. A similar conclusion was reached by Australia's National Breast Cancer Centre and National Cancer Control Initiative (2003) and the National Comprehensive Cancer Network in the United States (Distress Management Guidelines Panel, 2003). Of note, one trial found that use of an SSRI prevented the development of depression in patients vulnerable to interferon-induced depressive symptoms/depression (Musselman et al., 2001). There is no evidence suggesting greater efficacy of one drug over others (Pirl, 2004; Jacobsen et al., 2006; Williams and Dale, 2006).

It will be necessary to have more multicenter controlled randomized trials using larger patient cohorts studied over longer periods to better assess the potential efficacy of drugs that may be slow in achieving clinical effects. Trials should be limited to patients with clearly defined significant levels of anxious or depressive symptoms at baseline, such as severe adjustment disorder with anxious or depressive symptoms or anxiety disorder, post-traumatic stress disorder, or mood disorder, to ensure the opportunity to observe a reduction in symptoms. Studies also are needed to compare the efficacy of one drug over another for a targeted symptom. Given the efficacy of psychotherapeutic services and psychotropic drugs in cancer patients, trials comparing the effectiveness of medications alone, psychotherapy alone, and the two combined should be conducted, as has been done in cardiac patients. Moreover, there is a critical need to examine the use of SSRIs and anxiolytics in adolescents with cancer since currently there is virtually no information base to generalize to pediatric oncology.

Help in Managing Illness Comprehensively

Illness self-management is defined as an individual's "ability to manage the symptoms, treatment, physical and psychosocial consequences and lifestyle changes inherent in living with a chronic condition" (Barlow et al., 2002:178). In general, interventions designed to support illness self-management include providing basic information about the illness and its treatment; providing education and coaching in skills needed to manage the illness, control symptoms, and interact with the health care system; and increasing patient self-efficacy (Lev et al., 2001). Education and coaching are generally tailored to the needs and learning styles of individual patients, encourage patients' active participation in their care, and involve some form of problem-solving assistance. These basic elements of self-management support have often been combined with specific psychological or physical modalities, such as relaxation response or exercise. There is now considerable evidence for many chronic diseases other than cancer that interventions directed at improving patient knowledge, skills, and confidence in managing the illness improve outcomes (Chodosh et al., 2005). One of the best-studied illness self-management programs, found effective in randomized controlled trials, is the Chronic Disease Self-Management Program developed and offered by Stanford University School of Medicine (Stanford University School of Medicine, 2007). Self-management programs for a variety of chronic illnesses based on this model have been found to be effective in reducing pain and disability, lessening fatigue, decreasing needed visits to physicians and emergency rooms, and increasing self-reported energy and health for a variety of chronic illnesses, including heart disease, lung disease, stroke, and arthritis (Lorig et al., 2001; Bodenheimer et al., 2002; Lorig and Holman, 2003).[5,6]

The term "illness self-management" is most often associated with conditions such as diabetes mellitus for which lifestyle changes can significantly affect the severity and progression of the disease. For this reason, it might be thought that self-management may not apply to cancer care. The committee believes this would be an overly restrictive view of self-management behaviors. In the cancer care literature, many interventions have been designed to assist patients in coping with the various challenges presented by the illness and its treatment, such as physical symptoms (e.g., fatigue or nausea), psychological distress, sexual dysfunction, and interaction with multiple providers. These interventions share a common premise with self-management interventions for other chronic conditions—that patients (and their families) have a major role to play in addressing or managing these challenges, and their ability to fulfill this role competently can be improved by information, empowerment, and other support.

Self-management and self-care interventions aimed at improving physical function and quality of life in cancer patients have typically focused on the control of individual symptoms and generally have been individually administered by nurses, whereas self-management interventions in patients with conditions other than cancer have more often been conducted in groups. A limited number of interventions have targeted control of nausea (Winningham and MacVicar, 1988), fatigue (Dimeo et al., 1999,

---

[5]Stanford's model also is a required component of the Administration on Aging's public–private collaborative grant program for states and local communities, Empowering Older People to Take More Control of Their Health Through Evidence-Based Prevention Programs.

[6]Although many individuals with cancer have participated in the Stanford model of illness self-management through 700 "master trainers" in the United States and worldwide, the University of Louisiana Brown Cancer Center also held two workshops targeting cancer survivors that followed the Stanford model, and identified no areas needing modification for this group (Personal communication. Karen S. Newton, MPH, RD, Project Director, Chronic Illness Initiatives, University of Louisville Department of Family and Geriatric Medicine via Kate Lorig, RN, DrPH, Stanford Patient Education Research Center, September 5, 2006).

2004; Schwartz, 1999, 2000; Dimeo, 2001; Schwartz et al., 2001), pain (Miaskowski et al., 2004), and lymphedema (McKenzie and Kalda, 2003). These interventions (most often provided by nurses in the cancer care setting) have been variously termed psychoeducational, self-care, self-management support, and more recently, cognitive-behavioral interventions.[7] They have been administered to patients before therapy or the onset of symptoms as prevention, to those experiencing symptoms or distress, or to those who have completed therapy. They have included interventions provided by a nurse alone or complemented by computer programs, video presentations, and other tools. While there may be differences in the underlying theory, the interventions included under the four rubrics of psychoeducation, self-care, self-management support, and cognitive-behavioral interventions are all designed to increase an individual's skill in managing the illness and its effects. However, some approaches to illness self-management used with cancer patients have been delivered in combination with the provision of skilled physical nursing care, which has confounded interpretation of the effectiveness of the psychosocial component of care.

The PRO-SELF program, the most extensively tested strategy, targets various symptoms of cancer and its treatment and has been evaluated in multiple randomized trials (Larson et al., 1998; Dodd and Miaskowski, 2000; West et al., 2003; Kim et al., 2004; Miaskowski et al., 2004). The intervention involves nurses coaching patients and their families. The content includes information designed to assist patients "in managing the cancer treatment experience," including basic information about the disease and its treatment, symptoms, and approaches to symptom management. In addition to this information, patients receive coaching in the skills necessary to manage their symptoms—for example, mouth care for mucositis (Larson et al., 1998) or opioid use for pain (Miaskowski et al., 2004)—and problem-solving assistance. Studies of this strategy found significantly reduced pain intensity and more appropriate use of opioids (Miaskowski et al., 2004). Given and colleagues (2006) tested a cognitive-behavioral intervention that included classes focused on self-management, problem-solving, and communication with providers. Those receiving the experimental intervention reported significantly fewer severe symptoms at 10 and 20 weeks' follow-up. In randomized controlled trials, related interventions have been shown to improve mood and vigor among patients with malignant melanoma (Boesen et al., 2005), reduce psychological distress after radiotherapy (Stiegelis et al., 2004), reduce fatigue and improve functional status among cancer survivors (Gielissen et al., 2006), and improve sexual function and reduce worry among patients with prostate cancer (Giesler et al., 2005).

McCorkle and colleagues have developed and studied interventions in

---

[7]This is another example of the terminology problem discussed earlier in this chapter.

which nurses help cancer patients and their family caregivers manage the impacts of the illness and its treatment. Delivered in the home by advanced practice nurses, the interventions generally involve assessment of physical, psychosocial, and functional health status; teaching, support, and counseling; the provision of hands-on skilled nursing care if needed; assistance in accessing community resources; and coordination with other health care providers and settings. In a series of randomized trials, these interventions helped patients with lung cancer maintain independence longer and reduced rehospitalizations (McCorkle et al., 1989), improved mental health status among patients with solid tumors (McCorkle et al., 1994), reduced distress among the spouses of dying patients with lung cancer (McCorkle et al., 1998), and improved survival among postsurgical cancer patients (McCorkle et al., 2000).

Efforts to give patients with cancer and their families the information, skills, and confidence needed to manage the physical, psychosocial, and communication challenges associated with cancer and its care appear to be warranted by the literature. Progress in this area could be accelerated by the development of a taxonomy of interventions that, if used by researchers, would help identify the components that contribute most to effectiveness.

Assistance in Changing Behaviors to Minimize Impacts of Disease

Concurrent with the success of contemporary cancer therapies in curing cancer or extending life expectancy and with the recognition that behavior change can contribute to the prevention of some cancers, investigations of lifestyle interventions aimed at promoting health in cancer survivors have increased in number and priority. Such interventions are aimed at preventing the recurrence of cancer and improving overall health by addressing, for example, tobacco and alcohol use, dietary practices, physical activity, weight reduction, sun protection, and participation in disease surveillance programs. Behavior change in several of these areas has been achieved through such interventions as advice from physicians, counseling from peers or trained clinical educators, and exercise training (Demark-Wahnefried et al., 2006). Although the optimal methods for helping patients achieve lasting behavior change are not fully known, the clear health advantages of not smoking and adhering to diet and exercise guidelines, along with the availability of some evidence to guide clinicians in helping patients make beneficial changes in their health-related behaviors, support the need to undertake such efforts. Progress made to date in modifying behaviors to promote health in patients with cancer is reviewed below.

Tobacco control   Approximately 20 percent of adults with a history of cancer continue to smoke (Hewitt et al., 2003). Thus, tobacco control initiatives targeting cancer patients are critical to reducing or preventing the risk of cardiovascular, pulmonary, and neoplastic sequelae that can be associated with specific cancer treatments and aging. A limited number of randomized controlled trials have evaluated smoking cessation interventions in patients with cancer (Gritz et al., 1993; Wewers et al., 1994; Griebel et al., 1998; Browning et al., 2000; Sanderson Cox et al., 2002; Schnoll et al., 2003, 2005; Emmons et al., 2005). These interventions generally employ cognitive-behavioral counseling administered by health educators, nurses (Wewers et al., 1994; Griebel et al., 1998; Browning et al., 2000), dentists (Gritz et al., 1993), physicians (Gritz et al., 1993; Schnoll et al., 2003), or peers (Emmons et al., 2005). The interpretation of study results is limited by a variety of factors, however, including low statistical power (Stanislaw and Wewers, 1994; Wewers et al., 1994; Griebel et al., 1998; Browning et al., 2000), small sample size (Stanislaw and Wewers, 1994; Wewers et al., 1994; Griebel et al., 1998), high attrition rates (Gritz et al., 1993), and lack of long-term follow-up (Stanislaw and Wewers, 1994; Griebel et al., 1998; Schnoll et al., 2005). Consequently, results overall provide little or no evidence to support the effectiveness of behaviorally based smoking cessation interventions. Gritz and colleagues (1993) observed no difference in continuous abstinence rates at 12-month follow-up in patients with head and neck cancers randomized to receive standard advice to quit or surgeon-delivered smoking cessation counseling. Another study likewise found that quit rates did not differ among cancer patients who received standard smoking cessation counseling and those who received a brief smoking cessation intervention from their physician (Schnoll et al., 2003). In a third study, childhood cancer survivors randomized to receive peer-delivered smoking counseling with telephone follow-up were twice as likely to quit smoking as those who received self-help materials. However, the quit rate at 12-month follow-up for both groups was relatively modest (15 versus 9 percent), and the incremental cost of the intervention was substantial ($5,371 per additional quit) (Emmons et al., 2005).

Collectively, the available results of intervention trials in cancer populations, the well-established health risks associated with cancer and its treatment, and the morbidity associated with tobacco use support the need for more research aimed at developing effective, sustainable tobacco control interventions for cancer patients that take behavioral, psychological, and economic factors into account. In the interim, clinicians caring for patients with a past or present diagnosis of cancer should assess their smoking status and counsel those who smoke about the increased health risks they incur in doing so. This recommendation is based on the finding that among the population at large (i.e., without regard to having a particular diagnosis), individual face-to-face counseling by a trained therapist or nurse or brief advice from a physician can be effective in reducing smoking (Lancaster and Stead, 2004, 2005; Rice and Stead, 2004).

Diet and physical activity   Diet and physical activity are important health behaviors that affect the risk of both cancer and cardiovascular disease. Common health conditions such as overweight/obesity, cardiovascular disease, and osteopenia/osteoporosis may develop as a primary effect of specific cancer treatments or as a secondary effect of cancer on functional status, and dietary interventions offer the potential to reduce such cancer-related morbidity and promote overall health in vulnerable patients. Dietary interventions targeting patients with cancer have been evaluated in 11 prospective controlled trials that focused on either weight reduction (de Waard et al., 1993; Loprinzi et al., 1996; Djuric et al., 2002), fat restriction (Boyar et al., 1988; Chlebowski et al., 1992; Rose et al., 1993; Kristal et al., 1997), or specific nutrient intake (Nordevang et al., 1992; Pierce et al., 1997; Hebert et al., 2001; Pierce et al., 2004). Intervention methods have involved primarily resource-intensive, individualized counseling sessions delivered by trained nutritionists, although some studies have relied on trained volunteer staff (Kristal et al., 1997) or commercial weight loss programs such as Weight Watchers (Djuric et al., 2002). In addition to individualized instruction, some interventions have used such approaches as group sessions or telephone counseling (Pierce et al., 2004). Study results indicate that these interventions are largely effective in promoting dietary change as determined by dietary intake (Chlebowski et al., 1992; Nordevang et al., 1992; Pierce et al., 1997, 2004; Hebert et al., 2001), body weight (Boyar et al., 1988; Chlebowski et al., 1992; de Waard et al., 1993; Rose et al., 1993; Loprinzi et al., 1996; Kristal et al., 1997; Hebert et al., 2001; Djuric et al., 2002), and hormonal status (Boyar et al., 1988; Rose et al., 1993). Notably, some studies were limited by high attrition rates, which in most cases were similar among treatment and control participants (Chlebowski et al., 1992; Kristal et al., 1997; Pierce et al., 1997; Djuric et al., 2002). Moreover, evidence supporting the sustainability of the positive impact of interventions beyond 1 year is limited (Chlebowski et al., 1992). Several ongoing multisite trials are aimed at evaluating maintenance of the effects of dietary interventions and the relationship to survival outcomes. Preliminary results of the Women's Intervention Nutrition Study demonstrate significant reductions in dietary fat and weight in 290 women randomized to individual dietary instruction versus controls (Chlebowski et al., 1992). Investigators coordinating the Women's Healthy Eating and Living Study Intervention Nutrition Study similarly observed significant increases in intake of vegetables, fruits, and fiber that was confirmed by nutrient biomarkers among patients with breast cancer randomized to receive individualized dietary telephone counseling (Pierce et al., 2004). Continued follow-up of these groups will provide important information about the impact of dietary interventions on cancer-free survival.

The benefits of regular physical activity include improvements in physical functioning, cardiorespiratory fitness, strength, flexibility, weight status, lean muscle mass, mood, and quality of life (McTiernan et al., 1998; Courneya and Friedenreich, 1999; Pinto and Maruyama, 1999; Courneya, 2003; Fairey et al., 2003; Schwartz, 2004; Knols et al., 2005). A number of studies of exercise interventions have been conducted among patients with cancer, with the overall goals of ameliorating cancer-related symptoms (Winningham and MacVicar, 1988; Courneya et al., 2003b; McKenzie and Kalda, 2003) and improving physical functioning (MacVicar et al., 1989; Winningham et al., 1989; Berglund et al., 1994b; Dimeo et al., 1997a, 2003, 2004; Segal et al., 2001; Burnham and Wilcox, 2002; Courneya et al., 2003a,c; Jones et al., 2004; Fairey et al., 2005; Pinto et al., 2005). Of these studies, 34 involved randomized or controlled clinical trials that employed various exercise modalities, including cardiovascular (Winningham and MacVicar, 1988; MacVicar et al., 1989; Winningham et al., 1989; Dimeo et al., 1997a, 1998, 2003; Mock et al., 1997, 2001; Schwartz, 1999, 2000; Na et al., 2000; Schwartz et al., 2001; Segal et al., 2001; Courneya et al., 2003a), resistance (Cunningham et al., 1986; Segal et al., 2003), and/ or flexibility training (Kolden et al., 2002; Adamsen et al., 2003). Exercise interventions are generally described as "training programs" that vary in the nature of the training provided. Most are supervised by an exercise physiologist or similarly trained staff, but some are not. Some are delivered in a group setting, some are home-based, and some have both components. Some are described as self-paced.

Outcomes measured for exercise interventions include fatigue, quality of life, emotional distress, immunological parameters, aerobic capacity, and muscle strength. The majority of studies have found positive physiological and psychological outcomes as assessed by levels of fatigue (Mock et al., 1997; Schwartz, 1999; Mock, 2001; Schwartz et al., 2001; Segal et al., 2003), quality-of-life and psychological factors (Mock et al., 1997, 2001; Dimeo et al., 1999; Schwartz, 1999; Segal et al., 2001; Kolden et al., 2002; Adamsen et al., 2003; Courneya et al., 2003a), immunological parameters (Dimeo et al., 1997a,b, 2003; Na et al., 2000), aerobic capacity (MacVicar et al., 1989; Winningham et al., 1989; Dimeo et al., 1997a, 1998, 1999, 2003; Mock et al., 1997, 2001; Schwartz, 1999; Schwartz et al., 2001; Segal et al., 2001; Kolden et al., 2002; Adamsen et al., 2003; Courneya et al., 2003a), and muscle strength (Kolden et al., 2002; Adamsen et al., 2003; Segal et al., 2003). Exercise interventions have been found effective in improving oxygen capacity, fitness, strength, flexibility, and global health (MacVicar et al., 1989; Berglund et al., 1994b; Dimeo et al., 1997b; Segal et al., 2001, 2003; Burnham and Wilcox, 2002; Courneya et al., 2003c; McKenzie and Kalda, 2003). Several of these investigations observed increased engagement in social activities and reduction in sleep disturbance in addition to improved physiological outcomes (MacVicar et al., 1989;

Berglund et al., 1994b). Anthropometric benefits reported following exercise interventions include positive effects on weight and adiposity as gauged by waist and hip measurements (Winningham et al., 1989; Burnham and Wilcox, 2002). One study demonstrated significant improvement in such biomarkers as blood pressure, heart rate, hemoglobin, and circulating hormone levels in patients with breast cancer participating in a home-based physical activity intervention (Pinto et al., 2005). Another found a favorable effect of exercise on biomarkers associated with the metabolic syndrome, including insulin-like growth factor and insulin-like growth factor-binding protein 3 (Fairey et al., 2003).

It should be noted, however, that many trials of exercise interventions had methodological shortcomings, including nonrandom treatment assignments and small sample sizes. Also, patients with breast cancer were the predominant diagnostic group targeted for study, and the generalizability of those findings to patients with other cancer diagnoses is not clear. Nonetheless, collective results suggest that exercise is associated with many benefits for the cancer survivor, although a positive impact on survival has not been established. Future trials are needed to elucidate the optimal type and intensity of exercise for patients with cancer, particularly those with unique vulnerabilities resulting from cancer-related therapies, such as limb-sparing surgery or anthracycline chemotherapy. Moreover, because regular physical activity and healthy dietary practices are both important to weight maintenance, continued follow-up in ongoing trials will be important to determine the effectiveness of addressing energy balance through multicomponent behavioral interventions targeting both exercise and dietary modification (Demark-Wahnefried et al., 2002, 2003a,b; Rock and Demark-Wahnefried, 2002).

Provision of Material and Logistical Resources

Receiving treatment for cancer in medical settings, complying with prescribed treatments while at home, caring for oneself or a family member, and performing important family and social roles despite illness require patients and caregivers to have certain material and logistical resources. These include transportation, lodging for patients and caregivers when they must travel long distances for outpatient therapy, child care, wigs and prostheses (breast, limb, other), and supplies for managing the side effects of cancer and its treatment (e.g., compression bandages or sleeves for lymphedema control, ostomy supplies). As noted earlier in this chapter, informal sources of support can often provide many of these services, such as transportation or child care. When the service is covered by insurance or a patient has other financial means, material resources can be purchased. When informal supports and/or financial resources are limited, however, services are needed from other, formal sources. As noted in Chapter 1, the American Cancer Society and CancerCare both report that they frequently provide assistance in securing transportation to health-related appointments, supplies needed for health care, medical equipment, wigs, and prosthetics.

The effect on health or health care of providing these material and logistical resources has been the focus of limited research, likely for multiple reasons. First, as noted earlier in the chapter, some of these services have such long-standing and wide acceptance as humane services that there has been little question as to whether they "work." Transportation, for example, has long been acknowledged as a necessary resource for the receipt of health care, as is evident from its inclusion as a covered service since the inception of the Medicaid program. Moreover, the provision of many of these resources poses less physical risk than a new medication or other clinical treatment, thus attracting less attention as a priority focus for scare research dollars. Some of these services also have been perceived as "human services" rather than "health services" because they are not directly curative or biomedical in intent or origin, and are frequently provided through voluntary human services agencies as opposed to health care providers under third-party reimbursement. In addition, some of these resources may be perceived as "cosmetic" and thus of lower priority than life-saving medical treatments (Healey, 2003). When these services have been examined, the question often has been how to deliver them (often limited in availability) more efficiently and appropriately and how to prioritize their delivery to those in greatest need.

Among the sparse research that has sought to determine the effects on health or health care of providing logistical or material resources, one study documented that when individuals with cancer lacked transportation, treatment was foregone (Guidry et al., 1997). And studies of people with a variety of chronic diseases have found that environmental barriers such as cost and logistical obstacles interfere with the ability to manage their illness (Bayliss et al., 2003; Vincze et al., 2004). The absence of research on other types of support (e.g., use of breast prostheses generally and of different types) has in itself been identified as adversely affecting the quality of life of women after surgery for breast cancer (Healey, 2003).

The committee notes that the absence of research is not evidence of an intervention's ineffectiveness. Moreover, the frequent provision of many of these services to patients and families by voluntary agencies (detailed in a table presented later in this chapter) indicates that these services likely help patients and their caregivers meet health-related psychosocial needs. The provision of transportation, supplies, and other logistical and material support when needed also can logically be assumed to decrease patient distress and increase the ability of both patients and caregivers to manage illness and its consequences.

Help in Managing Disruptions in Family, School, and Work Life

As described in Chapters 1 and 2, cancer and its treatment and sequelae can limit the ability of patients and families to perform their usual personal roles and their roles in the family and the larger society. Unaddressed, these limitations can lead to emotional and mental health problems for both patient and family, and the inability to accomplish developmental tasks, such as attaining educational goals and establishing and maintaining social relationships, and to perform meaningful work inside and/or outside of the family. A number of services are aimed at addressing these problems. These include services to assist patients who are disabled in performing routine activities of daily living; to assist patients in dealing with cognitive impairments and educational difficulties; to support families and other caregivers in dealing with the emotional, physical, and other stresses of caregiving; and to provide patients and their families with legal protections afforded by such laws as the Americans with Disabilities Act and the Family and Medical Leave Act. As is true for the services described above, evidence in support of the effectiveness of these services varies.

Assistance with activities of daily living Personal care services (e.g., services to help patients bathe, dress, use the toilet, and groom themselves), as well as homemaker and chore services, are designed to help compensate for temporary or permanent inability to perform these tasks due to fatigue, pain, or loss of function. These services are often provided by families and other sources of informal support (Hayman et al., 2001) and, as with the material and logistical resources described above, are often available to some extent as well through the Medicaid and Medicare programs, the Older Americans Act, and free-standing home health agencies reimbursed through third-party insurers or out-of-pocket purchase by consumers. Also as with the provision of material and logistical resources, these services have long-standing and wide acceptance, and the committee did not review evidence for their effectiveness.

Cognitive and educational assistance As described in Chapter 1, cognitive impairment—manifest, for example, in a decreased ability to pay attention and concentrate, short-term memory loss, diminished language ability, decreased information processing speed, and diminished visual–motor integration and spatial abilities—has been well documented in children and adults treated for cancer (Anderson-Hanley et al., 2003; IOM and NRC, 2003; Matsuda et al., 2005; Stewart et al., 2006). The nature of this impairment may differ depending on the patient, the type of cancer, and the treatment regimen. Cognitive impairment associated with treatment for breast cancer, for example, appears to occur in fewer than half of patients and is mild and transient, although when present, it may take years to resolve (Matsuda et al., 2005). On the other hand, the cognitive impairment associated with brain tumors and acute lymphoblastic leukemia (the most common childhood cancers) appears to be more severe and persistent, likely because of the radiation and chemotherapy specifically targeting the central nervous system that are part of the treatment protocols for these cancers and the more vulnerable condition of the rapidly developing brains of children.

Very little research has tested approaches to reducing the cognitive impairment associated with treatment for cancer[8] in adults (McDougall, 2001). There is a need for well-designed longitudinal studies with baseline and ongoing measures of cognitive impairment using objective and sensitive measurement tools and approaches. These studies should also control for an array of confounding variables, such as depression, age, hormonal levels, and other treatments. Such studies would facilitate better understanding of the mechanisms, types, and severity and duration of cognitive impairment in adults, an essential precursor to the development of effective prevention, treatment, and rehabilitation interventions (Anderson-Hanley et al., 2003; Matsuda et al., 2005).

The development of services to address cognitive impairment in children has progressed somewhat further, and there is some early theoretical and empirical support for cognitive remediation, ecological or environmental interventions, and pharmacotherapy. Cognitive remediation involves identifying the patient's specific cognitive deficits and then implementing interventions to help reduce these deficits and enable the patient to relearn through retraining and practicing salient cognitive tasks. Ecological or environmental interventions involve modifying the learning context and the methods used by the individual to acquire information and demonstrate knowledge. In school settings, for example, this could involve providing preferential seating, allowing additional time to take examinations, using true/false and multiple-choice tests rather than essay questions, and providing written handouts rather than requiring a child to copy material from the board (Butler and Mulhern, 2005). With respect to pharmacotherapy, methylphenidate, a medication used to treat children with attention-deficit disorder has shown some slight but encouraging preliminary results in children with cancer (Mulhern et al., 2004). Much more research is needed before interventions with quantified efficacy can be identified. In the interim, ecological interventions are unlikely to present significant risks to children and should be pursued; they can be included as part of school re-entry or reintegration programs, but these programs as yet have not been well

---

[8]In contrast, more research evidence exists for the effectiveness of cognitive rehabilitation in individuals with cognitive impairment due to stroke and traumatic brain injury, which is more clearly mapped and better understood (see Cicerone et al., 2005, and Tate et al., 2006).

studied (Prevatt et al., 2000). Cognitive testing should also be undertaken to help identify areas in need of remediation.

Family and caregiver support   Because of the importance of caregivers as a source of social support to patients and the threats to their health posed by the physical, emotional, and other stresses associated with caregiving, a variety of services have been developed to support them in this role and to relieve some of their stress. These include provision of education about the illness and how to respond effectively to illness-related problems, caregiver support groups that provide emotional support and information, initiatives to increase patients' competence in providing self-care, psychotherapy, respite care services, and combinations of some of these services (Sorensen et al., 2002). Two systematic literature reviews of such interventions generally yielded mixed and nonsignificant findings. These reviews encompass a relatively small number of studies (with typically small sample sizes) involving various types of interventions, including stress and activity management programs, problem-solving interventions, and telephone counseling, and measuring a variety of outcomes. Some studies found improved coping and confidence (Kotkamp-Mothes et al., 2005) or reduced distress or increased satisfaction for caregivers (Harding and Higginson, 2003). Positive results were most likely for self-reported improvement in coping skills and knowledge.

A review of additional individual studies found varied and overall weak results on an array of outcomes. Psychoeducational interventions showed a positive impact on caregiver stress and problem solving (Bucher et al., 2001; Manne et al., 2004) that was statistically significant only for studies with larger populations (e.g., Pasacreta and McCorkle, 2000). Similarly, caregivers in studies that focused on problem-solving and educational interventions reported improved confidence in problem solving, but the study designs limit generalizability because of either nonrandomization of subjects or problems with selective attrition from studies. Studies using psychobehavioral interventions have shown modest impacts on selected variables, such as caregiver response to symptoms (Given et al., 2006).

There is some evidence for the effectiveness of interventions targeting caregivers of patients without regard to cancer diagnosis. Although in general it appears that the provision of information alone has little or no impact on most behaviors and outcomes (Bhogal et al., 2003; Forster et al., 2006), education in combination with other interventions (e.g., support groups or counseling) has shown modest effects on outcomes such as caregivers' self-reported comfort or stress reduction. Combination programs including such services as behavioral interventions, nursing care, and exercise also have been shown to have modest effects on some outcome variables (Roberts et al., 2000; Bennet, 2002; Sorensen et al., 2002). Combination programs for elders with dementia, including respite, psychoeducation, counseling, and emotional support, have resulted in increased caregiver satisfaction and in some studies, delayed institutionalization (Knight et al., 1993; McNally et al., 1999; Gitlin et al., 2003). On the other hand, two studies found that respite care for caregivers of patients with Alzheimer's disease did not result in reduced stress and burden of lasting duration for caregivers (McNally et al., 1999; Lee and Cameron, 2006). The generalizability of these findings to interventions targeting cancer patients is unclear; a meta-analysis of a variety of caregiver support interventions found that caregivers of patients with dementia benefited less from such intervention than did others (Sorensen et al., 2002).

Overall, it appears that these types of educational, problem-solving, and supportive interventions can improve some aspects of caregiver satisfaction or self-reported sense of mastery, but few have shown actual improvements in problem-solving abilities, pain management, or other more objective measures of reduced caregiver burden. This body of work suffers from the failure to use standardized outcome measures, limited randomization of patients and caregivers to intervention groups, lack of longitudinal designs that would allow for measurement of longer-term effects, and analysis that fails to control for selective attrition. Nevertheless, the key role caregivers play in delivering essential social support and providing hands-on health care and logistical support to patients clearly points to the need for oncology providers to assess caregivers' capabilities and stresses and work jointly with them and patients to identify and secure resources likely to be helpful in the caregiving role. As more research on support for caregivers is conducted, clinicians will have better insights into how best to provide such support.

Legal protections and services   Help in obtaining protections and rights such as those afforded by the Americans with Disabilities Act, the Family and Medical Leave Act, and the Individuals with Disabilities Education Act can help prevent or ameliorate disruptions in family, school, and work life. Legal instruments such as power of attorney, legal guardianship for minors, mechanisms for disposition of assets, and legal representation in other matters are also important (Fleishman et al., 2006). Although legal service is another area in which there is scarce research on effectiveness, the New York Legal Assistance Group, a nonprofit organization offering free civil legal services to poor and near-poor individuals and families living in New York City, examined the impact of legal services on the lives of 51 of its clients with cancer.[9] In response to a survey, these clients reported that

---

[9]As of 2005, the New York Legal Assistance Group had provided legal services to more than 500 individuals with cancer (Fleishman et al., 2006).

receipt of legal services reduced their worries (83 percent), improved their financial situation (51 percent), positively affected their family and loved ones (33 percent), helped them follow their treatment regimen (23 percent), and enabled them to keep medical appointments (22 percent) (Retkin et al., 2007).

Help in Managing Financial Demands and Insurance

As described in Chapter 1, cancer imposes substantial financial burdens. A number of services are aimed at relieving these burdens, including financial planning or counseling, insurance counseling (e.g., health, disability), other benefits eligibility assessment/counseling (e.g., Supplemental Security Income, Social Security Disability Income), help in managing day-to-day financial activities such as bill paying, and sometimes monetary awards. Once again, research on the effects of these services is limited, but nonprofit organizations such as the American Cancer Society and CancerCare report that help with financial and insurance problems is a frequently needed and provided service. The New York Legal Assistance Group also reports helping cancer patients arrange debt repayment with their creditors; secure benefits from federal financial assistance programs such as food stamps, Social Security Disability Income, Supplemental Security Income, and long- or short-term disability programs; and secure other insurance benefits. Clients with cancer who received these financial services cited significantly improved financial circumstances, reporting, for example, that receipt of these services "made me able to live with a roof over my head and food to eat" (Retkin et al., 2007:7).

READY AVAILABILITY OF KEY SERVICES

As described in Chapter 1, patients vary in the extent to which they need the psychosocial health services described in this chapter. Given the evidence described in Chapter 2, failing to address these needs can adversely affect the health and health care of patients. Thus all oncology providers should identify patients with psychosocial needs and take steps to ensure that they receive the services necessary to address them.

Psychosocial health services are provided by multiple sectors of the U.S. economy through different types of providers (see Table 6-3, *Some Availability of Psychosocial Services in Health and Human Services Sectors and from Informal Supports*, in Chapter 6). Depending on each patient's situation (e.g., geographic location, financial resources, health insurance status), some services are more accessible than others. For example, a shortage of mental health professionals with specific types of training (e.g., in child mental health) is a long-recognized problem in certain parts of the country, especially in rural and other geographically remote areas (IOM, 2006). However, the committee found the *ready and nationwide availability of a number of key psychosocial health services to patients with cancer.* Table 3-2 highlights information services and Table 3-3 other key psychosocial health services available nationwide at no cost to patients. Information such as this may be helpful to cancer care providers as they seek to provide their patients with information on sources of psychosocial health services. The next two chapters address how such providers can identify patients with psychosocial problems and help them receive the psychosocial health services they need.

TABLE 3-2 Selected[a] Nationwide Sources of Free Patient Information on Cancer and Cancer-Related Services

Program	Information Available On	How to Access
American Cancer Society (ACS) Cancer Reference Information	Specific cancers, treatment, and psychosocial services	www.cancer.org/docroot/cri/cri_0.asp 1-800-ACS-2345 (toll free)
American Institute of Cancer Research	Nutrition, diet, and exercise to combat cancer	www.aicr.org 1-800-843-8114 (toll free) Its online Nutrition Hotline allows survivors to e-mail a personal nutrition and diet question to a registered dietician
Asian and Pacific Islander National Cancer Survivors Network	Information on where to obtain psychosocial services, and languages spoken by sources of the services	www.apiahf.com/devsearch/report.asp
Association of Cancer Online Resources	Types of cancer, treatment options, clinical trials, and locating support groups	www.acor.org
Bladder Cancer Advocacy Network	Bladder cancer, other organizations with information on bladder cancer and that offer support services, finding clinical trials	www.bcan.org 1-888-901-BCAN (toll free)

continued

TABLE 3-2 Continued

Program	Information Available On	How to Access
Bloch Cancer Foundation	Sources of information about cancer, treatments, and fighting cancer	www.blochcancer.org 1-800-433-0464 (toll free)
Brain Tumor Society	General overview of brain tumors (symptoms, diagnosis, pathology, subtypes of brain tumors) and information on treatment options; complementary and alternative medicine; and finding brain tumor centers, financial and insurance resources, and support groups	www.tbts.org 1-800-770-8287 (toll free)
C3: Colorectal Cancer Coalition	Diagnosis, treatment options, dealing with side effects, and support services and resources	www.fightcolorectalcancer.org
Cancer Research and Prevention Foundation	General overview of various types of cancer, treatment options, and emerging therapies	www.preventcancer.org 1-800-227-2732 (toll free)
CancerCare	Diagnoses, treatment types, and multiple psychosocial support services	www.cancercare.org 1-800-813-HOPE (toll free)
Candlelighters Childhood Cancer Foundation	Treatments, finding support groups, financial assistance, cancer-related news, and where to find treatment clinics	www.candlelighters.org 1-800-366-2223 (toll free)
Colon Cancer Alliance	Colorectal rectal cancer, treatment, clinical trials, finding support services	www.ccalliance.org 1-877-422-2030 (toll free)
Colorectal Cancer Network	Colorectal cancer, treatment options, clinical trials, and finding treatment centers and support	www.colorectal-cancer.net
CureSearch	Information on childhood cancers, treatments, side effects, hospitals, and clinical trials Provides a directory of national and local support services	www.curesearch.org 1-800-458-6223 (toll free)
Facing Our Risk for Cancer Empowerment *(Breast Cancer)*	Telephone hotline matching patients to peer counselors and information about breast cancer	www.facingourrisk.org 1-866-824-7475 (toll free)

TABLE 3-2 Continued

Program	Information Available On	How to Access
fertileHope	Reproductive aspects of cancer and cancer treatment, parenthood options for persons at risk for infertility, clinical trials Finding doctors/clinics specializing in fertility treatments Locating support services	www.fertilehope.org 1-888-994-4673 (toll free) info@fertilehope.org
International Association of Laryngectomees	Locating a speech therapist or pathologist by state Directory of laryngectomee suppliers	www.larynxlink.com
International Myeloma Foundation	Myeloma, treatment options, managing side effects of treatment and myeloma symptoms, finding clinical trials, locating support groups	www.myeloma.org Telephone hotline: Toll free at 1-800-452-CURE or 1-800-452-2873, 9:00 am–4:00 pm PST Contact via email: TheIMF@ myeloma.org
Kidney Cancer Association	Kidney cancer, types of surgical treatment, therapies for advanced kidney cancer, finding clinical trials, finding support groups, other cancer organizations, information on patient self-empowerment Message board containing information on nutrition, diet, health insurance, financial resources	www.akca.us www.nkca.org Nurse hotline: 1-866-400-5151 (toll free), Monday–Friday, 9:00 am–4:00 pm PST
Lance Armstrong Foundation	Different types of cancer and their treatments; physical, practical, and emotional concerns; clinical trials; and resource directories	www.livestrong.org One-on-one help: 1-866-235-7205 (toll free)

continued

TABLE 3-2 Continued

Program	Information Available On	How to Access
The Leukemia and Lymphoma Society	Information on leukemia, lymphoma, and other blood cancers; finding support groups; developments in treatments; decision-support tools; and clinical trial updates	Online chat with information specialist: www.leukemia-lymphoma.org; Monday–Friday, 10:00 am–5:00 pm ET Telephone inquiries (Information Resource Center [IRC]): 1-800-955-4572, Monday–Friday, 9:00 am–6:00 pm EST. IRC information specialists are social workers, nurses, and health educators
Look Good . . . Feel Better Program	Appearance-related/cosmetic tips; e.g., skin care and make-up; hair care; hair loss; wig choice, styling, and care Locating a Look Good Feel Better Program in patients' areas	www.lookgoodfeelbetter.org 1-800-395-LOOK phone access 24 hours/day, 7 days/week, in English, Spanish, and other languages (toll free)
Lung Cancer Alliance	Lung cancer, treatment options, clinical trials, finding support groups, other resources	www.lungcanceralliance.org Hotline: 1-800-298-2436 (toll free)
The Lustgarten Foundation for Pancreatic Cancer Research	Pancreatic cancer and treatment Patient And Caregiver Education (PACE) program assists individuals to access information and support resources they need to make informed decisions PACE is staffed by a full-time, licensed social worker, who addresses patient inquiries, conducts searches for individualized information and clinical trials, and provides referrals as needed	www.lustgartenfoundation.org 1-866-789-1000 (toll free)
Lymphoma Foundation of America	Finding lymphoma specialists How to get a second opinion	www.lymphomahelp.org 1-800-385-1060 (toll free)

TABLE 3-2 Continued

Program	Information Available On	How to Access
Lymphoma Research Foundation	Different types of lymphoma, treatment options, clinical trials, and finding peer support	www.lymphoma.org Helpline: 1-800-500-9976 (toll free), helpline@lymphoma.org
Melanoma Research Foundation	Melanoma, tests, and questions to ask patient's doctor List of melanoma centers by region	www.melanoma.org 1-800-MRF-1290 (toll free)
Multiple Myeloma Research Foundation	Information on symptoms, diagnosis, prognosis, and stages; finding support groups; treatment options; matching clinical trials	www.multiplemyeloma.org Information on clinical trials: Speak with a clinical trial specialist at 1-800-506-9044. Available Monday–Friday, 8:30 am–6:00 pm ET Locating clinical trials online: www.multiplemyeloma.org/ clinical_trials/4.09.php
National Cancer Institute (NCI)	Different types of cancers; treatments; strategies for coping with fatigue, pain, emotional concerns; and clinical trials Information specialists are available to answer a range of questions in "real time" about cancer including most recent treatment advances and can take as much time as needed for thorough and personalized responses	www.cancer.gov Telephone inquiries: 1-800-4-CANCER (1-800-422-6237) TTY: 1-800-332-8615 Monday–Friday, 9:00 am–4:30 pm local time (toll free) Online web inquiries via: https://cissecure.nci.nih.gov/ livehelp/welcome.asp Email inquiries via: cancergovstaff@mail.nih.gov

continued

TABLE 3-2 Continued

Program	Information Available On	How to Access
National Coalition for Cancer Survivorship	Online publications on types of health insurance and coverage; employment rights; advice on communicating with your doctor Information on palliative care and symptom management, diet/nutrition, clinical trials, importance of exercise Finding cancer centers; support groups; other cancer organizations	www.canceradvocacy.org To order hard copies of publications, call toll-free at 1-877-NCCS-YES or 1-877-622-7937
National Lung Cancer Partnership	General information about lung cancer and resources to help navigate the challenges posed by lung cancer, including information on clinical trials and support services	www. nationallungcancerpartnership. org
National Lymphedema Network	Lymphedema, causes, symptoms, and treatment Treatment centers, suppliers, and manual lymphatic drainage therapists Finding emotional support groups, penpals, and netpals	www.lymphnet.org 1-800-541-3259 (toll free)
National Ovarian Cancer Coalition (NOCC)	Ovarian cancer and clinical trials Finding NOCC state chapters for support and educational programs Database for finding gynecologic oncologists	www.ovarian.org 1-888-OVARIAN (toll free)
National Prostate Cancer Coalition	General facts and information about prostate cancer; screening; risk factors; staging; side effects; information on diet/nutrition; treatment options	www.fightprostatecancer.org
Needy Meds	Programs that help with the cost of medicine and other health care expenses	www.needymeds.com

TABLE 3-2 Continued

Program	Information Available On	How to Access
North American Brain Tumor Coalition	Brain tumor facts, public policy issues affecting brain tumor health care	www.nabraintumor.org
The Oral Cancer Foundation	Oral cancer, treatment, rehabilitation, dental issues, and emotional issues	www.oralcancerfoundation.org
Ovarian Cancer National Alliance	Ovarian cancer, symptoms, stages, diagnosis, approaches to treatment, and finding a clinical trial	www.ovariancancer.org 1-866-399-6262 (toll free) ocna@ovariancancer.org
Pancreatic Cancer Action Network (PanCAN)	Types of pancreatic cancer, treatment options, side effects of treatment, diet and nutrition, pancreatic cancer specialists and cancer centers, clinical trials, location of educational symposiums in the United States about pancreatic cancer Offers Patient and Liaison Services (PALS), a comprehensive, call-in information program for patients, families, and health professionals	www.pancan.org 1-877-272-6226 (toll free) Email pals@pancan.org to connect with a PALS Associate Monday–Friday, 8:00 am–5:00 pm PST
People Living With Cancer (sponsored by the American Society of Clinical Oncology (ASCO))	Cancer, types of cancer, diagnosis, finding an oncologist, treatment, coping, managing side effects, survivorship, clinical trials Finding emotional support services, financial assistance, treatment	www.plwc.org 1-888-651-3038 (toll free) contactus@plwc.org help@plwc.org privacy@plwc.org
Planet Cancer (targeted to young adults with cancer)	Practical advice on dealing with side effects and coping with cancer, news/articles on cancer research	www.planetcancer.org contactus@planetcancer.org
Prostate Cancer Foundation	Prostate cancer, treatment options, side effects, nutrition, and other lifestyle practices to improve health	www.prostatecancerfoundation.org 1-800-757-2873 (toll free) info@prostatecancerfoundation.org

continued

TABLE 3-2 Continued

Program	Information Available On	How to Access
Sarcoma Foundation of America	Types of sarcomas, symptoms, diagnosis; treatment options; links to other sarcoma organizations; information on clinical trials	www.curesarcoma.org
Shop Well With You	Customized clothing tips arranged by cancer-related treatments and side-effects	www.shopwellwithyou.org
	Directory of cancer-specific products such as swimsuits and head coverings and where items can be located	
	Guidance on how to use clothing and accessories to maintain a positive body-image during and after treatment	
	Articles and books on body-image, clothing, cancer, and wellness	
The Skin Cancer Foundation	Various types of skin cancer, treatment, and health care after treatment	www.skincancer.org 1-800-754-6490 (toll free)
	Finding a skin cancer physician	info@skincancer.org
Support for People with Oral and Head and Neck Cancer	Oral, head, and neck cancers; and treatments, clinical trials, rehabilitation and resources to improve or manage symptoms of cancer or its treatment	www.spohnc.org 1-800-377-0928 (toll free) info@spohnc.org
	Developments in treating head and neck cancer	
Susan G. Komen for the Cure	Breast cancer, treatment, care after treatment, support services, and research	www.komen.org 1-800-462-9273 (toll free)
The Testicular Cancer Resource Center	Testicular cancer, treatment, clinical follow-up after treatment, coping, experts in testicular cancer, and life after treatment	http://tcrc.acor.org Email questions: dougbank@ alum.mit.edu

TABLE 3-2 Continued

Program	Information Available On	How to Access
Thyroid Cancer Survivors' Association, Inc.	Thyroid cancer, treatment, nutrition and diet, finding a specialist and support groups	www.thyca.org 1-877-588-7904 (toll free) thyca@thyca.org
US Too *(Prostate Cancer)*	Prostate cancer, treatment options, post-treatment issues, clinical trials	www.ustoo.org Hotline: 1-800-808-7866 (toll free)
Women's Cancer Network	Various types of cancers, treatment, symptom management, care issues affecting women with cancer, clinical trials, and finding an oncologist	www.wcn.org 1-800-444-4441 (toll free)
Y-ME National Breast Cancer Organization, Inc.	Breast cancer, treatment, side effects, clinical trials, coping, and quality of life issues	Brochures by mail (English and Spanish) www.y-me.org 24-hour, toll-free, national hotline staffed by trained survivors: 1-800-221-2141 (English) 1-800-986-9505 (Spanish) Interpreters available for 150 languages Free, monthly, 1-hour teleconferences on breast cancer issues with presentation by a medical professional followed by a question and answer session

[a]The committee recognizes that there are many more organizations that provide free information services to cancer patients, and regrets the inability to acknowledge all of them in this report. The organizations included here are intended to illustrate the breadth of information services available at no cost to patients and should not be viewed as a complete list.

TABLE 3-3 Selected[a] Psychosocial Services (Other Than Information) Available at No Cost to Individuals/Families with Cancer

Psychosocial Service	Program	How to Access	Locations Available	Capacity
Counseling	**American Psychosocial Oncology Society** Counseling—telephone referral	www.apos-society.org 1-866-276-7443 (toll free)	In all 50 states	Helpline served 186 callers in 2006
Counseling	**CancerCare** Counseling—face-to-face, online, telephone	www.cancercare.org 1-800-813-HOPE (toll free)	In all 50 states	42,680 individuals from all 50 states received counseling, education, support group, referral or financial assistance in FY2005 (unduplicated count)
Counseling	**Lymphoma Foundation of America** *(Lymphoma)* Counseling—one-on-one telephone and peer counseling	www.lymphomahelp.org 1-800-385-1060 (toll free)	In all 50 states	In 2005, provided counseling to 1,300 patients
Decision support	**ACS' Reach to Recovery** *(Breast Cancer)* Decision support by providing information through face-to-face visits or telephone conversations	www.cancer.org/docroot/ESN/content/ESN_3_1x_Reach_to_Recovery_5.asp 1-800-ACS-2345 (toll free)	In all 50 states	
Decision support	**Living Beyond Breast Cancer** *(Breast Cancer)* Informed decision making—education conferences and teleconferences	www.lbbc.org 1-888-753-5222 (toll free)	In all 50 states	Three large conferences annually

Decision support	**Pancreatic Cancer Action Network** (*Pancreatic Cancer*) Decision support—information from trained professional via telephone or e-mail	www.pancan.org 1-877-272-6226 (toll free)	In all 50 states	In 2006, provided decision support to 6,655 people via e-mail or telephone
Education	**ACS' I Can Cope Program** Community or online classes on cancer management, treatment, financial concerns, community resources, nutrition, emotional matters, and communication skills	www.cancer.org/docroot/ESN/content/ESN_3_1X_I_Can_Cope.asp 1-800-ACS-2345 (toll free)		
Education	**ACS' Look Good . . . Feel Better Program** Group or one-on-one program providing beauty tips and cosmetologic assistance to help patients cope with skin changes and hair loss and other effects of cancer treatment	www.lookgoodfeelbetter.org 1-800-395-LOOK (toll free)		
Education	**American Institute of Cancer Research** Advice and information on health questions and nutrition answered by a dietitian	www.aicr.org 1-800-843-8114 (toll free)	In all 50 states	Phone advice to approximately 35 callers/month Approximately 100 email responses per month

continued

TABLE 3-3 Continued

Psychosocial Service	Program	How to Access	Locations Available	Capacity
Education	**Bladder Cancer Advocacy Network** (*Bladder Cancer*) Telephone workshops	www.bcan.org	In all 50 states	
Education	**Brain Tumor Society (BTS)** One-day seminars, annual conferences, and symposium	www.tbts.org	3 one-day seminars in 3 U.S. cities	Averages approximately 100 people at each seminar
Education	**CancerCare** Education—cancer types, treatment options, quality-of-life concerns	www.cancercare.org 1-800-813-HOPE (toll free)	In all 50 states	42,680 individuals from all 50 states received counseling, education, support group, referral or financial assistance in FY2005 (unduplicated count) An additional 45,300 unduplicated individuals participated in telephone education workshops
Education	**Gilda's Club Worldwide** Lectures and workshops to cancer patients and their families on how to live with cancer. Topics include stress reduction, nutrition, and practical issues	www.gildasclub.org 1-888-GILDA-4-U (toll free)	Freestanding Gilda's Clubs in 19 cities in the United States	In 2006, 172,000 member visits to Gilda's Clubs across the United States (not including guests and visitors)

continued

Education	**International Myeloma Foundation (IMF)** Seminars and symposia for patients and families on topics including managing side effects, becoming a better patient, and understanding lab results	www.myeloma.org 1-800-452-2873 (toll free)	4–6 seminars/ symposia yearly in different regions of the United States	Approximately 200–250 people attend each seminar/symposia each year
Education	**Kidney Cancer Association** Patient/survivor conference on topics including kidney cancer pathology and types of treatment and therapy	www.nkca.org	2–3 patient/ survivor conferences in the United States yearly; three conferences will be held in 2007	95 people registered for January 2007 Patient/Survivor Conference
Education	**The Leukemia and Lymphoma Society** Provides education and information targeted to patients, survivors, and caregivers. Topics include treatment options and how to strengthen coping and decision-making skills	www.leukemia-lymphoma.org	Chapters in all 50 states	

TABLE 3-3 Continued

Psychosocial Service	Program	How to Access	Locations Available	Capacity
Education	**Living Beyond Breast Cancer** *Support services.* News on educational breast cancer conferences and workshops in the country	www.lbbc.org 1-888-753-5222 (toll free)	Conferences/ workshops mostly in Philadelphia area. National conferences annually in varied cities	
Education	**Lymphoma Foundation of America** *(Lymphoma)* Education programs—quality of life issues; topics include art therapy, healing, and support for caregivers	www.lymphomahelp.org 1-800-385-1060 (toll free)	Educational programs at multiple locations in the country	
Education	**Lymphoma Research Foundation** *(Lymphoma)* Education workshops, webcasts/ podcasts, teleconferences, and forums discussing a range of topics including treatment options and support issues	www.lymphoma.org 1-800-500-9976 (toll free) helpline@lymphoma.org	State chapters across the United States	As of 2007 to date, 10,554 patients, survivors and loved ones have received education

Education	**Men Against Breast Cancer** (*Breast Cancer*) Workshops giving information and practical advice for patients and families	info@ menagainstbreastcancer. org 1-866-547-6222	In all 50 states	Performed education workshops in 15 states including Washington, DC 75 people will be attending conference in 2007
Education	**Multiple Myeloma Research Foundation** Seminars for patients and caregivers on latest research developments	www.multiplemyeloma. org	In 2007, three seminars to be held in Boston, Philadelphia, and Palo Alto, CA	In 2006, symposia in Atlanta, Cleveland, Houston, Los Angeles, and New York averaged 124 attendees each
Education	**National Coalition for Cancer Survivorship** Self-learning audio program that educates cancer patients on developing skills, such as communicating, negotiating, problem-solving, and decision-making skills, to help them better cope with cancer	www. cancersurvivaltoolbox.org	In all 50 states	Distributed approximately 30,000 cancer Survivor Toolboxes as a CD set in 2005 and 2006

continued

TABLE 3-3 Continued

Psychosocial Service	Program	How to Access	Locations Available	Capacity
Education	**Pancreatic Cancer Action Network** *(Pancreatic Cancer)* Educational workshops and conferences	www.pancan.org 1-877-272-6226 (toll free)	In 2006 held symposia in Chicago, New York, and Los Angeles; five symposia scheduled for 2007	Approximately 170 attendees at each 2006 symposium
Education	**Thyroid Cancer Survivors' Association, Inc.** *(Thyroid Cancer)* Educational workshops	www.thyca.org 1-877-588-7904 (toll free) thyca@thyca.org	Chapters in 36 cities and towns in the United States	Annual conference draws over 400 participants. Workshops have a total of 200–400 participants depending on how many workshops take place in a particular year Holding five free 1-day regional workshops, plus an annual 3-day International Thyroid Cancer Survivors' Conference, in 2007
Education	**US Too** *(Prostate Cancer)* Education workshops—in-person and telephone	www.ustoo.org 1-800-808-7866 (toll free)	Over 300 state chapters across the United States	

Education	**The Wellness Community** Education workshops	www. thewellnesscommunity.org 1-888-793-WELL (toll free)	21 Wellness Communities and 28 satellite centers in the United States	186,000 unique visitors to the Virtual Wellness Community
Education	**Y-ME National Breast Cancer Organization, Inc.** (*Breast Cancer*) Education teleconferences	www.y-me.org 1-800-221-2141 (toll free)	16 Y-ME local affiliates in various regions of the United States	
Emotional support	**ACS' Cancer Survivors Network** Finding support groups, relaxation classes, cancer-related community events, cancer books and articles	www.acscsn.org		
Emotional support	**ACS' Man-to-Man Program** (*Prostate Cancer*) Personal visits and telephone emotional support and information on prostate cancer	www.cancer.org/docroot/ ESN/content/ESN_3_1X_ Man_to_Man_36.asp 1-800-ACS-2345 (toll free)		

continued

TABLE 3-3 Continued

Psychosocial Service	Program	How to Access	Locations Available	Capacity
Emotional support	**ACS' Reach to Recovery** (*Breast Cancer*) Emotional support—face-to-face or telephone	www.cancer.org/docroot/ ESN/content/ESN_3_1x_ Reach_to_Recovery_5.asp 1-800-ACS-2345 (toll free)		
Emotional support	**Association of Cancer Online Resources** Emotional support—online chat	www.oncochat.org	In all 50 states	
Emotional support	**Bloch Cancer Foundation** Emotional support—telephone, peer matching	www.blochcancer.org 1-800-433-0464 (toll free)	In all 50 states	In 2006, received nearly 3,700 calls and e-mails from people requesting information and/or a match with a survivor of the same type of cancer

Matched more than 1,100 people with one or more of the nearly 500 cancer survivors around the country who volunteer for Bloch Cancer Foundation |
| Emotional support | **Bladder Cancer Advocacy Network** (*Bladder Cancer*) Online emotional support group | www.bcan.org | In all 50 states | |

Emotional support	**Brain Tumor Society** COPE Program is a matching program that provides emotional support by email or telephone	www.tbts.org To participate in the COPE Program, call toll free at 1-800-770-TBTS (8287), ext 25, or e-mail support@tbts.org	In all 50 states	31 people matched in 2006
Emotional support	**Cancer Hope Network** Emotional support—one-on-one	1-877-467-3638 (toll free)	In all 50 states	Currently provides about 2,000 peer-to-peer matches per year
Emotional support	**Cancer Information and Counseling Line (Affiliate of AMC Cancer Research Center)** General information, emotional support through telephone counseling to cancer patients and their families	1-800-525-3777 (toll free) cicl@amc.org	In all 50 states	
Emotional support	**Colon Cancer Alliance** *(Colon Cancer)* Emotional support—peer-to-peer matching program	www.ccalliance.org 1-877-422-2030 (toll free)	38 state chapters in the United States	
Emotional support	**Facing Our Risk for Cancer Empowerment** *(Breast Cancer)* Emotional support through online chat and telephone hotline matching patients to peer counselors	www.facingourrisk.org 1-866-824-7475 (toll free)	In all 50 states	200–300 matches per year

continued

128

TABLE 3-3 Continued

Psychosocial Service	Program	How to Access	Locations Available	Capacity
Emotional support	**Gilda's Club Worldwide** Lectures and workshops to cancer patients and their families on how to live with cancer. Topics include stress reduction, nutrition, and practical issues	www.gildasclub.org 1-888-GILDA-4-U (toll free)	Freestanding Gilda's Clubs in 19 cities in the United States	In 2006, 172,000 member visits to Gilda's Clubs across the United States (not including guests and visitors)
Emotional support	**Lance Armstrong Foundation (LAF)** Emotional support and counseling	www.livestrong.org 1-866-235-7205 1-800-620-6167 (clinical trial)	In all 50 states	In February 2007, 647 patients contacted Livestrong. Of those, 373 referred to CancerCare, 257 referred to Patient Advocate Foundation, and 82 were matched to clinical trials
Emotional support	**The Leukemia and Lymphoma Society** Emotional support—in-person, online chat, or peer-to-peer support	www.leukemia-lymphoma.org	Chapters in all 50 states	
Emotional support	**Living Beyond Breast Cancer** (*Breast Cancer*) Emotional support—one-on-one via telephone	www.lbbc.org 1-888-753-5222 (toll free)	In all 50 states	Helps approximately 600 women per year

| Emotional support | **Lung Cancer Alliance** *(Lung Cancer)* Emotional support—telephone peer-to-peer (Phone Buddy Program), online community | www.lungcanceralliance. org 1-800-298-2436 (toll free) | In all 50 states | Telephone referral hotline fields 5,000 calls and responds to at least another 2,000 requests for information via e-mail a year; at least 75% of the 5,000 calls are referred to other organizations for support, financial assistance, etc.

Online emotional support community currently has over 1,100 registered users and over 2 million hits to the site a month

Phone Buddy Program has made 350 individual matches in 2006 |
Emotional support	**Lymphoma Foundation of America** *(Lymphoma)* Emotional support—in-person groups	www.lymphomahelp.org 1-800-385-1060 (toll free)	In all 50 states	
Emotional support	**Lymphoma Research Foundation** *(Lymphoma)* Emotional support—one-on-one peer support program	www.lymphoma.org 1-800-500-9976 (toll free) helpline@lymphoma.org	State chapters across the United States	Based on service delivered during the first half of 2007, an estimated 576 patients and caregivers will be matched for peer support as of 2007
Emotional support	**National Ovarian Cancer Coalition** *(Ovarian Cancer)* Telephone peer-to-peer emotional support and information on ovarian cancer	www.ovarian.org 1-888-682-7426 (toll free)	80 licensed divisions in 42 U.S. states	

continued

TABLE 3-3 Continued

Psychosocial Service	Program	How to Access	Locations Available	Capacity
Emotional support	**Oral Cancer Foundation** (*Oral Cancer*) Emotional support—online peer-to-peer support	www. oralcancerfoundation.org	In all 50 states	
Emotional support	**Pancreatic Cancer Action Network** (*Pancreatic Cancer*) Emotional support—telephone or e-mail	www.pancan.org 1-877-272-6226 (toll free)	In all 50 states	In 2006, provided emotional support to 6,655 people
Emotional support	**Planet Cancer** Emotional support—retreats and online	www.planetcancer.org	Online support—in all 50 states Retreats held annually	
Emotional support	**Pregnant With Cancer** Emotional support—peer-to-peer via telephone or e-mail	www.pregnantwithcancer. org 1-800-743-4471 (toll free)	In all 50 states	Makes approximately 100 matches a year; have approximately 50,000 unique visitors to the Pregnant With Cancer website annually
Emotional Support	**Starlight Starbright Children's Foundation** Finding regional offices across the United States for accessing emotional support and education	www.slsb.org		

Emotional support	**Support for People with Oral and Head and Neck Cancer** (*Head and Neck Cancer*) Emotional support—matching peer-to-peer	www.spohnc.org 1-800-377-0928 (toll free) info@spohnc.org	54 chapters in cities/towns across the United States	From 2004–2007 made approximately 200 matches per year
Emotional Support	**Testicular Cancer Resource Center** (*Testicular Cancer*) Emotional support groups—e-mail for cancer patients and caregivers	www.tcrc.acor.org	In all 50 states	
Emotional support	**Thyroid Cancer Survivors' Association, Inc.** (*Thyroid Cancer*) Emotional support—e-mail or face-to-face	www.thyca.org 1-877-588-7904 (toll free) thyca@thyca.org	Chapters in 36 cities and towns in the United States	Approximately 11,000 annually receive help from e-mail and face-to-face emotional support Website receives over 250,000 visits each month
Emotional support	**Ulman Cancer Fund for Young Adults** Emotional support—e-mail peer groups	www.ulmanfund.org 1-888-393-FUND (toll free)	Sponsors 8 support groups nationally in 6 different cities	
Emotional support	**US Too** (*Prostate Cancer*) Emotional support groups—in-person and online	www.ustoo.org 1-800-808-7866 (toll free)	Over 300 state chapters across the United States	

continued

TABLE 3-3 Continued

Psychosocial Service	Program	How to Access	Locations Available	Capacity
Emotional support	**The Wellness Community** Emotional support groups—online and in-person	www.thewellnesscommunity.org 1-888-793-WELL (toll free)	21 Wellness Communities and 28 satellite centers in the United States	In 2005: Served more than 216,000 people: 30,000 in support groups and other face-to-face programs 186,000 unique visitors to the Virtual Wellness Community
Emotional support	**Women's Cancer Network** Emotional support—online postings	www.wcn.org	In all 50 states	
Emotional support	**Y-ME National Breast Cancer Organization, Inc.** (*Breast Cancer*) Emotional support—matching cancer patients or family members with survivors	www.y-me.org 1-800-221-2141 (toll free)	16 Y-ME local affiliates in various regions of the United States	
Financial assistance	**Brain Tumor Society** CARES Financial Assistance Program provides grants up to $2,000 per family, per year for specific non-medical costs related to a primary brain tumor diagnosis such as transportation, home health assistance related to brain tumor diagnosis, home adaptation related to brain tumor diagnosis, and child care	www.tbts.org 1-800-770-8287 (toll free)	In all 50 states	102 grants awarded in 2006

Financial assistance	**CancerCare** Financial assistance	www.cancercare.org 1-800-813-HOPE (toll free)	In all 50 states	In FY 2006, 3,482 patients received $1,812,206 for unmet financial needs such as child care, home care, and living expenses; in the first 8 months of fiscal year 2007, 2,069 received $727,745 in such financial assistance
Financial assistance	**Hill-Burton Program** Free or reduced cost health care services to eligible patients	www.hrsa.gov/hillburton/default.htm 1-800-638-0742 (toll free)	In all states except IN, NE, NV, RI, UT, WY; As of April 2007, 260 obligated Hill-Burton Facilities	
Financial assistance	**The Leukemia and Lymphoma Society** Financial assistance for services such as specific approved drugs for treatment/control of leukemia, Hodgkin and non-Hodgkin lymphoma, and myeloma; processing, typing, screening, and cross-matching of blood components for transfusions; transportation to a treatment center or family support group; x-ray therapy; also offers financial assistance for insurance co-payments	www.leukemia-lymphoma.org	Chapters in all 50 states	

continued

TABLE 3-3 Continued

Psychosocial Service	Program	How to Access	Locations Available	Capacity
Financial assistance	**Lymphoma Research Foundation** Financial assistance for U.S. lymphoma patients to help pay for treatment-related expenses	www.lymphoma.org 1-800-500-9976 (toll free)	In all 50 states	Approximately 81 grants awarded yearly
Financial assistance	**Supplemental Security Income (SSI)** Financial assistance for medically determinable needy aged (65 years old or older), blind, or disabled persons	1-800-772-1213 (toll free)	In all 50 states	An estimated 53,376 individuals under 65 years old were receiving SSI benefits because of cancer diagnosis in December 2003 (IOM, 2006)
Financial assistance and counseling	**Lance Armstrong Foundation (LAF)** Financial counseling	www.livestrong.org 1-866-235-7205 (toll free) 1-800-620-6167 (clinical trial)	In all 50 states	In February 2007, 647 patients contacted Livestrong. Of those 373 were referred to CancerCare, 257 were referred to Patient Advocate Foundation, and 82 were matched to clinical trials

continued

Financial assistance and counseling	**Patient Advocate Foundation (PAF)** Assistance resolving obstacles to health care access including those related to pre-authorization of treatment; appeals processes with insurers; coordination of benefits; expedited applications to Social Security Disability, Medicaid, and Medicare programs; and mediation to resolve medical debt crisis. Case management provided to uninsured patients to negotiate medical care from point of detection through completion of treatment. A Co-Pay Relief Program provides financial assistance to patients.	www.patientadvocate.org 1-800-532-5274 (toll free) help@patientadvocate.org	In all 50 states
Housing	**ACS' Hope Lodge** Temporary housing for patients during treatment	www.cancer.org/docroot/ SHR/content/SHR_2.1_x_ Hope_Lodge.asp 1-800-ACS-2345	22 locations in 18 states including Puerto Rico

TABLE 3-3 Continued

Psychosocial Service	Program	How to Access	Locations Available	Capacity
Legal advice/ assistance	**Cancer Legal Resource Center** Hotline that matches cancer patients and survivors to volunteer attorneys for information when possible; hotline also provides information and resources on cancer-related legal issues	www.lls.edu/academics/ candp/clrc.html 866-THE-CLRC (toll free)	In all 50 states, Puerto Rico, and U.S. Virgin Islands	Receives approximately 3,500 calls per year Reaches an additional 17,000 people per year through community outreach and educational seminars
Legal advice/ assistance	**Lymphoma Foundation of America** *(Lymphoma)* Legal expert referral; representation on job security and patient rights	www.lymphomahelp.org 1-800-385-1060 (toll free)	In all 50 states	In 2005, made 24–36 referrals
Transportation	**ACS' Road to Recovery** Roundtrip transportation for cancer patients from home to treatment center	www.cancer.org/ docroot/COM/content/ div_Southeast/COM_4_ 2x_Road_to_Recovery_ Service_Program. asp?sitearea=COM 1-800-ACS-2345 (toll free)		

Transportation	CancerCare	www.cancercare.org 1-800-813-HOPE (toll free)	In all 50 states	14,919 patients provided $3,005,679 in financial grants in FY2006 to pay for transportation
Caregiver support	**National Family Caregiver Support Program** Provides caregivers of older adults (60 years old or older) and grandparents (60 years old or older) of grandchildren no older than 18 years old with information on services available; individual counseling, organization of support groups, and caregiver training; respite care; and supplemental services on a limited basis	www.aoa.gov/prof/aoaprog/caregiver/caregiver.asp	In all 50 states	3.8 million individuals received information about caregiver programs and services 436,000 caregivers received assistance in accessing services Almost 180,000 caregivers received counseling and training services 70,000 received respite 50,000 caregivers received supplemental services
Logistical support	**U.S. Administration on Aging** Supportive services to older citizens and caregivers; services include transportation to medical appointments and financial counseling	www.aoa.gov	In all 50 states	

continued

TABLE 3-3 Continued

Psychosocial Service	Program	How to Access	Locations Available	Capacity
Wigs and prosthesis	**Y-ME National Breast Cancer Organization, Inc.** *(Breast Cancer)* Provides free wigs and prosthesis	www.y-me.org 1-800-221-2141 (toll free)	16 Y-ME local affiliates in various regions of the United States	

[a]The committee recognizes that there are many more organizations that provide free psychosocial services to cancer patients, and regrets the inability to acknowledge all of them and all services provided in this report. The organizations included here are intended to illustrate the breadth of psychosocial services available at no cost to patients and should not be viewed as a complete list of organizations or services.

REFERENCES

Adamsen, L., J. Midtgaard, M. Rorth, N. Borregaard, C. Andersen, M. Quist, T. Moller, M. Zacho, J. K. Madsen, and L. Knutsen. 2003. Feasibility, physical capacity, and health benefits of a multidimensional exercise program for cancer patients undergoing chemotherapy. *Support Care Cancer* 11(11):707–716.

AHRQ (Agency for Healthcare Research and Quality). 2002. *Management of cancer symptoms: Pain, depression, and fatigue.* Evidence report/technology assessment no. 61 (AHRQ publication no. 02-E032). Rockville, MD: AHRQ.

Alter, C., S. Fleishman, A. Kornblith, J. C. Holland, D. Biano, R. Levenson, V. Vinciguerra, and K. R. Rai. 1996. Supportive telephone intervention for patients receiving chemotherapy: A pilot study. *Psychosomatics* 37(5):425–431.

Anderson-Hanley, C., M. L. Sherman, R. Riggs, V. B. Agocha, and B. E. Compas. 2003. Neuropsychological effects of treatments for adults with cancer: A meta-analysis and review of the literature. *Journal of the International Neuropsychological Society* 9(7):967–982.

Andrykowski, M., and S. Manne. 2006. Are psychological interventions effective and accepted by cancer patients? I. Standards and levels of evidence. *Annals of Behavioral Medicine* 32(2):93–97.

Bandura, A. 1997. *Self-efficacy: The exercise of control.* New York: W.H. Freeman.

Barlow, J., C. Wright, J. Sheasby, A. Turner, and J. Hainsworth. 2002. Self-management approaches for people with chronic conditions: A review. *Patient Education and Counseling* 48(2):177–187.

Barlow, S. H., G. M. Burlingame, R. S. Nebeker, and E. Anderson. 2000. Meta-analysis of medical self-help groups. *International Journal of Group Psychotherapy* 50(1):53–69.

Barsevick, A. M., C. Sweeney, E. Haney, and E. Chung. 2002. A systematic qualitative analysis of psychoeducational interventions for depression in patients with cancer. *Oncology Nursing Forum* 29(1):73–84.

Bayliss, E. A., J. F. Steiner, D. H. Fernald, L. A. Crane, and D. S. Main. 2003. Description of barriers to self-care by persons with comorbid chronic diseases. *Annals of Family Medicine* 1(1):15–21.

Bennet, J. 2002. Maintaining and improving physical function in elders. *Annual Review of Nursing Research* 20:3–33.

Berglund, G., C. Bolund, U. L. Gustafsson, and P. O. Sjödén. 1994a. A randomized study of a rehabilitation program for cancer patients: The "starting again" group. *Psycho-Oncology* 3(2):109–120.

Berglund, G., C. Bolund, U. L. Gustafsson, and P. O. Sjödén. 1994b. One-year follow-up of the "starting again" group rehabilitation programme for cancer patients. *European Journal of Cancer Care* 30A(12):1744–1751.

Bhogal, S. K., R. W. Teasell, N. C. Foley, and M. R. Speechley. 2003. Community reintegration after stroke. *Topics in Stroke Rehabilitation* 10(2):107–129.

Bodenheimer, T., K. Lorig, H. Holman, and K. Grumbach. 2002. Patient self-management of chronic disease in primary care. *Journal of the American Medical Association* 288(19): 2469–2475.

Boesen, E., L. Ross, K. Frederiksen, B. Thomsen, K. Dahlstrom, G. Schmidt, J. Naested, C. Krag, and C. Johansen. 2005. Psychoeducational intervention for patients with cutaneous malignant melanoma: A replication study. *Journal of Clinical Oncology* 23(6): 1270–1277.

Boyar, A. P., D. P. Rose, J. R. Loughridge, A. Engle, A. Palgi, K. Laakso, D. Kinne, and E. L. Wynder. 1988. Response to a diet low in total fat in women with postmenopausal breast cancer: A pilot study. *Nutrition and Cancer* 11(2):93–99.

Browning, K. K., K. L. Ahijevych, P. Ross, Jr., and M. E. Wewers. 2000. Implementing the Agency for Health Care Policy and Research's smoking cessation guideline in a lung cancer surgery clinic. *Oncology Nursing Forum* 27(8):1248–1254.

Bucher, J. A., M. Loscalzo, J. Zabora, P. S. Houts, C. Hooker, and K. BrintzenhofeSzoc. 2001. Problem-solving cancer care education for patients and caregivers. *Cancer Practice* 9(2):66–70.

Burnham, T. R., and A. Wilcox. 2002. Effects of exercise on physiological and psychological variables in cancer survivors. *Medicine and Science in Sports and Exercise* 34(12): 1863–1867.

Butler, R. W., and R. K. Mulhern. 2005. Neurocognitive interventions for children and adolescents surviving cancer. *Journal of Pediatric Psychology* 30(1):65–78.

Campbell, H., M. R. Phaneuf, and K. Deane. 2004. Cancer peer support programs—do they work? *Patient Education and Counseling* 55(1):3–15.

Chlebowski, R. T., D. Rose, I. M. Buzzard, G. L. Blackburn, W. Insull, Jr., M. Grosvenor, R. Elashoff, and E. L. Wynder. 1992. Adjuvant dietary fat intake reduction in postmenopausal breast cancer patient management. The Women's Intervention Nutrition Study (WINS). *Breast Cancer Research and Treatment* 20(2):73–84.

Chodosh, J., S. C. Morton, W. Mojica, M. Maglione, M. J. Suttorp, L. Hilton, S. Rhodes, and P. Shekelle. 2005. Meta-analysis: Chronic disease self-management programs for older adults. *Annals of Internal Medicine* 143(6):427–438.

Cicerone, K. D., C. Dahlberg, J. F. Malec, D. M. Langenbahn, T. Felicetti, S. Kneipp, W. Ellmo, K. Kalmar, J. T. Giacino, J. P. Harley, L. Laatsch, P. A. Morse, and J. Catanese. 2005. Evidence-based cognitive rehabilitation: Updated review of the literature from 1998 through 2002. *Archives of Physical Medicine and Rehabilitation* 86(12):1681–1692.

Costa, D., I. Mogos, and T. Toma. 1985. Efficacy and safety of mianserin in the treatment of depression of women with cancer. *Acta Psychiatrica Scandinavica*. 320 (Supplementum):85–92.

Coulter, A., and J. Ellins. 2006. *Patient-focused interventions: A review of the evidence*. London: The Health Foundation and Picker Institute Europe.

Courneya, K. S. 2003. Exercise in cancer survivors: An overview of research. *Medicine and Science in Sports and Exercise* 35(11):1846–1852.

Courneya, K. S., and C. M. Friedenreich. 1999. Physical exercise and quality of life following cancer diagnosis: A literature review. *Annals of Behavioral Medicine* 21(2):171–179.

Courneya, K. S., C. M. Friedenreich, H. A. Quinney, A. L. Fields, L. W. Jones, and A. S. Fairey. 2003a. A randomized trial of exercise and quality of life in colorectal cancer survivors. *European Journal of Cancer Care* 12(4):347–357.

Courneya, K. S., C. M. Friedenreich, R. A. Sela, H. A. Quinney, R. E. Rhodes, and M. Handman. 2003b. The group psychotherapy and home-based physical exercise (grouphope) trial in cancer survivors: Physical fitness and quality of life outcomes. *Psycho-Oncology* 12(4):357–374.

Courneya, K. S., J. R. Mackey, G. J. Bell, L. W. Jones, C. J. Field, and A. S. Fairey. 2003c. Randomized controlled trial of exercise training in postmenopausal breast cancer survivors: Cardiopulmonary and quality of life outcomes. *Journal of Clinical Oncology* 21(9):1660–1668.

Coyne, J., S. Lepore, and S. Palmer. 2006. Efficacy of psychosocial interventions in cancer care: Evidence is weaker than it first looks. *Annals of Behavioral Medicine* 32(2):104–110.

Cunningham, B. A., G. Morris, C. L. Cheney, N. Buergel, S. N. Aker, and P. Lenssen. 1986. Effects of resistive exercise on skeletal muscle in marrow transplant recipients receiving total parenteral nutrition. *JPEN: Journal of Parenteral and Enteral Nutrition* 10(6):558–563.

Davison, K., J. Pennebaker, and S. Dickerson. 2000. Who talks? The social psychology of illness support groups. *American Psychologist* 55(2):205–217.

de Waard, F., R. Ramlau, Y. Mulders, T. de Vries, and S. van Waveren. 1993. A feasibility study on weight reduction in obese postmenopausal breast cancer patients. *European Journal of Cancer Prevention* 2(3):233–238.

Demark-Wahnefried, W., A. J. Kenyon, P. Eberle, A. Skye, and W. E. Kraus. 2002. Preventing sarcopenic obesity among breast cancer patients who receive adjuvant chemotherapy: Results of a feasibility study. *Clinical Exercise Physiology* 4(1):44–49.

Demark-Wahnefried, W., E. C. Clipp, C. McBride, D. F. Lobach, I. Lipkus, B. Peterson, D. Clutter Snyder, R. Sloane, J. Arbanas, and W. E. Kraus. 2003a. Design of fresh start: A randomized trial of exercise and diet among cancer survivors. *Medicine and Science in Sports and Exercise* 35(3):415–424.

Demark-Wahnefried, W., M. C. Morey, E. C. Clipp, C. F. Pieper, D. C. Snyder, R. Sloane, and H. J. Cohen. 2003b. Leading the way in exercise and diet (project lead): Intervening to improve function among older breast and prostate cancer survivors. *Controlled Clinical Trials* 24(2):206–223.

Demark-Wahnefried, W., B. Pinto, and E. R. Gritz. 2006. Promoting health and physical function among cancer survivors: Potential for prevention and questions that remain. *Journal of Clinical Oncology* 24(32):5125–5130.

Devine, E. C., S. K. Westlake, E. C. Devine, and S. K. Westlake. 1995. The effects of psycho-educational care provided to adults with cancer: Meta-analysis of 116 studies. *Oncology Nursing Forum* 22(9):1369–1381.

Dimeo, F. C. 2001. Effects of exercise on cancer-related fatigue. *Cancer* 92(Supplement 6): 1689–1693.

Dimeo, F., S. Fetscher, W. Lange, R. Mertelsmann, and J. Keul. 1997a. Effects of aerobic exercise on the physical performance and incidence of treatment-related complications after high-dose chemotherapy. *Blood* 90(9):3390–3394.

Dimeo, F. C., M. H. Tilmann, H. Bertz, L. Kanz, R. Mertelsmann, and J. Keul. 1997b. Aerobic exercise in the rehabilitation of cancer patients after high dose chemotherapy and autologous peripheral stem cell transplantation. *Cancer* 79(9):1717–1722.

Dimeo, F., B. G. Rumberger, and J. Keul. 1998. Aerobic exercise as therapy for cancer fatigue. *Medicine and Science in Sports and Exercise* 30(4):475–478.

Dimeo, F. C., R. D. Stieglitz, U. Novelli-Fischer, S. Fetscher, and J. Keul. 1999. Effects of physical activity on the fatigue and psychologic status of cancer patients during chemotherapy. *Cancer* 85(10):2273–2277.

Dimeo, F., S. Schwartz, T. Fietz, T. Wanjura, D. Boning, and E. Thiel. 2003. Effects of endurance training on the physical performance of patients with hematological malignancies during chemotherapy. *Support Care Cancer* 11(10):623–628.

Dimeo, F. C., F. Thomas, C. Raabe-Menssen, F. Propper, and M. Mathias. 2004. Effect of aerobic exercise and relaxation training on fatigue and physical performance of cancer patients after surgery. A randomised controlled trial. *Support Care Cancer* 12(11):774–779.

Distress Management Guidelines Panel. 2003. Distress management clinical practice guidelines in oncology. *Journal of the National Comprehensive Cancer Network* 1(3):344–393.

Djuric, Z., N. M. DiLaura, I. Jenkins, L. Darga, C. K. Jen, D. Mood, E. Bradley, and W. M. Hryniuk. 2002. Combining weight-loss counseling with the weight watchers plan for obese breast cancer survivors. *Obesity Research* 10(7):657–665.

Dodd, M., and C. Miaskowski. 2000. The PRO-SELF program: A self-care intervention program for patients receiving cancer treatment. *Seminars in Oncology Nursing* 16(4): 300–308.

Donnelly, J., A. Kornblith, S. Fleishman, E. Zuckerman, G. Raptis, C. A. Hudis, N. Hamilton, D. Payne, M. J. Massie, L. Norton, and J. C. Holland. 2000. A pilot study of interpersonal psychotherapy by telephone with cancer patients and their partners. *Psycho-Oncology* 9(1):44–56.

Dunn, J., S. K. Steginga, N. Rosoman, and D. Millichap. 2003. A review of peer support in the context of cancer. *Journal of Psychosocial Oncology* 21(2):55–67.

Emmons, K. M., E. Puleo, E. Park, E. R. Gritz, R. M. Butterfield, J. C. Weeks, A. Mertens, and F. P. Li. 2005. Peer-delivered smoking counseling for childhood cancer survivors increases rate of cessation: The partnership for health study. *Journal of Clinical Oncology* 23(27):6516–6523.

Epstein, R. M., and R. L. Street. 2007. *Patient-centered communication in cancer care: Promoting healing and reducing suffering.* NIH Publication No. 07-6225. Bethesda, MD: National Cancer Institute.

Evans, R., and R. Connis. 1995. Comparison of brief group therapies for depressed cancer patients receiving radiation treatment. *Public Health Reports* 110(3):306–311.

Eysenbach, G. 2003. The impact of the internet on cancer outcomes. *CA: A Cancer Journal for Clinicians* 53(6):356–371.

Eysenbach, G., J. Powell, M. Englesakis, C. Rizo, and A. Stern. 2004. Health related virtual communities and electronic support groups: Systematic review of the effects of online peer to peer interactions. *British Medical Journal* 328(7449):1166.

Fairey, A. S., K. S. Courneya, C. J. Field, G. J. Bell, L. W. Jones, and J. R. Mackey. 2003. Effects of exercise training on fasting insulin, insulin resistance, insulin-like growth factors, and insulin-like growth factor binding proteins in postmenopausal breast cancer survivors: A randomized controlled trial. *Cancer Epidemiology, Biomarkers & Prevention* 12(8):721–727.

Fairey, A. S., K. S. Courneya, C. J. Field, G. J. Bell, L. W. Jones, and J. R. Mackey. 2005. Randomized controlled trial of exercise and blood immune function in postmenopausal breast cancer survivors. *Journal of Applied Physiology* 98(4):1534–1540.

Fisch, M., P. Loehrer, J. Kristeller, S. Passik, S. H. Jung, J. Shen, M. A. Arquette, M. J. Brames, and L. H. Einhorn. 2003. Fluoxetine versus placebo in advanced cancer outpatients: A double-blinded trial of the Hoosier Oncology Group. *Journal of Clinical Oncology* 21(10):1937–1943.

Fleishman, S. B., R. Retkin, J. Brandfield, and V. Braun. 2006. The attorney as the newest member of the cancer treatment team. *Journal of Clinical Oncology* 24(13):2123–2126.

Forster, A., J. Smith, J. Young, P. Knapp, A. House, and J. Wright. 2006. Information provision for stroke patients and their caregivers. *Cochrane Database of Systematic Reviews* (3):CD001919.

Gielissen, M., S. Verhagen, F. Witjes, and G. Bleijenberg. 2006. Effects of cognitive behavior therapy in severely fatigued disease-free cancer patients compared with patients waiting for cognitive behavior therapy: A randomized controlled trial. *Journal of Clinical Oncology* 24(30):4882–4887.

Giesler, R., B. Given, C. Given, S. Rawl, Monahan, D. Burns, F. Azzouz, K. Reuille, S. Weinrich, M. Koch, and V. Champion. 2005. Improving the quality of life of patients with prostate carcinoma: A randomized trial testing the efficacy of a nurse-driven intervention. *Cancer* 104(4):752–762.

Gill, D., and S. Hatcher. 2006. Antidepressants for depression in medical illness. *Cochrane Database of Systematic Reviews* (3):CD001312.

Gitlin, L. N., S. H. Belle, L. D. Burgio, S. J. Czaja, D. Mahoney, D. Gallagher-Thompson, R. Burns, W. W. Hauck, S. Zhang, R. Schulz, M. G. Ory, and REACH Investigators. 2003. Effect of multicomponent interventions on caregiver burden and depression: The reach multisite initiative at 6-month follow-up. *Psychology and Aging* 18(3):361–374.

Given, B., C. Given, A. Sikorskii, S. Jeon, P. Sherwood, and M. Rahbar. 2006. The impact of providing symptom management assistance on caregiver reaction: Results of a randomized trial. *Journal of Pain & Symptom Management* 32(5):433–443.

Glassman, A., C. O'Conner, R. Califf, K. Swedberg, P. Schwartz, J. T. Bigger, K. R. Krishnan, L. T. van Zyl, J. R. Swenson, M. S. Finkel, C. Landau, P. A. Shapiro, C. J. Pepine, J. Mardekian, W. M. Harrison, D. Barton, and M. McIvor. 2002. Sertraline treatment of major depression in patients with acute MI or unstable angina. *Journal of the American Medical Association* 288(6):701–709.

Goel, V., C. A. Sawka, E. C. Thiel, E. H. Gort, and A. M. O'Connor. 2001. Randomized trial of a patient decision aid for choice of surgical treatment for breast cancer. *Medical Decision Making* 21(1):1–6.

Goodwin, P. J. 2005. Support groups in advanced breast cancer: Living better if not longer. *Cancer* 104(Supplement 11):2596–2601.

Goodwin, P. J., M. Leszcz, M. Ennis, J. Koopmans, L. Vincent, H. Guther, E. Drysdale, M. Hundleby, H. M. Chochinov, M. Navarro, M. Speca, and J. Hunter. 2001. The effect of group psychosocial support on survival in metastatic breast cancer. *New England Journal of Medicine* 345(24):1719–1726.

Greer, S., S. Moorey, J. Baruch, M. Watson, B. M. Robertson, A. Mason, L. Rowden, M. G. Law, and J. M. Bliss. 1992. Adjuvant psychological therapy for patients with cancer: A prospective randomized trial. *British Medical Journal* 304(6828):675–680.

Griebel, B., M. E. Wewers, and C. A. Baker. 1998. The effectiveness of a nurse-managed minimal smoking-cessation intervention among hospitalized patients with cancer. *Oncology Nursing Forum* 25(5):897–902.

Gritz, E. R., C. R. Carr, D. Rapkin, E. Abemayor, L. C. Chang, W. K. Wong, T. R. Belin, T. Calcaterra, K. T. Robbins, G. Chonkich, J. Beumer, and P. H. Ward. 1993. Predictors of long-term smoking cessation in head and neck cancer patients. *Cancer Epidemiology, Biomarkers and Prevention* 2(3):261–270.

Guidry, J., L. Aday, D. Zhang, and R. Winn. 1997. Transportation as a barrier to cancer treatment. *Cancer Practice* 5(6):361–366.

Harding, R., and I. J. Higginson. 2003. What is the best way to help caregivers in cancer and palliative care? A systematic literature review of interventions and their effectiveness. *Palliative Medicine* 17(1):63–74.

Hayman, J. A., K. M. Langa, M. U. Kabeto, S. J. Katz, S. M. DeMonner, M. E. Chernew, M. B. Slavin, and A. M. Fendrick. 2001. Estimating the cost of informal caregiving for elderly patients with cancer. *Journal of Clinical Oncology* 19(13):3219–3225.

Healey, I. R. 2003. External breast prostheses: Misinformation and false beliefs. Can we do better to help women after mastectomy? *Medscape General Medicine* 5(3).

Hebert, J. R., C. B. Ebbeling, B. C. Olendzki, T. G. Hurley, Y. Ma, N. Saal, J. K. Ockene, and L. Clemow. 2001. Change in women's diet and body mass following intensive intervention for early-stage breast cancer. *Journal of the American Dietetic Association* 101(4):421–431.

Heeringen, K. V., and M. Zivkov. 1996. Pharmacological treatment of depression in cancer patients. A placebo-controlled study of mianserin. *British Journal of Psychiatry* 169(4):440–443.

Helgeson, V. S., S. Cohen, R. Schultz, and J. Yasko. 2000. Group support interventions for women with breast cancer: Who benefits from what? *Health Psychology* 19(2): 107–114.

Helgeson, V. S., S. J. Lepore, and D. T. Eton. 2006. Moderators of the benefits of psychoeducational interventions for men with prostate cancer. *Health Psychology* 25(3):348–354.

Hewitt, M., J. H. Rowland, and R. Yancik. 2003. Cancer survivors in the United States: Age, health, and disability. *Journal of Gerontology* 58(1):82–91.

Holland, J., G. Morrow, A. Schmale, L. Degoratis, M. Stefanek, S. Berenson, P. J. Carpenter, W. Breitbart, and M. Feldstein. 1991. A randomized clinical trial of alprazolam versus progressive muscle relaxation in cancer patients with anxiety and depressive symptoms. *Journal of Clinical Oncology* 9(6):1004–1011.

Holland, J., S. Romano, J. Heiligenstein, R. Tepner, and M. Wilson. 1998. A controlled trial of fluoxetine and desipramine in depressed women with advanced cancer. *Psycho-Oncology* 7(4):291–300.

Hoybye, M., C. Johansen, and T. Tjornhoj-Thomsen. 2005. Online interaction. Effects of storytelling in an internet breast cancer support group. *Psycho-Oncology* 14(3):211–220.

IOM (Institute of Medicine). 2001. *Crossing the quality chasm: A new health system for the 21st century.* Washington, DC: National Academy Press.

IOM. 2006. *Improving the quality of health care for mental and substance-use conditions.* Washington, DC: The National Academies Press.

IOM. 2007. *Learning what works best: The nation's need for evidence on comparative effectiveness in health care.* http://www.iom.edu/Object.File/Master/43/390/Comparative%2 0Effectiveness%20White%20Paper%20(F).pdf (accessed June 11, 2007).

IOM and NRC (National Research Council). 2003. *Childhood cancer survivorship: Improving care and quality of life.* M. Hewitt, S. L. Weiner, and J. V. Simone, eds. Washington, DC: The National Academies Press.

IOM and NRC. 2006. *From cancer patient to cancer survivor: Lost in transition.* M. Hewitt, S. Greenfield, and E. Stovall, eds. Washington, DC: The National Academies Press.

Jacobsen, P., K. Donovan, Z. Swaine, and I. Watson. 2006. Management of anxiety and depression in adult cancer patients: Toward an evidence-based approach. In *Oncology: An evidence-based approach.* Edited by A. Chang, P. Ganz, D. Hayes, T. Kinsella, H. Pass, J. Schiller, R. Stone, and V. Strecher. New York: Springer-Verlag. Pp. 1552–1579.

Jones, L. W., K. S. Courneya, A. S. Fairey, and J. R. Mackey. 2004. Effects of an oncologist's recommendation to exercise on self-reported exercise behavior in newly diagnosed breast cancer survivors: A single-blind, randomized controlled trial. *Annals of Behavioral Medicine* 28(2):105–113.

Kazdin, A. 2000. *Psychotherapy for children and adolescents: Directions for research and practice.* New York: Oxford University Press.

Kim, J., M. Dodd, C. West, S. Paul, N. Facione, K. Schumacher, D. Tripathy, P. Koo, and C. Miaskowski. 2004. The pro-self pain control program improves patients' knowledge of cancer pain management. *Oncology Nursing Forum* 31(6):1137–1143.

Kissane, D., M. McKenzie, S. Bloch, C. Moskowitz, D. P. McKenzie, and I. O'Neill. 2006. Family focused grief therapy: A randomized, controlled trial in palliative care and bereavement. *American Journal of Psychiatry* 163(7):1208–1218.

Kissane, D., B. Grabsch, D. Clarke, G. C. Smith, A. W. Love, S. Bloch, R. D. Snyder, and Y. Li. 2007. Supportive-expressive group therapy for women with metastatic breast cancer: Survival and psychosocial outcome from a randomized controlled trial. *Psycho-Oncology* 16(4):277–286.

Klerman, G. L. 1989. Mood disorders: Introduction. In *Treatments of psychiatric disorders: A task force report of the American Psychiatric Association.* Vol. 3. Edited by American Psychiatric Association. Washington, DC: American Psychiatric Association. Pp. 1726–1745.

Knight, B. G., S. M. Lutzky, and F. Macofsky-Urban. 1993. A meta-analytic review of interventions for caregiver distress: Recommendations for future research. *Gerontologist* 33(2):240–248.

Knols, R., N. K. Aaronson, D. Uebelhart, J. Fransen, and G. Aufdemkampe. 2005. Physical exercise in cancer patients during and after medical treatment: A systematic review of randomized and controlled clinical trials. *Journal of Clinical Oncology* 23(16):3830–3842.

Kolden, G. G., T. J. Strauman, A. Ward, J. Kuta, T. E. Woods, K. L. Schneider, E. Heerey, L. Sanborn, C. Burt, L. Millbrandt, N. H. Kalin, J. A. Stewart, and B. Mullen. 2002. A pilot study of group exercise training (GET) for women with primary breast cancer: Feasibility and health benefits. *Psycho-Oncology* 11(5):447–456.

Kotkamp-Mothes, N., D. Slawinsky, S. Hindermann, and B. Strauss. 2005. Coping and psychological well being in families of elderly cancer patients. *Critical Reviews in Oncology-Hematology* 55(3):213–229.

Kristal, A. R., A. L. Shattuck, D. J. Bowen, R. W. Sponzo, and D. W. Nixon. 1997. Feasibility of using volunteer research staff to deliver and evaluate a low-fat dietary intervention: The American Cancer Society Breast Cancer Dietary Intervention Project. *Cancer Epidemiology, Biomarkers and Prevention* 6(6):459–467.

Lancaster, T., and L. F. Stead. 2004. Physician advice for smoking cessation. *Cochrane Database of Systematic Reviews* (4):CD000165.

Lancaster, T., and L. F. Stead. 2005. Individual behavioural counselling for smoking cessation. *Cochrane Database of Systematic Reviews* (2):CD001292.

Larson, P., C. Miaskowski, L. MacPhail, M. Dodd, D. Greenspan, S. Dibble, S. Paul, and R. Ignoffo. 1998. The pro-self mouth aware program: An effective approach for reducing chemotherapy mucositis. *Cancer Nursing* 21(4):263–268.

Leach, L. S., and H. Christensen. 2006. A systematic review of telephone-based interventions for mental disorders. *Journal of Telemedicine and Telecare* 12(3):122–129.

Lee, H., and M. Cameron. 2006. Respite care for people with dementia and their carers. *Cochrane Database of Systematic Reviews* (1).

Lev, E. L., K. M. Daley, N. E. Conner, M. Reith, and C. Fernandez. 2001. An intervention to increase quality of life and self-care self-efficacy and decrease symptoms in breast cancer patients. *Scholarly Inquiry for Nursing Practice: An International Journal* 15(3):277–294.

Lieberman, M. A., and B. A. Goldstein. 2005. Self-help on-line: An outcome evaluation of breast cancer bulletin boards. *Journal of Health Psychology* 10(6):855–862.

Loprinzi, C. L., L. M. Athmann, C. G. Kardinal, J. R. O'Fallon, J. A. See, B. K. Bruce, A. M. Dose, A. W. Miser, P. S. Kern, L. K. Tschetter, and S. Rayson. 1996. Randomized trial of dietician counseling to try to prevent weight gain associated with breast cancer adjuvant chemotherapy. *Oncology* 53(3):228–232.

Lorig, K. R., and H. Holman. 2003. Self-management education: History, definition, outcomes, and mechanisms. *Annals of Behavioral Medicine* 26(1):1–7.

Lorig, K. R., P. Ritter, A. L. Stewart, D. S. Sobel, B. W. Brown, A. Bandura, V. M. Gonzalez, D. D. Laurent, and H. R. Holman. 2001. Chronic disease self-management program: 2-year health status and health care utilization outcomes. *Medical Care* 39(11):1217–1223.

Lundberg, G. D. 2002. Resolved: Psychosocial interventions can improve clinical outcomes in organic disease: Discussant comments. *Psychosomatic Medicine* 64(4):568–570.

Lustman, P., L. Griffith, J. A. Gavard, and R. Clouse. 1992. Depression in adults with diabetes. *Diabetes Care* 15(11):1631–1639.

Ly, K. L., J. Chidgey, J. Addington-Hall, M. Hotopf, K. L. Ly, J. Chidgey, J. Addington-Hall, and M. Hotopf. 2002. Depression in palliative care: A systematic review. Part 2. Treatment. *Palliative Medicine* 16(4):279–284.

MacVicar, M. G., M. L. Winningham, and J. L. Nickel. 1989. Effects of aerobic interval training on cancer patients' functional capacity. *Nursing Research* 38(6):348–351.

Manne, S., J. Babb, W. Pinover, E. Horwitz, and J. Ebbert. 2004. Psychoeducational group intervention for wives of men with prostate cancer. *Psycho-Oncology* 13(1):37–46.

Manne, S., J. Ostroff, T. Norton, K. Fox, L. Goldstein, and G. Grana. 2006. Cancer-related relationship communication in couples coping with early stage breast cancer. *Psycho-Oncology* 15(3):234–247.

Marcus, A. C., K. M. Garrett, D. Cella, L. B. Wenzel, M. J. Brady, L. A. Crane, M. W. McClatchey, B. C. Kluhsman, and M. Pate-Willig. 1998. Telephone counseling of breast cancer patients after treatment: A description of a randomized controlled trial. *Psycho-Oncology* 7(6):470–482.

Markowitz, J., G. Klerman, S. Perry, K. Clougherty, L. Josephs. 1993. Interpersonal psychotherapy for depressed HIV-seropositive patients. In *New applications of interpersonal psychotherapy*. Edited by G. Klerman and M. Weissman. Washington, DC: American Psychiatric Press. Pp. 199–224.

Matsuda, T., T. Takayama, M. Tashiro, Y. Nakamura, Y. Ohashi, and K. Shimozuma. 2005. Mild cognitive impairment after adjuvant chemotherapy in breast cancer patients— evaluation of appropriate research design and methodology to measure symptoms. *Breast Cancer* 12(4):279–287.

McArdle, J., W. George, C. McArdle, D. C. Smith, A. R. Moodie, A. V. Hughson, and G. D. Murray. 1996. Psychological support for patients undergoing breast cancer surgery: A randomized study. *British Medical Journal* 312(7034):813–816.

McCorkle, R., J. Benoliel, G. Donaldson, F. Georgiadou, C. Moinpour, and B. Goodell. 1989. A randomized clinical trial of home nursing care of lung cancer patients. *Cancer* 64(6):1375–1382.

McCorkle, R., C. Jepson, L. Yost, E. Lusk, D. Malone, L. Braitman, K. Buhler-Wilerson, and J. Daly. 1994. The impact of post-hospital home care on patients with cancer. *Research in Nursing and Health* 17(4):243–251.

McCorkle, R., L. Robinson, I. Nuamah, E. Lev, and J. Benoliel. 1998. The effects of home nursing care for patients during terminal illness on the bereaved's psychological distress. *Nursing Research* 47(1):2–10.

McCorkle, R., N. Strumpf, I. Nuamah, D. Adler, M. Cooley, C. Jepson, E. Lusk, and M. Torosian. 2000. A specialized home care intervention improves survival among older post-surgical cancer patients. *Journal of the American Geriatrics Society* 48(12):1707–1713.

McDougall, G. J. 2001. Memory improvement program for elderly cancer survivors. *Geriatric Nursing* 22(4):185–190.

McGinty, K. L., S. A. Saeed, S. C. Simmons, and Y. Yildirim. 2006. Telepsychiatry and e-mental health services: Potential for improving access to mental heath care. *Psychiatry Quarterly* 77(4):335–342.

McKenzie, D. C., and A. L. Kalda. 2003. Effect of upper extremity exercise on secondary lymphedema in breast cancer patients: A pilot study. *Journal of Clinical Oncology* 21(3):463–466.

McNally, S., Y. Ben-Shlomo, S. Newman. 1999. The effects of respite care on informal carers' well-being: A systematic review. *Disability and Rehabilitation* 21(1):1–14.

McPherson, C. J., I. J. Higginson, and J. Hearn. 2001. Effective methods of giving information in cancer: A systematic literature review of randomized controlled trials. *Journal of Public Health Medicine* 23(3):227–234.

McTiernan, A., C. Ulrich, C. Kumai, D. Bean, R. Schwartz, J. Mahloch, R. Hastings, J. Gralow, and J. D. Potter. 1998. Anthropometric and hormone effects of an eight-week exercise-diet intervention in breast cancer patients: Results of a pilot study. *Cancer Epidemiology, Biomarkers and Prevention* 7(6):477–481.

Meyer, T. J., and M. M. Mark. 1995. Effects of psychosocial interventions with adult cancer patients: A meta-analysis of randomized experiments. *Health Psychology* 14(2): 101–108.

Miaskowski, C., M. Dodd, C. West, K. Schumacher, S. M. Paul, D. Tripathy, and P. Koo. 2004. Randomized clinical trial of the effectiveness of a self-care intervention to improve cancer pain management. *Journal of Clinical Oncology* 22(9):1713–1720.

Mock, V. 2001. Evaluating a model of fatigue in children with cancer. *Journal of Pediatric Oncology Nursing* 18(2 Supplement 1):13–16.

Mock, V., K. H. Dow, C. J. Meares, P. M. Grimm, J. A. Dienemann, M. E. Haisfield-Wolfe, W. Quitasol, S. Mitchell, A. Chakravarthy, and I. Gage. 1997. Effects of exercise on fatigue, physical functioning, and emotional distress during radiation therapy for breast cancer. *Oncology Nursing Forum* 24(6):991–1000.

Mock, V., M. Pickett, M. E. Ropka, E. Muscari Lin, K. J. Stewart, V. A. Rhodes, R. McDaniel, P. M. Grimm, S. Krumm, and R. McCorkle. 2001. Fatigue and quality of life outcomes of exercise during cancer treatment. *Cancer Practice* 9(3):119–127.

Moorey, S., S. Greer, M. Watson, J. D. R. Baruch, B. M. Robertson, A. Mason, L. Rowden, R. Tunmore, M. Law, and J. M. Bliss. 1994. Adjuvant psychological therapy for patients with cancer: Outcome at one year. *Psycho-Oncology* 3(1):39–46.

Moynihan, C., J. Bliss, J. Davidson, L. Burchell, and A. Horwich. 1998. Evaluation of adjuvant psychological therapy in patients with testicular cancer: Randomized controlled trial. *British Medical Journal* 316(7129):429–435.

Mulhern, R. K., R. B. Khan, S. Kaplan, S. Helton, R. Christensen, M. Bonner, R. Brown, X. Xiong, S. Wu, S. Gururangan, and W. E. Reddick. 2004. Short-term efficacy of methylphenidate: A randomized, double-blind, placebo-controlled trial among survivors of childhood cancer. *Journal of Clinical Oncology* 22(23):4743–4751.

Musselman, D., D. Lawson, J. F. Gumnick, A. Manatunga, S. Penna, R. Goodkin, K. Greiner, C. B. Nemeroff, and A. H. Miller. 2001. Paroxetine for the prevention of depression induced by high-dose interferon alfa. *New England Journal of Medicine* 344(13):961–966.

Na, Y. M., M. Y. Kim, Y. K. Kim, Y. R. Ha, and D. S. Yoon. 2000. Exercise therapy effect on natural killer cell cytotoxic activity in stomach cancer patients after curative surgery. *Archives of Physical Medicine and Rehabilitation* 81(6):777–779.

National Breast Cancer Centre and National Cancer Control Initiative. 2003. *Clinical practice guidelines for the psychosocial care of adults with cancer.* Camperdown, NSW, Australia: National Breast Cancer Centre.

Neumann, P. J., N. Divi, M. T. Beinfeld, B.-S. Levine, P. S. Keenan, E. F. Halpern, and G. S. Gazelle. 2005. Medicare's national coverage decisions, 1999–2003: Quality of evidence and review. *Health Affairs* 24(1):243–254.

Newell, S., R. Sanson-Fisher, and N. Savolainen. 2002. Systematic review of psychological therapies for cancer patients: Overview and recommendations for future research. *Journal of the National Cancer Institute* 94(8):558–584.

Nezu, A., C. Nezu, S. Felgoise, K. S. McClure, and P. S. Houts. 2003. Project Genesis: Assessing the efficacy of problem-solving therapy for distressed adult cancer patients. *Journal of Consulting and Clinical Psychology* 71(6):1036–1048.

Nordevang, E., E. Callmer, A. Marmur, and L. E. Holm. 1992. Dietary intervention in breast cancer patients: Effects on food choice. *European Journal of Clinical Nutrition* 46(6):387–396.

Pai, A. L. H., D. Drotar, K. Zebracki, M. Moore, and E. Youngstrom. 2006. A meta-analysis of the effects of psychological interventions in pediatric oncology on outcomes of psychological distress and adjustment. *Journal of Pediatric Psychology* 31(9):978–988.

Pajares, F. 2002. *Overview of social cognitive theory and of self-efficacy. Emory University.* http://www.emory.edu/EDUCATION/mfp/eff.html (accessed October 8, 2004).

Pasacreta, J., and R. McCorkle. 2000. Cancer care: Impact of interventions on caregiver outcomes. *Annual Review of Nursing Research* 18:127–148.

Patenaude, A., and M. Kupst. 2005. Psychosocial functioning in pediatric cancer. *Journal of Pediatric Psychology* 30(1):9–27.

Pierce, J. P., S. Faerber, F. A. Wright, V. Newman, S. W. Flatt, S. Kealey, C. L. Rock, W. Hryniuk, and E. R. Greenberg. 1997. Feasibility of a randomized trial of a high-vegetable diet to prevent breast cancer recurrence. *Nutrition and Cancer* 28(3):282–288.

Pierce, J. P., V. A. Newman, S. W. Flatt, S. Faerber, C. L. Rock, L. Natarajan, B. J. Caan, E. B. Gold, K. A. Hollenbach, L. Wasserman, L. Jones, C. Ritenbaugh, M. L. Stefanick, C. A. Thomson, and S. Kealey. 2004. Telephone counseling intervention increases intakes of micronutrient- and phytochemical-rich vegetables, fruit and fiber in breast cancer survivors. *The Journal of Nutrition* 134(2):452–458.

Pinto, B. M., and N. C. Maruyama. 1999. Exercise in the rehabilitation of breast cancer survivors. *Psycho-Oncology* 8(3):191–206.

Pinto, B. M., G. M. Frierson, C. Rabin, J. J. Trunzo, and B. H. Marcus. 2005. Home-based physical activity intervention for breast cancer patients. *Journal of Clinical Oncology* 23(15):3577–3587.

Pirl, W. F. 2004. Evidence report on the occurrence, assessment, and treatment of depression in cancer patients. *Journal of the National Cancer Institute Monographs* 32:32–39.

Plante, W. A., D. Lobato, R. Engel. 2001. Review of group interventions for pediatric chronic conditions. *Journal of Pediatric Psychology* 26(7):435–453.

Prevatt, F. F., R. W. Heffer, and P. A. Lowe. 2000. A review of school reintegration programs for children with cancer. *Journal of School Psychology* 38(5):447–467.

Rassmussen, A., M. Lunde, D. Poulsen, K. Sørensen, S. Qvitzau, and P. Bech. 2003. A double-blind, placebo-controlled study of sertraline in the prevention of depression in stroke patients. *Psychosomatics* 44(3):216–221.

Razavi, D., J. Allilaire, M. Smith, A. Salimpour, M. Verra, B. Desclaux, P. Saltel, I. Piollet, A. Gauvain-Piquard, C. Trichard, B. Cordier, R. Fresco, E. Guillibert, D. Sechter, J. P. Orth, M. Bouhassira, P. Mesters, and P. Blin. 1996. The effect of fluoxetine on anxiety and depression symptoms in cancer patients. *Acta Psychiatrica Scandinavica* 94(3):205–210.

Razavi, D., N. Kormoss, A. Collard, C. Farvacques, and N. Delvaux. 1999. Comparative study of the efficacy and safety of trazodone versus clorazepate in the treatment of adjustment disorders in cancer patients: A pilot study. *The Journal of International Medical Research* 27(6):264–272.

Rehse, B., and R. Pukrop. 2003. Effects of psychosocial interventions on quality of life in adult cancer patients: Meta analysis of 37 published controlled outcome studies. *Patient Education & Counseling* 50(2):179–186.

Relman, A. S., and M. Angell. 2002. Resolved: Psychosocial interventions can improve clinical outcomes in organic disease (con). *Psychosomatic Medicine* 64(4):558–563.

Retkin, R., J. Brandfield, and C. Bacich. 2007. *Impact of legal interventions on cancer survivors*. New York: LegalHealth—A Division of the New York Legal Assistance Group.

Rice, V. H., and L. F. Stead. 2004. Nursing interventions for smoking cessation. *Cochrane Database of Systematic Reviews* (1):CD001188.

Roberts, J., G. Browne, A. Gafni, M. Varieur, P. Loney, and M. D. Ruijter. 2000. Specialized continuing care models for persons with dementia: A systematic review of the research literature. *Canadian Journal on Aging* 19(1):109–126.

Rock, C. L., and W. Demark-Wahnefried. 2002. Nutrition and survival after the diagnosis of breast cancer: A review of the evidence. *Journal of Clinical Oncology* 20(15):3302–3316.

Rodin, G., N. Lloyd, M. Katz, E. Green, J. A. Mackay, R. K. S. Wong, and Supportive Care Guidelines Group of Cancer Care Ontario Program in Evidence-based Care. 2007. The treatment of depression in cancer patients: A systematic review. *Supportive Care in Cancer* 15(2):123–136.

Rose, D. P., J. M. Connolly, R. T. Chlebowski, I. M. Buzzard, and E. L. Wynder. 1993. The effects of a low-fat dietary intervention and tamoxifen adjuvant therapy on the serum estrogen and sex hormone-binding globulin concentrations of postmenopausal breast cancer patients. *Breast Cancer Research and Treatment* 27(3):253–262.

Ruskin, P. E., M. Silver-Aylaian, M. A. Kling, S. A. Reed, D. D. Bradham, J. R. Hebel, D. Barrett, F. Knowles, and P. Hauser. 2004. Treatment outcomes in depression: Comparison of remote treatment through telepsychiatry to in-person treatment. *American Journal of Psychiatry* 161(8):1471–1476.

Sanderson Cox, L., C. A. Patten, J. O. Ebbert, A. A. Drews, G. A. Croghan, M. M. Clark, T. D. Wolter, P. A. Decker, and R. D. Hurt. 2002. Tobacco use outcomes among patients with lung cancer treated for nicotine dependence. *Journal of Clinical Oncology* 20(16):3461–3469.

Schnoll, R. A., B. Zhang, M. Rue, J. E. Krook, W. T. Spears, A. C. Marcus, and P. F. Engstrom. 2003. Brief physician-initiated quit-smoking strategies for clinical oncology settings: A trial coordinated by the eastern cooperative oncology group. *Journal of Clinical Oncology* 21(2):355–365.

Schnoll, R. A., R. L. Rothman, D. B. Wielt, C. Lerman, H. Pedri, H. Wang, J. Babb, S. M. Miller, B. Movsas, E. Sherman, J. A. Ridge, M. Unger, C. Langer, M. Goldberg, W. Scott, and J. Cheng. 2005. A randomized pilot study of cognitive-behavioral therapy versus basic health education for smoking cessation among cancer patients. *Annals of Behavioral Medicine* 30(1):1–11.

Schulberg, H., W. Katon, G. Simon, and A. J. Rush. 1998. Treating major depression in primary care practice: An update of the Agency for Health Care Policy and Research guidelines. *Archives of General Psychiatry* 55(12):1121–1127.

Schwartz, A. L. 1999. Fatigue mediates the effects of exercise on quality of life. *Quality of Life Research* 8(6):529–538.

Schwartz, A. L. 2000. Daily fatigue patterns and effect of exercise in women with breast cancer. *Cancer Practice* 8(1):16–24.

Schwartz, A. L. 2004. Physical activity after a cancer diagnosis: Psychosocial outcomes. *Cancer Investigation* 22(1):82–92.

Schwartz, A. L., M. Mori, R. Gao, L. M. Nail, and M. E. King. 2001. Exercise reduces daily fatigue in women with breast cancer receiving chemotherapy. *Medicine and Science in Sports and Exercise* 33(5):718–723.

Segal, R., W. Evans, D. Johnson, J. Smith, S. Colletta, J. Gayton, S. Woodard, G. Wells, and R. Reid. 2001. Structured exercise improves physical functioning in women with stages I and II breast cancer: Results of a randomized controlled trial. *Journal of Clinical Oncology* 19(3):657–665.

Segal, R. J., R. D. Reid, K. S. Courneya, S. C. Malone, M. B. Parliament, C. G. Scott, P. M. Venner, H. A. Quinney, L. W. Jones, M. E. D'Angelo, and G. A. Wells. 2003. Resistance exercise in men receiving androgen deprivation therapy for prostate cancer. *Journal of Clinical Oncology* 21(9):1653–1659.

Sheard, T., and P. Maguire. 1999. The effect of psychological interventions on anxiety and depression in cancer patients: Results of two meta-analyses. *British Journal of Cancer* 80(11):1770–1780.

Simon, G. E., W. Katon, E. Lin, C. Rutter, W. G. Manning, M. Von Korff, P. Ciechanowski, E. J. Ludman, and B. A. Young. 2007. Cost-effectiveness of systematic depression treatment among people with diabetes mellitus. *Archives of General Psychiatry* 64(1):65–72.

Sorensen, S., M. Pinquart, D. Habil, and P. Duberstein. 2002. How effective are interventions with caregivers: An updated meta-analysis. *The Gerontologist* 42(3):356–372.

Spiegel, D., J. Bloom, and I. Yalom. 1981. Group support for patients with metastatic cancer. A randomized outcome study. *Archives of General Psychiatry* 38(5):527–533.

Spirig, R. 1998. Support groups for people living with HIV/AIDS: A review of literature. *Journal of the Association of Nurses in AIDS Care* 9(4):43–55.

Stanford University School of Medicine. 2007. *Chronic disease self-management program.* http://patienteducation.stanford.edu/programs/cdsmp.html (accessed January 17, 2007).

Stanislaw, A. E., and M. E. Wewers. 1994. A smoking cessation intervention with hospitalized surgical cancer patients: A pilot study. *Cancer Nursing* 17(2):81–86.

Stein, K., M. Golant, and G. Greer. 2007. Emerging models of web-based cancer support services. *Psycho-Oncology* 16(Supplement 3):S30.

Stewart, A., C. Bielajew, B. Collins, M. Parkinson, and E. Tomiak. 2006. A meta-analysis of the neuropsychological effects of adjuvant chemotherapy treatment in women treated for breast cancer. *The Clinical Neuropsychologist* 20(1):76–89.

Stiegelis, H., M. Hagedoorn, R. Sanderman, F. Bennenbroek, B. Buunk, A. V. D. Bergh, G. Botke, and A. Ranchor. 2004. The impact of an informational self-management intervention on the association between control and illness uncertainty before and after radiotherapy. *Psycho-Oncology* 13(4):248–259.

Tate, R. L., A. Moseley, M. Perdices, S. McDonald, L. Togher, R. Schultz, S. Savage, and K. Winders. 2006. Update on Cicerone's systematic review of cognitive rehabilitation: The psycBITE perspective. *Archives of Physical Medicine and Rehabilitation* 87(3):446.

Thaxton, L., J. G. Emshoff, and O. Guessous. 2005. Prostate cancer support groups: A literature review. *Journal of Psychosocial Oncology* 23(1):25–40.

Ussher, J., L. Kirsten, P. Butow, and M. Sandoval. 2006. What do cancer support groups provide which other supportive relationships do not? The experience of peer support groups for people with cancer. *Social Science and Medicine* 62(10):2565–2576.

Vincze, G., J. C. Barner, and D. Lopez. 2004. Factors associated with adherence to self monitoring of blood glucose among people with diabetes. *The Diabetes Educator* 30(1):112–125.

Wald, T. G., R. G. Kathol, R. Noyes, B. T. Carroll, and G. H. Clamon. 1993. Rapid relief of anxiety in cancer patients with both alprazolam and placebo. *Psychosomatics* 34(4):324–332.

Weis, J. 2003. Support groups for cancer patients. *Supportive Care in Cancer* 11(12):763–768.

Wells, K., J. Golding, and M. Burnam. 1988. Psychiatric disorder in a sample of the general population with and without chronic medical conditions. *American Journal of Psychiatry* 145(8):976–981.

West, C. M., M. J. Dodd, S. M. Paul, K. Schumacher, D. Tripathy, P. Koo, and C. Miaskowski. 2003. The PRO-SELF(c): Pain control program—an effective approach for cancer pain management. *Oncology Nursing Forum Online* 30(1):65–73.

Wewers, M. E., J. M. Bowen, A. E. Stanislaw, and V. B. Desimone. 1994. A nurse-delivered smoking cessation intervention among hospitalized postoperative patients—influence of a smoking-related diagnosis: A pilot study. *Heart Lung* 23(2):151–156.

Williams, R. B., and N. Schneiderman. 2002. Resolved: Psychosocial interventions can improve clinical outcomes in organic disease (pro). *Psychosomatic Medicine* 64(4):552–557.

Williams, R. B., N. Schneiderman, A. Relman, and M. Angell. 2002. Resolved: Psychosocial interventions can improve clinical outcomes in organic disease—rebuttals and closing arguments. *Psychosomatic Medicine* 64(4):564–567.

Williams, S., and J. Dale. 2006. The effectiveness of treatment for depression/depressive symptoms in adults with cancer: A systematic review. *British Journal of Cancer* 94(3):372–390.

Winefield, H. R. 2006. Support provision and emotional work in an internet support group for cancer patients. *Patient Education & Counseling* 62(2):193–197.

Winningham, M. L., and M. G. MacVicar. 1988. The effect of aerobic exercise on patient reports of nausea. *Oncology Nursing Forum* 15(4):447–450.

Winningham, M. L., M. G. MacVicar, M. Bondoc, J. I. Anderson, and J. P. Minton. 1989. Effect of aerobic exercise on body weight and composition in patients with breast cancer on adjuvant chemotherapy. *Oncology Nursing Forum* 16(5):683–689.

Zabalegui, A., S. Sanchez, P. D. Sanchez, and C. Juando. 2005. Nursing and cancer support groups. *Journal of Advanced Nursing* 51(4):369–381.

4

A Model for Delivering
Psychosocial Health Services

CHAPTER SUMMARY

Many different providers of health services—some in oncology, some delivering health care for other complex health conditions—recognize that psychosocial problems can have both direct and indirect effects on health and have developed interventions to address them. Some of these interventions are derived from theoretical or conceptual frameworks; some are based on research findings; and some have undergone empirical testing. The best have all three characteristics. When viewed together, these interventions evidence common elements that point to a model for the effective delivery of psychosocial health services. The components of this model include (1) identifying patients with psychosocial health needs that are likely to affect their health or health care, and developing with patients appropriate plans for (2) linking patients to appropriate psychosocial health services, (3) supporting patients in managing their illness, (4) coordinating psychosocial with biomedical health care, and (5) following up on care delivery to monitor the effectiveness of services and determine whether any changes are needed. Effective patient–provider communication is central to all of these components.

EFFECTIVE DELIVERY OF PSYCHOSOCIAL HEALTH CARE

The committee conducted a search[1] to identify empirically validated models of the effective delivery of psychosocial health services. This search

---

[1]This search involved reviewing peer-reviewed literature, seeking recommendations from experts in the delivery of cancer and other complex health care (experts contacted are listed in Appendix B), and investigating models otherwise identified by the committee.

yielded a number of models tested and found to be effective in delivering these services and improving health. These models are described in Annex 4-1 at the end of this chapter and are listed in Table 4-1, which highlights components common to many or all of them: (1) identifying patients with psychosocial health needs that are likely to affect their ability to receive health care and manage their illness, and developing with patients appropriate plans for (2) linking patients to appropriate psychosocial health services, (3) supporting them in managing their illness, (4) coordinating psychosocial with biomedical health care, and (5) following up on care delivery to monitor the effectiveness of services and determine whether any changes are needed. Table 4-1 also includes practice guidelines, produced through systematic reviews of evidence, that identify approaches for the effective delivery of psychosocial health services, along with the consensus-based guidelines for Distress Management developed by the National Comprehensive Cancer Network (NCCN)—an alliance of 21 leading U.S. cancer centers. The various ways in which these programs carry out some of these functions also are listed in the table and elaborated on in the text that follows.

Evidence derived from the models listed in Table 4-1 (summarized in Annex 4-1) strongly suggests that a *combination of activities* rather than any single activity by itself (e.g., screening, case management, illness self-management) is needed to deliver appropriate psychosocial health care effectively to individuals with complex health conditions. This conclusion also is supported by the findings of several systematic reviews of psychosocial care. For example, not surprisingly, screening by itself is less effective than screening with follow-up. The U.S. Preventive Services Task Force, for instance, recommends screening for depression in adults in clinical practices only when practices have systems in place to ensure effective follow-up treatment and ongoing monitoring. This recommendation reflects research finding that only small benefits result from screening by itself, but larger benefits when screening is accompanied by effective follow-up (U.S. Preventive Services Task Force, 2002). Consistent with this finding, a review of studies of interventions to improve the management of depression in primary care settings found that those with the most multidimensional approaches (such as case management combined with clinician education and structured links to connect primary and specialty medical care) were most likely to achieve desired outcomes (Gilbody et al., 2003). Another systematic review of randomized controlled trials designed to improve the use of needed health and social services after hospital discharge found that interventions emphasizing follow-up on the results of a needs assessment showed more positive results than needs assessment alone (Richards and Coast, 2003).

In this chapter, the committee recommends a unifying model for plan-

155

TABLE 4-1 Models for Delivering Psychosocial Health Services and Their Common Components

Model	Common Components[a]					
	Identification of Patients with Psychosocial Health Needs	Care Planning to Address Those Needs	Mechanisms to Link Patients to Psychosocial Health Services	Support for Illness Self-Management	Mechanisms for Coordinating Psychosocial and Biomedical Care	Follow-up on Care Delivery
Building Health Systems for People with Chronic Illnesses (Palmer and Somers, 2005)	Risk and eligibility screening Needs assessment	Yes	Care management[b]	Yes	Multidisciplinary team care Pooled funding	Outcome measurement
Chronic Care Model (ICIC, 2007)	No	Yes	Linkage to community resources Case management for complex cases	Yes	Clinical information systems Team care	Use of information systems to accomplish this Planned or structured follow-up visits
Clinical Practice Guidelines for Distress Management (NCCN, 2007a)	Screening for distress Needs assessment	Yes	Social work and referral services	No	Coordination of oncology team	Yes

continued

TABLE 4-1 Continued

Model	Common Components[a]					
	Identification of Patients with Psychosocial Health Needs	Care Planning to Address Those Needs	Mechanisms to Link Patients to Psychosocial Health Services	Support for Illness Self-Management	Mechanisms for Coordinating Psychosocial and Biomedical Care	Follow-up on Care Delivery
Clinical Practice Guidelines for the Psychosocial Care of Adults with Cancer (National Breast Cancer Centre and National Cancer Control Initiative, 2003)	Screening for anxiety/depression	No	Development of referral pathways and networks Coordinator of care designated by patient	No	Multidisciplinary team care Coordinator of care designated by patient	Yes
Collaborative Care of Depression in Primary Care (Katon, 2003)	Use of standardized screening and diagnostic tools for depression	Yes	Structured, formal arrangement for psychiatric consultation	Yes	Case conferences Mental health specialists located within primary care sites	Surveillance of medication use and patient outcomes
Improving Supportive and Palliative Care for Adults with Cancer (NICE, 2004)	Needs assessment	Yes	Yes	Identified as part of rehabilitation services	Multiple strategies including, e.g., multidisciplinary teams, information systems, patient-held records	Yes

Partners in Care (Wells et al., 2004)	Screening for probable depression; Follow-up assessment	Treatment plan formulated with patient	Yes	Manualized patient education and activation interventions and tools	Yes	Yes
Project IMPACT Collaborative Care Model (Unutzer et al., 2002)	Structured assessment to confirm diagnosis	Yes	Case management; Formal arrangement for psychiatry consultation	Yes	Multidisciplinary team care and team meetings; Clinical information systems	Yes
Promoting Excellence in End-of-Life Care Program (Byock et al., 2006)	Comprehensive psychosocial assessment	Advance care planning	Varies by site	Patient/family education	Varies by site	Yes
Three Component Model (3CM™) (Anonymous, 2004, 2006)	Screening for depression and diagnostic assessment	Yes	Case management	Yes	Formal agreements between primary care providers and consulting psychiatrists	Outcome measurement and follow-up using standardized instruments

[a]Sometimes an intervention (such as use of a case manager) performs more than one function, such as linking individuals to needed service and coordinating their psychosocial and biomedical care. When a model clearly states that this is the case, or when it appears to be the case, an intervention is listed in more than one column.

[b]*Case* management and *care* management are sometimes used interchangeably, although different program developers sometimes give a conceptual basis for their particular terminology. In this chart, the wording of the referenced document is used and refers generally to the assignment of an individual (a case or care manager) who is responsible for linking an individual to needed services; coordination of some aspects of their care; and/or following up to assure the service delivery, service effectiveness, or to monitor changing patient needs or status.

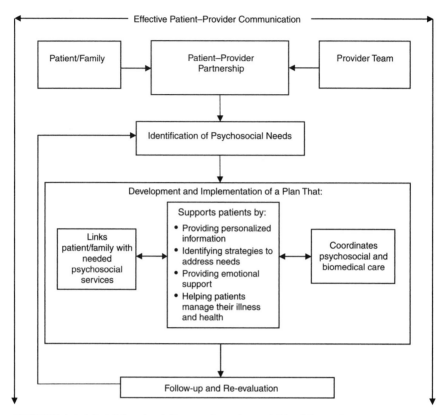

FIGURE 4-1 Model for the delivery of psychosocial health services.

ning and delivering psychosocial health care for patients with cancer. This model is based on the evidence yielded by the models listed in Table 4-1, evidence suggesting added value from multiple components of effective care delivery, and evidence (presented below) supporting the contributions of many of these individual components to the effective provision of psychosocial health care. The committee's model, illustrated in Figure 4-1, integrates the five common components identified above. Although these components individually are in some cases supported by research findings, in other cases there may not be strong evidence of their effectiveness as stand-alone interventions. Nonetheless, the committee recommends their inclusion based on their presence in the reviewed models and with the understanding that a lack of research findings is not necessarily synonymous with ineffectiveness.[2] We also note that effective patient–provider communication is central to the success of all five components of the model. The model is described in detail below.

A UNIFYING MODEL FOR CARE DELIVERY

Effective Patient–Provider Communication

At the heart of the committee's model is a well-functioning patient–provider partnership, characterized, in large part, by effective communication. Communicating effectively means that patients are able to receive and understand information about their illness and health care, and clearly express their needs for assistance and the values and personal resources that will shape the health care system's response to these needs. Patients should be comfortable with asking questions of all their care providers and equally comfortable with responding to questions posed to them. They should be competent and at ease as a member of their own health care team, which will make decisions about the best strategy for addressing their illness. Patients with language barriers, cognitive deficits, or other impediments to communication should receive assistance in overcoming these barriers to effective communication.

In many instances, members of the patient's family also are involved in this communication. In pediatric cases, a family member may be the primary communicator and participant in planning care; with adults, some patients may also have limited capacity to communicate. Even when adult patients are able to communicate, as discussed in Chapters 1 and 2, family members are key caregivers, especially for older adults. Treatment planning and planning for managing the effects of illness requires communication with the patient's caregivers as well as with the patient. When patients do not have the capacity to participate actively themselves, there needs to be an explicit substitute who is legally and psychologically able to act as the patient's advocate.

Care providers similarly should possess the communication skills necessary to be effective clinicians and supportive partners in care—a hallmark of high-quality health care (IOM, 2001) and health care professionals (IOM, 2003). These communication skills include establishing a good interpersonal relationship with the patient (Arora, 2003). Key aspects of

---

[2]For example, an intervention may be so obviously helpful (e.g., providing transportation to help those without means to get to their appointments to do so) that it (rightly) has not been a priority for research (see Chapter 3), or a research design may not have been sufficient to detect the outcome of interest.

effective patient–clinician communication identified in the National Cancer Institute (NCI) report *Patient-Centered Communication in Cancer Care* include (1) fostering healing relationships, (2) exchanging information, (3) responding to emotions, (4) managing uncertainty, (5) making decisions, and (6) enabling patient self management (Epstein and Street, 2007). As described in Chapter 1, however, these attributes are not commonly found in cancer care today.

Current Patient–Provider Communication

Most patients, including those with cancer, say they want more information from their physicians (Guadagnoli and Ward, 1998; Wong et al., 2000; Gaston and Mitchell, 2005; Kahán et al., 2006; Kiesler and Auerbach, 2006). Patients report being dissatisfied with the limited information they receive and when they receive it. Clinicians often have a limited understanding of patients' information needs, knowledge, and concerns. As a result, they fail to provide the type or amount of information patients need and communicate in language that patients often do not understand (Kerr et al., 2003a,b; Kahán et al., 2006; Epstein and Street, 2007). Clinicians' delivery of bad news is particularly problematic. Conversely, patients do not always disclose relevant information about their symptoms or concerns (Epstein and Street, 2007).

Further, the majority of patients (ranging in studies from 60 to 90 percent) say that they prefer either an active or shared/collaborative role in decisions made during office visits (Mazur and Hickman, 1997; Guadagnoli and Ward, 1998; Dowsett et al., 2000; Wong et al., 2000; Gattellari et al., 2001; Bruera et al., 2002; Davison et al., 2002, 2003; Keating et al., 2002; Davison and Goldenberg, 2003; Janz et al., 2004; Gaston and Mitchell, 2005; Katz et al., 2005; Mazur et al., 2005; Ramfelt et al., 2005; Siminoff et al., 2005; Flynn et al., 2006; Hack, 2006). However, studies show that physicians substantially underestimate patients' desire for an active or shared role in their care (Bruera et al., 2002; Janz et al., 2004; Kahán et al., 2006).

Some physicians, particularly female and primary care physicians, have a more participatory or collaborative style with patients (Kaplan et al., 1996; Cooper-Patrick et al., 1999; Roter et al., 2002; Street et al., 2003). Lower levels of participatory decision making among physicians have been associated with several patient characteristics, including age, education, and minority status (Kaplan et al., 1996; Cooper-Patrick et al., 1999; Adams et al., 2001; Xu et al., 2004), although these patient characteristics do not account for the majority of the variation in conversational behavior among either physicians or patients during office visits (Kaplan et al., 1995; Benbassat et al., 1998). There is evidence that physicians and patients mutually influence each other's conversational behavior (Robinson and Roter, 1999; Del Piccolo et al., 2002; Street et al., 2003, 2005; Butow et al., 2004; Janz et al., 2004; Maly et al., 2004; Gordon et al., 2005; Kindler et al., 2005; Adler, 2007) and that physicians may take their cues in part from patients, who typically exhibit relatively passive behavior during office visits (Gordon et al., 2005, 2006a,b; Street and Gordon, 2006). Such passivity characterizes even physicians when they become patients. The average patient asks five or fewer questions during a 15-minute office visit, and many ask no questions (Brown et al., 1999, 2001; Sleath et al., 1999; Cegala et al., 2000; Butow et al., 2002; Bruera et al., 2003; Kindler et al., 2005). Among the most passive patients are those above age 60, those with more severe illness or multiple comorbid conditions (including psychological distress), those who are less well educated, and males (Butow et al., 2002; Sleath and Rubin, 2003; Street et al., 2003; Maliski et al., 2004; Gaston and Mitchell, 2005; Flynn et al., 2006; Gordon et al., 2006b; Siminoff et al., 2006a). Minorities also have been noted to be more passive in physician–patient interactions (Gordon et al., 2005; Street et al., 2005; Siminoff et al., 2006a; Gordon et al., 2006b). Moreover, a systematic review of randomized controlled trials and uncontrolled studies of interventions designed to improve the provision of information and encourage participation in decision making by patients with advanced cancer found that although almost all patients expressed a desire for full information, only about two-thirds wished to participate actively in decision making about their care (Gaston and Mitchell, 2005).

Correspondence between patients' preferred role in decision making and their actual role during office visits with physicians, although intuitively compelling, has relatively little empirical support as a factor affecting patient outcomes and quality of care. However, such correspondence has been linked with reduced anxiety (Gattellari et al., 2001; Kahán et al., 2006) and depression (Schofield and Butow, 2003), satisfaction with treatment choices (Keating et al., 2002), and more appropriate treatment choices (Siminoff et al., 2006b). The NCI report *Patient-Centered Communication in Cancer Care* articulates a comprehensive research agenda for better understanding and intervening to improve patient–provider communication (Epstein and Street, 2007).

The Importance of Communication

There is reason to be concerned about findings of poor communication and lack of patient involvement. A substantial body of evidence indicates that effective physician–patient communication is positively related to patients' health outcomes (Kaplan et al., 1989; Stewart, 1995; Piccolo et al., 2000; Heisler et al., 2002; Engel and Kerr, 2003; Kerr et al., 2003a,b;

Schofield and Butow, 2003; Maliski et al., 2004). Patients of physicians who involve them in treatment decisions during office visits have better health outcomes than those of physicians who do not (Kaplan et al., 1995; Adams et al., 2001; Gattellari et al., 2001; Hack et al., 2006). Physicians' participatory decision-making style also is positively related to the quality and outcomes of patient care generally (Guadagnoli and Ward, 1998), including continuity of care (Kaplan et al., 1996), health outcomes (Adams et al., 2001; van Roosmalen et al., 2004), decreased psychological distress (Zachariae et al., 2003), trust in the physician (Berrios-Rivera et al., 2006; Gordon et al., 2006a,b), more preventive health services (Woods et al., 2006), better communication with physicians (Thind and Maly, 2006), and satisfaction with care (Kaplan et al., 1996; Adams et al., 2001). Similar benefits are found specifically in cancer care (Arora, 2003).

Interventions to Improve Communication

Many clinicians have identified a need for stronger communication skills for themselves, their patients, and families. Interventions to improve physician–patient communication have targeted either physicians or patients; few have targeted both simultaneously (Epstein and Street, 2007).

Training physicians to negotiate with patients has been found to increase patient involvement in treatment decisions (Timmermans et al., 2006). A substantial literature also documents the effects of interventions aimed at improving patients' participation in their care (Epstein and Street, 2007). Such interventions include those aimed at improving patients' participation in multiple decisions over multiple visits with physicians (e.g., question asking, decision elicitation, and negotiation skills), enhancing the presentation of options, tailoring risk information, and providing testimonials describing outcomes of treatment to help patients participate in single or discrete decisions and improve information seeking (question asking).

The means used to deliver these interventions also vary widely. "Coached care" for chronic disease makes use of patient medical records, guidelines for clinical care management reviewed with patients before office visits, and coaching in using information to participate effectively with physicians. This approach has been linked with improved physiological and functional patient outcomes and increased patient participation in physician–patient communication among patients with chronic disease (Greenfield et al., 1988; Kaplan et al., 1989; Rost et al., 1991; Keeley et al., 2004). Decision aids to assist patients in choosing among treatment options have been shown to decrease decisional conflict, increase satisfaction with treatment decisions (Whelan et al., 2004), and decrease adjuvant therapy for low-risk patients with breast cancer (Peele et al., 2005; Siminoff et al., 2006b).

An extensive literature documents the beneficial effects of interactive videos presenting treatment options, tailored risk information, and patient testimonials describing outcomes of treatment. Benefits include improved functional outcomes, increased confidence in treatment, and increased satisfaction with decision making (Flood et al., 1996; Liao et al., 1996; Barry et al., 1997). Following similar interventions, others have noted changes in patients' treatment choices, favoring less invasive treatment (Mazur and Merz, 1996). O'Connor and colleagues (1995) note that these types of decision aids, compared with usual care, yield improvements in patients' knowledge of their disease and its treatment, more realistic expectations, less decisional conflict, more active participation in office visits, and less indecision about options. No effect on patient anxiety was observed. Videos with or without supporting materials have been shown to enhance patients' understanding of treatment options (Onel et al., 1998) and physician–patient communication during office visits (Frosch et al., 2001; Brown et al., 2004a). In a review of small media interventions, counseling and small-group education sessions, or a combination of these approaches, Briss and colleagues (2004) found that while such interventions increased patients' knowledge about their disease and the accuracy of their risk perceptions, whether such interventions lead to increased patient participation in treatment decisions has been less well studied.

Other interventions to improve patient participation in care, such as the use of question-prompt sheets, audiotaping of visits, or more basic decision aids, have been linked with greater patient involvement in treatment decisions (Butow et al., 1994; Guadagnoli and Ward, 1998; Cegala et al., 2000; Maly et al., 2004; Gaston and Mitchell, 2005).

Conclusions

Despite strong evidence for the importance of effective patient–provider communication and patients' participation in decision making in achieving better health care outcomes, such communication is not yet the norm. As described above and in Chapter 1, physician–patient communication is generally inadequate, and patients are poorly prepared for communicating effectively (whether this involves simple information-seeking skills or more active involvement in treatment decisions). Physicians, too, are poorly prepared to elicit patients' information needs and preferences for involvement in their care. There is a need for more creative and intensive interventions to enhance patient–physician communication and support patient decision making, targeting in particular those most at risk (e.g., older adults, those of lower socioeconomic status, and those with comorbid conditions including psychosocial distress and decreased cognition). Many approaches are being tested to meet this need. These approaches require more rigorous evaluation, especially in less well-organized health care settings.

NCI's state-of-the-science report on patient-centered communication in cancer care (Epstein and Street, 2007) can inform clinical practice, as well as research. This report finds that most skill-building interventions targeting clinicians consist of formal training as part of medical education or continuing education programs (e.g., a 3-day course on communication skills) to increase clinician knowledge and improve communication behaviors. Very little research has focused on changing clinical practices and health care systems. With respect to clinician education and training programs, the report finds that the most effective communication skill-building programs are those that are carried out over a long period of time, use multiple teaching methods, allow for practice, provide timely feedback, and allow clinicians to work in groups with skilled facilitators. The report also finds that because clinicians develop routines for interacting with patients early in their careers, communication training should occur early in professional education. Clinicians should seek out such opportunities for communication training as part of their continuing education activities. Training is available from such sources as the Institute for Healthcare Communication (http://www. healthcarecomm.org/index.php) to improve knowledge, skills, and clinical practice in communication with patients.

With respect to improved patient communication, use of tools to support communication and formal strategies to teach communication techniques to patients have been found effective in improving communication with clinicians. These tools and techniques include encouraging patients to write down their questions and concerns prior to meeting with clinicians; providing written "prompts" to patients that serve as reminders of key questions or issues; and providing information and decision aids about the illness, treatment, and health through booklets, videos, coaching sessions, and use of diaries (Epstein and Street, 2007). Patient advocacy organizations can play an important role in strengthening the patient side of the patient–provider partnership through the provision of such tools and training. An example is the Cancer Survival Toolbox (available free of charge), which teaches people with cancer how to obtain information, make decisions, solve problems, and generally communicate more effectively with health care providers (Walsh-Burke et al., 1999; NCCS, 2007).

Identifying Patients with Psychosocial Health Needs

Identifying psychosocial health needs is the essential precursor to meeting those needs. This can occur in several ways: (1) patients may volunteer information about these needs in their discussions with health care providers; (2) providers may ask about psychosocial health needs during structured or unstructured clinical conversations with the patient; (3) providers may screen patients using validated instruments; and (4) providers may perform an in-depth psychosocial assessment of patients after or independently of screening. These approaches vary considerably in their reliability and their sensitivity in uncovering patients' needs.

Relying on patients to volunteer information or on providers to elicit it in the course of standard care both are unlikely to be adequate. A study of the ability of medical oncologists and nurses in the United States to recognize on their own the psychosocial problems of their oncology patients found that these providers frequently failed to detect depression at all and when they did, greatly underestimated its seriousness (Passik et al., 1998; McDonald et al., 1999). This finding parallels data on the low rate of detection of depression in primary care settings when depression screening tools are not used. And while there is evidence for the effectiveness of structured clinical interviews in detecting some psychosocial needs (e.g., for treatment of depression), this approach is criticized for the amount of time it takes and the requirement for specialized (costly) personnel to conduct the interviews (Trask, 2004). Patients' reluctance to volunteer information about their need for psychosocial services (Arora, 2003) can also impede the detection of problems.

In contrast, several screening tools and in-depth needs assessment instruments have been found to be effective in reliably identifying individuals with psychosocial health needs. Screening involves the administration of a test or process to individuals who are not known to have or do not necessarily perceive that they have or are at risk of having a particular condition or need. It is used to identify those who are likely to have a condition of interest and should benefit from its detection and treatment. A screening instrument yields a yes or no answer as to whether an individual is at high risk. A positive screen should be followed by a more in-depth needs assessment. In some practices, needs assessment may be performed without a preceding screen.

Screening

Many screening instruments are brief and can be self-administered by the patient—sometimes in the waiting room before a visit with the clinician. Instruments range from the low-tech, requiring only paper and pencil, to the high-tech, using a computer-based touch screen; some of the latter instruments automatically compare responses with those given previously and generate an automatic report to the clinician. The success of many practices in using such screening tools counters generalizations that patients are unwilling to discuss psychosocial concerns. Still, as discussed below, too few clinicians employ these reliable methods routinely to identify patients with psychosocial health needs.

Current practice   Screening for psychosocial health needs using validated instruments is not routinely practiced in oncology. In a national survey[3] of

---

[3]Response rate = 47 percent.

1,000 randomly selected members of the American Society of Clinical Oncology, 14 percent of respondents reported screening for psychosocial distress using a standardized tool. A third reported that they did not routinely
screen for distress. Of the 65 percent that did routinely screen, 78 percent
did so using some combination of asking direct questions (61 percent), such
as "How are you coping?", "Are you depressed?", or "How do you feel?";
observing patients' moods (57 percent); taking their history (53 percent);
talking to family members (44 percent); or other methods. Similarly, of 15
organizations responding to a survey of 18 member institutions of NCCN,
only 8 reported that they routinely screened for distress in at least some of
their patients. Of these 8, 3 screened as part of a patient interview, 2 used
a self-report measure, and 3 used both. Only 3 routinely screened all of
their patients; the majority screened only certain groups of patients, such as
those undergoing bone marrow transplantation or those with breast cancer
(Jacobsen and Ransom, 2007).

Reasons given by individual oncologists for not screening include a lack
of time, a perception of limited referral resources, a belief that patients are
unwilling or resistant to discussing distress, and uncertainty about identifying and treating distress.[4] Reasons given by member institutions of NCCN
for not screening include screening not considered necessary or worthwhile
(one institution), not enough resources to address those identified by a
screener as needing care (one institution), and insufficient resources to both
screen and address identified needs (one institution). The other institutions
reported that they were currently in the process of pilot testing procedures
for routine screening for distress (Jacobsen and Ransom, 2007).

The above concerns may not be justified. The experiences of those who
have developed or now use screening tools show that screening need not
take much time and that patients are willing to communicate their distress.
Further, research shows that physicians', nurses', and other personnel's individual assessments of the levels of stress experienced by patients or their
family members are less accurate than a standardized instrument (Hegel
et al., 2006). Although there remain some unresolved issues in screening
that could be addressed by further research (see Chapter 8), the research
and implementation examples reviewed below and in Chapter 5 demonstrate that screening can be both an effective and a feasible mechanism
for identifying individuals with psychosocial health needs. The variation
among existing validated screening instruments can facilitate the inclusion of screening in routine clinical practice by accommodating the differing interests and resources of various clinical sites. Patient Care Monitor
(PCM), for example, is automated and part of a comprehensive patient
assessment, care, and education system. Other instruments, such as the

---

[4]Personal communication, William F. Pirl, MD, January 4, 2007.

Distress Thermometer, require nothing more than paper and pencil. Most are administered by patients themselves. Although some must be purchased commercially and require a licensing agreement and fee, others are available at no cost.

Screening tools   In addition to having strong predictive value,[5] effective screening tools should be brief and feasible for routine use in various clinical settings. Such tools are available for screening patient populations and identifying individuals with some types of psychosocial health care needs. For example, a number of screening tools for detecting mental health problems, such as anxiety, depression, adjustment disorders, or post-traumatic stress disorder (PTSD) or post-traumatic stress syndrome (PTSS), have been tested with cancer survivors in different oncology settings and found to meet these criteria. The Brief Symptom Inventory (BSI)©-18, for example, measures depression, anxiety, and overall psychological distress level in approximately 4 minutes (Derogatis, 2006). Its reliability, validity, sensitivity, and specificity have been documented in tests involving more than 1,500 cancer patients with more than 35 different cancer diagnoses (Zabora et al., 2001), as well as adult survivors of childhood cancer (Recklitis et al., 2006). The Hospital Anxiety and Depression Scale (HADS) also is useful in screening individuals with cancer or other illnesses for psychological distress because its 14-item, self-report questionnaire omits measures of fatigue, pain, or other somatic expressions of psychological distress that could instead be symptoms of physical illness and confound the interpretation of screening results (Zigmond and Snaith, 1983). Other useful psychological screening tools include, for example, the Brief Zung Self-Rating Depression Scale; Rotterdam Symptom Checklist; Beck Depression Inventory-Short Form (Trask, 2004); PTSD Checklist-Civilian Version (Andrykowski et al., 1998); Patient Health Questionnaire (PHQ), SF (Short Form)-8; 4-item Primary Care PTSD Screen (Hegel et al., 2006); and PHQ-9 (Lowe et al., 2004).

However, in addition to unresolved questions about the appropriate use and interpretation of the results obtained with these psychological screening tools (Trask, 2004; Mitchell and Coyne, 2007), their varying foci necessitate either administering multiple tools—infeasible for most clinical

---

[5]Screening instruments are never 100 percent accurate and should be distinguished from diagnostic tools and processes. All screening instruments detect false positives (people without the condition whom the instrument falsely identifies as having the condition) and the converse (false negatives). Consequently, a measure of all screening tools is their predictive value—how accurately they identify those who actually have the condition(s) of interest (the instrument's sensitivity) and identify those who do not (the instrument's specificity).

settings[6]—or choosing among them. No guidance exists with respect to which tools should be used for the different types of patients seen in various clinical settings. Moreover, these tools do not screen for the broader array of psychosocial health needs. If, for example, an individual has inadequate social support or financial resources but perceives this situation as the norm or does not experience clinically significant anxiety or depression, these screening instruments may not identify this individual as having psychosocial health needs. In a small study of distress in 50 candidates for bone marrow transplantation, patient reports of distress were found to be accounted for only in part by depression and/or anxiety, suggesting that patients' experiences of distress "were not adequately captured by simple measures of anxiety and depression (the HADS)" and that the "patient definition of distress is qualitatively different from symptoms of anxiety and depression" (Trask et al., 2002:923). Other studies also have observed variable results from the use of different screening instruments (Hegel et al., 2006).

Thus, there is a need for psychosocial screening instruments that can accurately and efficiently detect a comprehensive range of health-related psychosocial problems—including difficulties with logistical or material needs (e.g., transportation or insurance), inadequate social supports, behavioral risk factors, and emotional problems such as anxiety or depression. Although few in number, instruments that can be used to screen for a broader array of psychosocial needs exist. These instruments vary somewhat in their content and approach, which may reflect their different purposes and conceptual bases (as well as the absence of a shared understanding of health-related psychosocial stress and psychosocial health services, as discussed in Appendix B). Although additional testing of these instruments would be beneficial, the validity, reliability, and feasibility of some are sufficiently established that many oncology practices now routinely screen all of their patients for psychosocial health needs using such instruments as those described below.

The Distress Thermometer uses a visual analogue scale displayed on a picture of a thermometer to screen for any type of psychological distress. Individuals are instructed to circle the number (from zero [no distress] to 10 [extreme distress]) that best describes how much distress they have experienced over the past week (NCCN, 2006). The single-item, paper-and-pencil Distress Thermometer is self-administered in less than a minute. Testing

---

[6]Although the Comprehensive Breast Cancer program of Dartmouth-Hitchcock Medical Center routinely screens all newly diagnosed breast cancer patients using multiple instruments, including the Distress Thermometer, PHQ, Primary Care PTSD Screen, screens for alcohol (CAGE questionnaire) and tobacco use, the Medical Outcomes Short Form (SF-8), and a self report version of the Charlson Comorbidity index. Personal communication from E. Dale Collins, MD, Director, Comprehensive Breast Program, Dartmouth-Hitchcock Medical Center, March 1, 2007. See also Hegel et al., 2006.

in individuals with different types of cancer at multiple cancer centers has shown that a rating of 4 or higher correlates with significant distress and that the instrument affords good sensitivity and specificity (Jacobsen et al., 2005). Testing has also revealed concordance with the HADS and BSI (Roth et al., 1998; Trask et al., 2002; Akizuki et al., 2003; Hoffman et al., 2004; Jacobsen et al., 2005). In guidelines issued by NCCN, a 35-item **Problem List** provided on the same page as the thermometer asks patients to identify separately the types of problems they have (e.g., financial, emotional, work-related, spiritual, family, physical symptoms) (NCCN, 2006). This tool can help identify psychosocial problems that are not linked to psychological distress, as well as those that are. The Problem List does not ask about behaviors such as smoking, alcohol or drug use, exercise, or diet or about cognitive problems that could interfere with illness self-management. The Distress Thermometer is available at no cost from NCCN. No data are available on the extent of its use overall, although three member cancer centers of NCCN report using it (Jacobsen and Ransom, 2007).

The **Patient Care Monitor (PCM) 2.0** is an automated, 86-item screening tool that reviews psychological status, problems in role functioning, and overall quality of life, as well as physical symptoms and functioning. Designed to screen for patient problems frequently encountered by practicing oncologists, it is completed by the patient using a computer-based tablet and pen prior to each visit with the clinician. The questionnaire takes an average of 11 minutes to complete. Once completed, it is sent automatically via secure wireless connection to a central server at the practice site; responses are compared with those given previously; and the results are printed out for review by the clinician prior to the visit with the patient. Scores for distress and despair/depression are automatically generated and included in the PCM report. Measures of the instrument's validity and reliability for use with adults have been favorable in testing among multiple convenience samples of patients in one large oncology practice (Fortner et al., 2003; Schwartzberg et al., 2007). PCM has not undergone tests of its sensitivity and specificity; however, a threshold for follow-up assessment has been established using normalized T scores derived from a normative database created from data submitted by licensed users. At present, a score of 65 is more than 1 standard deviation beyond the mean and represents the top 5 percent for either distress or despair/depression. Patients with scores of 65 or higher are strongly recommended to receive further assessment. PCM is a component of the PACE (Patient Assessment, Care, and Education) product, commercially available from the Supportive Care Network, and has a Spanish version. As of January 2007, it was in use by more than 110 oncology practices in the United States.

The *Psychosocial Assessment Tool*© (**PAT**) 2.0 was developed for use with families of children newly diagnosed with cancer to assess the patient's level of risk for psychosocial health problems during treatment. Risk factors for which it screens pertain to family structure and resources, social support, children's knowledge of their disease, school attendance, children's emotional and behavioral concerns, marital/family problems, family beliefs, and other family stressors (Kazak et al., 2001). PAT differs from the Distress Thermometer and PCM in that it was developed for children and for one-time use, although the developers report interest in its periodic use.[7]

The first version of PAT was pilot tested with 107 families and found to be feasible for routine use as a self-report instrument completed by families (Kazak et al., 2001). The 2.0 version includes modifications to improve clarity, ease of use, and content and can be completed in approximately 10 minutes. In subsequent testing, total scores on PAT 2.0 were significantly correlated in the predicted direction with parents' acute distress, anxiety, and conflict and children's behavioral symptoms, as well as with lower family cohesion. Favorable construct, criterion-related, and convergent validity were found as compared with established tools for measuring children's behavior, parents' anxiety and acute stress, and family functioning, as well as with physician- and nurse-completed versions of PAT. Results of tests of internal consistency and test–retest reliability have also been favorable. Cut-off scores for identifying varying levels of need have been determined a priori on the basis of research on the original PAT. As of January 2007, PAT 2.0 was recommended only for research purposes, although its developers believe that upon publication of the most recent research findings, there will be interest in its clinical use and that it is suitable for such use.[8]

Psychosocial Screen for Cancer (PSSCAN) is a 21-item tool that measures perceived social support (instrumental, emotional, network size), desired social support, anxiety, depression, and quality of life. Developed by the British Columbia Cancer Agency (BCCA) of Canada, it has performed well on psychometric tests and tests of reliability and validity in three samples totaling almost 2,000 patients. PSSCAN is in clinical use in a few Canadian cancer centers, although BCCA is committed to its use by all new patients. It also is being used in Ireland and in some U.S. facilities. BCCA has formulated norms for a healthy population (based on a sample size of 800; manuscript in preparation) and has developed software for the tool's use on touch-screen computers. This software has been pilot tested with cancer patients and is ready for large-scale use. The questionnaire can be completed in less than 10 minutes by all patients (except those who do not read English or have severe problems with eye or motor control). The

---

[7]Personal communication, A. Kazak, Children's Hospital of Philadelphia, January 4, 2007.

[8]Personal communication, A. Kazak, Children's Hospital of Philadelphia, January 9, 2007.

software also autoscores all items on completion and prints a one-page summary of scored data for immediate staff use and incorporation into patient charts. Raw data are automatically deposited into an Excel data file for later processing with standard statistical packages. PSSCAN is available at no cost (Linden et al., 2005).[9]

Other screening tools also exist and have been subjected to or are in various stages of testing. Some of these are simple checklists to identify psychosocial health needs (Pruyn et al., 2004). Although there are reports on pilot tests of the feasibility of these checklists, they have not undergone further testing for their validity, reliability, or predictive value as screens. However, a review of six studies of the use of checklists to identify psychosocial health needs in cancer care found that use of these screening tools positively influenced health care providers to pay attention to psychosocial health needs, talk with their patients about these needs, and make referrals to providers of psychosocial health services (Kruijver et al., 2006).

Assessment

In the absence of a common definition of needs assessment and descriptions of how it relates to screening,[10] in this report psychosocial needs assessment is defined as the identification and examination of the psychological, behavioral, and social problems of patients that interfere with their ability to participate fully in their health care and manage their illness and its consequences. Needs assessment contrasts with screening in that the latter is a brief process for identifying the *risk* for having psychosocial health needs, while needs assessment is a more in-depth evaluation that confirms the *presence* of such needs and describes their nature. Needs assessment thus requires more time than screening.

Full understanding of each individual's psychosocial problems and resulting needs is frequently cited as an essential precursor to ensuring that cancer patients receive the necessary psychosocial health services (NICE,

---

[9]Personal communication, Wolfgang Linden, PhD, University of British Columbia, March 1 and 2, 2007.

[10]There appears to be no commonly accepted definition of the process of needs assessment across systematic reviews of the process (Thompson and Briggs, 2000; Gilbody et al., 2006a), reviews of tools for assessing the health needs of patients with cancer (Wen and Gustafson, 2004) and other conditions (Asadi-Lari and Gray, 2005), and clinical practice guidelines (NICE, 2004). Indeed, none of the preceding reviews includes a definition of needs assessment. Although this may be because the process is so well understood that it needs no definition, evidence suggests otherwise. Asadi-Lari and Gray (2005) pointedly note the sometimes interchangeable use of the terms "needs" and "health status" and "health-related quality of life" in some reviews. Discussion of how needs assessment relates to screening also is absent. At least one tool (Kazak et al., 2001) is simultaneously identified as a screening tool and assessment instrument.

2004), to providing good-quality health care overall, and to improving health-related quality of life (Wen and Gustafson, 2004). The United Kingdom's National Institute for Clinical Evidence recommends, for example, that "assessment and discussion of patients' needs for physical, psychological, social, spiritual, and financial support should be undertaken at key points (such as at diagnosis; at commencement, during, and at the end of treatment; at relapse; and when death is approaching)" (NICE, 2004:7). Needs assessments are theorized to facilitate communication between patients and providers about issues that are not otherwise raised (Wen and Gustafson, 2004).

A systematic review of randomized trials (Gilbody et al., 2002) and one cancer-specific randomized pilot project (Boyes et al., 2006) addressing needs assessment used by itself or with minimal follow-up (such as feedback of results to clinicians) found little support for the effectiveness of the process in improving psychosocial functioning. When combined with follow-up care planning and implementation of those plans, however, needs assessment was found to be effective in improving access to needed services in a systematic review of randomized controlled trials evaluating the effectiveness of interventions in improving access to services after hospital discharge[11] (Richards and Coast, 2003). In another systematic review and meta-analysis, systematic assessment of medical, functional, psychosocial, and environmental domains and follow-up implementation of an intervention plan were found to be effective in preventing functional decline in older adults (Stuck et al., 2002). Needs assessment was also identified as one essential ingredient in reduced hospital admissions or medical costs in a qualitative analysis of effective care coordination programs for Medicare (Chen et al., 2000). These findings are consistent with that of the committee that a combination of activities, rather than a single activity by itself (in this case, needs assessment), is needed for the effective delivery of appropriate psychosocial health care.

A systematic search by Wen and Gustafson (2004) for needs assessment instruments for patients with cancer revealed 17 patient and 7 family instruments (generally self-report) for which information was available on their reliability, validity, burden, and psychometric properties (see Table 4-2). These instruments varied greatly in the needs addressed,[12] the domains

---

[11]However, this review also found only "limited support" for the effectiveness of needs assessment when implementation of the recommended services was the responsibility of different providers.

[12]For example: physical, psychological, and medical interactions; sexual problems; coping information; activities of daily living; interpersonal communication; availability and continuity of care; physician competence; support networks; spiritual needs; child care; family needs; pain/symptom control; home services; and having a purpose.

covered, and the items included in similarly named domains (see Table 4-3). Reviewers also found a lack of evidence for the instruments' sensitivity to change over time, failure to examine their required reading levels, and failure to address the period after initial treatment for cancer. Despite these deficiencies and the need for further research (see Chapter 8), results of the two systematic reviews that examined the use of needs assessment instruments when processes for follow-up on identified needs were implemented, as well as the reasonableness of needs assessment as a means of identifying individuals who need psychosocial health services, argue for the usefulness of the process as a prelude to the planning and provision of such services. This conclusion also is supported by the models for delivering psychosocial health services contained in Table 4-1.

Planning Care to Address Identified Needs

Once psychosocial health needs have been identified, a plan should be developed that will assist the patient in managing his or her illness and maintaining the highest possible level of functioning and well-being. Nearly all of the models for delivering psychosocial health services reviewed by the committee (Table 4-1) identify care planning as a component of the intervention. This inclusion of planning may originate from (1) the long-standing practice of developing treatment or care plans as a part of routine medical, nursing, and other health care; (2) the logic of developing a plan for action before action is taken; and/or (3) the identification of care planning in some research as an essential to improving health care. Although care planning in itself has not been the subject of much health services research, some research identifies it as one ingredient in effective interventions to improve health care outcomes in adults with chronic illnesses (Chen et al., 2000; Stuck et al., 2002). Written plans developed jointly with the patient and containing clear goals are characteristic of care coordination initiatives that achieve reductions in hospital care and medical costs (Chen et al., 2000). Moreover, research has shown that people vary in their expression of the need for psychosocial support and in the types of support they prefer.

For these reasons, the committee believes that planning for the delivery of psychosocial health services is a logical step in meeting the need for such services. Advance planning is likely to facilitate the identification and implementation of interventions best suited to each patient's individual situation and to conserve resources not useful to the patient. Such planning for psychosocial health services should address mechanisms needed to effectively (1) link the patient with the needed services, (2) support the patient in managing his or her illness and its consequences, and (3) coordinate psychosocial and biomedical health care.

TABLE 4-2 Comparison of Needs Assessment Instruments (Wen and Gustafson, 2004)

Instrument	Purpose and Administration	Items and Domains	Question Format	Conceptual and Measurement Model
		Patient General		
CARES (Cancer Rehabilitation Evaluation System)	Find how cancer affects psychosocial, physical and behaviors Patient completes	93–132 items; 6 domains: physical, psychological, medical interaction, marital, sexual, miscellaneous	Five-point scale plus "do you want help (yes/no)?"	Competency-based model of coping
CARES-SF (Cancer Rehabilitation Evaluation System-Short Form)	Shortens the CARES for use with clinical trials Patient completes	38–57 items; 5 domains: physical, psychological, medical interaction, marital, sexual	Five-point scale plus "do you want help (yes/no)?"	
CPNS (Cancer Patient Need Survey)	Measures the importance of needs and the degree to which their needs are met Patient completes	51 items; 5 domains: coping, help, information, work, and cancer shock	"Importance": seven-point Likert scale; "how well met": seven-point Likert scale	
CPNQ (Cancer Patient Need Questionnaire)	Assesses unmet needs of people with cancer Patient completes	71 items; 5 domains: psychological needs, health info, ADLs, patient care/support, interpersonal communication	Five-point scale: "what is your level of need for help?"	

Validity		Reliability			
Content Validity	Construct Validity	Internal Consistency	Reproducibility	Responsiveness	Burden

Patient General

Literature; Interviews with patients and family; Expert review	Correlated with SCL-90, KPS, DAS; Good agreement with interviewers.	Domains α ranged from .88–.92	Subscales: r=.84–.95 87% agreement n=71, time=1 week		Time: 10–45 min; Reading level N/A; Acceptability: most found it easy to use
Selected from the CARES by experts	Correlated well with CARES, FLIC, KPS, DAS; Large sample sizes	Domains α ranged from .60–.84	Dimensions: r=.69–.92 81%–86% agreement n=120, time=10 days	Find physical, psychosocial change with time Correlated with FLIC @ 1, 7, 14 mo post-diagnosis	Time N/A; Reading level N/A; Acceptable N/A
Interviews with nurses, patients, and caregivers using Objective Content Test and Q-sort method		Overall: 0.91 Importance: .83–.93 How well met: .79–.95 Domain: α=.88–.92			Time: 2–45 min; Reading level N/A; Acceptability: reported no problems when used
Literature; Interviews; Expert review; Pilot test	Discriminant validity: able to distinguish patients with different disease stages	Domains α ranged from .78–.90	Intercorrelation all significant kappa >.4 n=124, time=10–14 days		Time: 20 min; Reading level: 4th or 5th grade; Acceptability: 25% non-completion rate

continued

TABLE 4-2 Continued

Instrument	Purpose and Administration	Items and Domains	Question Format	Conceptual and Measurement Model
SCNS (Supportive Care Needs Survey)	Assesses impact of cancer on lives of cancer patients Patient completes	61 items; 5 domains: psychological needs, health information, physical/daily living needs, patient care and support, and sexuality	Five-point scale: "what is your level of need for help?"	Factor analysis
HCS-PF (Home Care Study-Patient Form)	Assesses attitudes of terminally and chronically ill patients toward medical care Interview; patient may be able to complete	33 items; 2 domains *Satisfaction with:* care availability, care continuity, MD availability, MD competence, MD personality, MD communication, general satisfaction *Preference:* home care, decision-making	Agreement with five-point Likert scale	
NEQ (Need Evaluation Questionnaire)	Assess needs of hospitalized cancer patients in clinical setting Patient completes	23 items; 3 domains: helps diagnosis/prognosis, exam/treatment, communication and relations	Agreement with yes/no statement	Factor analysis
PNAT (Patient Needs Assessment Tool)	Screen cancer patients for physical and psychological functioning problems Part of clinician interview	16 items; 3 domains: physical, psychological, and social	Five-item impairment scale for each area within domain	

Validity		Reliability			
Content Validity	Construct Validity	Internal Consistency	Reproducibility	Responsiveness	Burden
Based on CPNQ; Expert review; Pilot test		Domain α ranged from .87–.97			Time: 20 min; Reading level: 5th grade; Acceptability: patients found it understandable, 35% non-completion
Based on scales by Zyranski and Ware; Pilot test	Poor discriminant validity	Domains α ranged from 0.10–0.75			Time: N/A; Reading level: N/A; Acceptability: N/A
Interviews; Pilot tests		Domains: α ranged from .69–.81	Cohen's kappa ranged from .54–.94 Time=1week		Time: 5 min; Reading level N/A; Acceptability: 63% of patients OK; 24% in-complete; 3% missing data
Literature; Clinical experience	Physical domain correlates with KPS; Psychological with GAIS, BSI MPAS, BDI Social with ISEL	Domains: α ranged from .85–.94	Interrater reliability: Friedman: .87, .76, .73; Spearman rank order: .59–.98		Time: 20–30 min.; Training level: low; Acceptablity: N/A

continued

TABLE 4-2 Continued

Instrument	Purpose and Administration	Items and Domains	Question Format	Conceptual and Measurement Model
PNI (Psychosocial Needs Inventory)	Measure the unmet psychosocial needs of cancer patients and their caregivers Patient and caregiver complete	48 items; 7 domains: related to health professionals, information needs, related to support networks, identify needs, emotional and spiritual, practical and childcare need	Five-point "Importance" scale Five-point "Satisfaction" scale	
PCNA (Prostate Cancer Needs Assessment)	Measures the importance and unmet needs of men with prostate cancer Patient completes	135 items; 3 domains: information, support, and care delivery	Ten-point "Importance" scale Ten-point "Extent Need Met" scale	
PINQ (Patient Information Need Questionnaire)	Measures the information need among cancer patients for the improvement of clinical practice and research Patient completes	17 items; 2 domains: disease-oriented and information about access to help and solution	Four-point scale	Factor analysis; Similar structure was found across Hodgkins; breast cancer patients and over time
DINA (The Derdiarian Informational Needs Assessment)	Measures the informational needs of cancer patients Interview	144 items; 4 domains: disease, personal, family, and social relationship	Check the need present and rate importance on 10-point scale	Theory of information seeking; Needs and hierarchy of needs

| Validity | | Reliability | | | |
Content Validity	Construct Validity	Internal Consistency	Reproducibility	Responsiveness	Burden
Literature; Interviews; Focus group	Discriminant validity: detected the differences among needs at four critical movements of cancer trajectory	α >.7 for each of the first six domains			Time: N/A; Read level: N/A; Acceptability: 59% non-response rate and the characteristic of the non-respondents was examined
Literature; Interviews using Critical Incident Technique and Nominal Group; Expert review	Correlated with overall satisfaction-with-care	Agreement on classification by three researchers working independently	R=.97 Time=2 weeks		Time: 43 min; Reading level: 7th grade; Acceptability: 11% non-completion
Literature; Interviews	Correlated with RSC, State-Anxiety Inventory and MMPI D-scale	Domains: α ranged from .88–.92; Inter-item correlation >0.2		Detected the changing needs of patients at three time points before and after first treatment	Time: N/A; Reading level: N/A; Acceptability: reasons to refuse: not wanting to be reminded of their illness, feeling too old, etc.
Expert review		Domain: α exceeded 0.9 for all domains	80%–100% agreement found using McNemar test time=15–20 min.	Detected difference between control group and experimental group	Time: N/A; reading level N/A; Acceptability: N/A

continued

TABLE 4-2 Continued

Instrument	Purpose and Administration	Items and Domains	Question Format	Conceptual and Measurement Model
INM (Information Needs Measure)	Assess the priority of informational needs of cancer patients Patient completes	9 information categories	Control preference scale; ranking of informational resources; prioritization of information needs	Based on the theoretical framework of Derdiarian
TINQ-BC (Toronto Informational Needs Questionnaire-Breast Cancer)	Identify information needed by women with recent breast cancer diagnosis to deal with illness Patient completes	51 items; 5 domains: diagnosis, tests, treatments, physical, psychosocial	Five-point "Importance" scale	
		Stage Specific		
PACA (Palliative Care Assessment)	Assess effectiveness of hospital's palliative care program Professional completes	12 items; 3 domains: symptom control, insight, and future placement	Four-point scale, except five-point scale for insight	

Validity		Reliability			
Content Validity	Construct Validity	Internal Consistency	Reproducibility	Responsiveness	Burden
Literature; Based on works by Derdiarian; Expert review		Kendall zeta: .95–.99 Kendall coefficient of agreement: .20–.35			Time: N/A; Reading level: N/A; Acceptability: N/A
Literature; Nurse opinions	Correlated with the information scale of HOS	Overall α=.97; Domains α ranged from .73–.93; Correlation of subscales to total scale: .38–.88			Time: 20 min; Reading level: N/A; Acceptability: OK
Stage Specific					
Interviews of patients	Symptom scores correlated with McCorkle symptom distress scale		Kappa ranged from .44–1	Sensitivity to detected statistically significant intervention effects	Time: few min.; Training level: N/A; Acceptability: N/A

continued

TABLE 4-2 Continued

Instrument	Purpose and Administration	Items and Domains	Question Format	Conceptual and Measurement Model
STAS (Support Team Assessment Schedule)	Assess quality of palliative care of multi-disciplinary cancer support teams Professional completes	17 items; 8 domains: pain/symptom control, insight, psychosocial, family needs, home services, planning affairs, support of other professionals, communication	Five-point Likert scale	
NEST (The Needs Near the End-of-Life Care Screening Tool)	Measure experiences of end-of-life patients and possibly assess impact of interventions Interview; patient completes if possible	135 items; 8 domains: patient-MD relations, social connection, caregiving need, psychological distress, spirituality, personal acceptance, have purpose, clinician communication	Five-point Likert scale	Frame for a good death; Factor analysis; Measurement invariance across sociodemographic strata; Item response theory on the short version

Caregiver

FAMCARE	Measure family satisfaction with advanced cancer care Family completes	20 items; 4 domains: information giving, care availability, physical care, pain control, and 2 other items	Five-point Likert "Satisfaction scale"	

| Validity | | Reliability | | | |
Content Validity	Construct Validity	Internal Consistency	Reproducibility	Responsiveness	Burden
Literature; Clinical experience	Correlated with patient and family score, Karnofsky score, Spitzer QOL index. Support team scores correlate with patient and family scores		Interrater reliability: 90% agreement except predictability	Detected improvement in palliative care Evaluated 2 palliative care support teams	Time: 2 min. for existing patients, 5 min. new patients; Training level: N/A; Acceptability: N/A
Literature; Interviews and focus groups; Symptom items from other scales; Pilot tests; Expert review		Domains: α ranged from 0.63–0.85 at baseline and 0.64–0.89 at follow up			Time: N/A; Reading level N/A; Acceptability: 69.2% patients found interview helpful
		Caregiver			
Interviews; Family ranking of items; Q-sort	Correlated with McCusker and with overall satisfaction with care questions	Overall α: 0.93; Domains: α ranged from .61–.88	R=.92 n=23, time <23 hrs		Time: 22 min; Reading level: N/A; Acceptability: N/A

continued

TABLE 4-2 Continued

Instrument	Purpose and Administration	Items and Domains	Question Format	Conceptual and Measurement Model
FIN (Family Inventory of Needs)	Measure needs of cancer patient's family and extent needs are met Family completes	20 items, 1 domain	Ten-point "importance" scale and met/ unmet check	Fulfillment theory; factor analysis
FIN-H (Family Inventory of Needs-Husbands)	Measure information needs of husbands of women with breast cancer Husband completes	30 items; 5 domains: surgical care needs, communication with MD, family relations, diagnosis/treatment specifics, husband's involvement	Five-point "Importance" subscale and three-point "Need Met" subscale	Factor analysis
HCNS (Home Caregiver Need Survey)	Measures the importance and satisfaction of the needs of caregivers Caregiver completes	90 items; 6 domains: information, household, patient care, personal, spiritual, and psychological	Seven-point "Importance" subscale and seven-point "Satisfaction" subscale	Lackey-Wingate model
HCS-CF (Home Care Study-Caretaker Form)	Assess attitude of terminally and chronically ill caretakers toward medical care of their patients Interview; patient may be able to complete	42 items; 2 domains: *Satisfaction with care:* availability, continuity, MD availability, MD competence, MD personality, MD communication, general satisfaction *Preference for:* home care, decision making	Agreement with five-point Likert scale	

Validity		Reliability			
Content Validity	Construct Validity	Internal Consistency	Reproducibility	Responsiveness	Burden
Literature; Items from original Critical Care Family Needs Inventory; Family review	Correlated with FAMCARE	Overall α for "importance" scale: 0.83			Time: "short"; Reading level: N/A; Acceptability: N/A
Based on FIN Pilot test		Overall α ranged from .90–.93; 73%–87% of items: item-total correlation 0.4–0.7	Importance subscale: r=0.82, Need Met subscale: r=.79 time: <24 hrs		Time: 16–30 min; Reading level: N/A; Acceptability: 12 husbands refused to complete
Statements from patients and home caregivers; Expert evaluation; Pilot test	Psychological, patient care, personal and household Domains correlated with KPSS	Overall α: 0.93, 0.98; Domains: α ranged from .85–.97		Detected changing caregiver needs at 3 time points	Time: 30 min; Reading: 5th grade level; Acceptability: caregivers OK
Based on scales by Zyranski and Ware; Pilot test	Good discriminant validity	Domains: α ranged from .50–.85			Time: N/A; Reading level: N/A; Acceptability: N/A

continued

TABLE 4-2 Continued

Instrument	Purpose and Administration	Items and Domains	Question Format	Conceptual and Measurement Model
NSS (Need Satisfaction Scale)	Assess the intensity and satisfaction of the needs of bereaved families	9 items	Five-point "Felt need" subscale and five-point "Met need" subscale	
	Family completes			
		Relative		
ISNQ (Information and Support Needs Questionnaire)	Assess information and support needs of women who have primary relative with breast cancer	29 items; 2 domains: information and support	Four-point "Importance" subscale and Four-point "Need Met" subscale	
	Self-complete			

NOTE: This table is from "Needs Assessment for Cancer Patients and Their Families." Kuang-Yi Wen and David H. Gustafson, *Health and Quality of Life Outcomes*, 2004, © 2004 Wen and Gustafson; licensee BioMed Central Ltd. The electronic version of it is an Open Access article: verbatim copying and redistribution of the article are permitted in all media for any purpose, provided this notice is preserved along with the article's original URL: http://www. hqlo.com/content//pdf/1477-7525-2-11.pdf.

Validity		Reliability			
Content Validity	Construct Validity	Internal Consistency	Reproducibility	Responsiveness	Burden
Literature; Expert review	Unmet needs correlated with overall satisfaction with care	Overall α: 0.84; "Felt need" subscale: 0.74; "Met need" subscale: 0.84			Time: 15 min; Reading level: N/A; Acceptability: N/A
		Relative			
Literature; Interviews		Domains: α ranged from .92–.95			Time: 37 min; Reading level: "middle" class; Acceptability: "several" reported it didn't apply

TABLE 4-3 Comparison of Domain Item Distribution Across Needs Assessment Instruments (Wen and Gustafson, 2004)

Instruments →	CARES	CARES-SF	CPNS	CPQ	SCNS	HCS-PF	NEQ	PNAT	PNI	PCNA
# Items → Domain ↓	93–132	38–57	51	71	61	33	23	16	48	135
Pain										
Symptom Ctrl										
Physical	26	10			9		6			
Cancer Shock			11							
Psychological	44	17			16	22	5			
Psychosocial										
Spiritual										
Insight										
Sexuality	8	3			3					
Personal										
Marital	18	6								
Caregiving needs										
Family										
Social							5			
Communication			2				•			
Planning										
Other Prof										
Information			10	10	15					64
Diagnostic Info						•				
Treatment Info						•				
Investigative Info										
Daily Living					7					
Work			5							
Household										
Activity Mgt										
Coping			16							
Future Placemt										
Sense of purpose										
Participation						3				
MD Interaction	11	4				2				
MD/Care Availability						8				
MD Competence						4				
Patient Care					8	8				
Continuity of C						4				
Home Care						4				
Access to Care						4				
Care delivery									35	
Support									36	
Financial										
Help			9							
Other	32	19			4					

NOTE: • unclear numbers of items.
SOURCE: This table is from "Needs Assessment for Cancer Patients and Their Families." Kuang-Yi Wen and David H. Gustafson, *Health and Quality of Life Outcomes*, 2004, © 2004 Wen and Gustafson; licensee BioMed Central Ltd. The electronic version of it is an

PINQ	DINA	INM	TINQ-BC	PACA	STAS	NEST	FAM CARE	FIN	FIN-H	HCNS	HCS-CF	NSS	ISNQ
17	144	9	51	10	17		20	20	30	89	42	20	29
				1	1		3				5		
				7	1								
			11										
			5			•				30			
					2								
			1			•				6			
				1	1								
		1											
•		1				•				11		20	
						•			6				
•		2	3		2								
•						•			6				
					3	•							
					1								
					2		6			14			
									4				18
9	•	1	9										
		2	16										
			7										
										12			
				1						5	7		
						•					2		
							3				8		
						•					4		
							6			16			
											4		
											4		
									9				
					1								
							2	20					
													11
					1								
8													
		2			1								

Linking Patients to Psychosocial Health Services

Several mechanisms used to link patients with psychosocial health services delivered by health and human service providers have empirical support, although the strength of this support varies. These mechanisms include structured referral arrangements and formal agreements with external providers, case management, and collocation and clinical integration of services. Use of care/system navigators is also being studied for its effectiveness in linking patients with needed services.

Structured Referral

Although referral to other organizational or individual providers is a common mechanism for linking individuals with psychosocial health services (see the models in Table 4-1, examples in Chapter 5, and services delivered by referred organizations in Tables 3-2 and 3-3 in Chapter 3), there has been little study of the general effectiveness of such referrals. Most studies of referral have addressed referrals between physicians. These and one Australian study of referrals of cancer patients to psychosocial services indicate high rates of failure to connect individuals to the referred providers, frequent failure of the referred individuals to accept the referred services, and failure to track the outcomes of referrals (Bickell and Young, 2001; Curry et al., 2002; Grimshaw et al., 2006). These findings are consistent with the low ranking accorded referral by others studying practices aimed at achieving care coordination (Friedmann et al., 2000) and the finding of low success of referral by itself in linking cancer patients to needed psychosocial health services in one study of health maintenance organizations (HMOs) (Eakin and Strycker, 2001). And oncology nurses participating in focus groups pertaining to the implementation of survivorship care plans stated that they do not typically have formalized mechanisms for making referrals to social work services (IOM, 2007). On the other hand, the high utilization of services provided by such organizations as the American Cancer Society (which do not themselves provide medical services and thus depend in part on referrals for their clients) indicates that referrals can successfully link patients to needed services.

The few studies of how to make referrals more effective in linking patients with needed services have addressed referrals from primary to specialty care. The results of these studies indicate that using structured referral forms and educating referrers are most likely to improve the referral process (Grimshaw et al., 2006). Having formal agreements in place with those to whom referrals are made can also help (Friedmann et al., 2000). Tracking or following up on the actual receipt of referred services in cancer care is also recommended (Bickell and Young, 2001; Curry et al., 2002).

Referring patients to external providers is likely to continue to be a primary mechanism for linking patients with needed psychosocial health services because it requires fewer organizational and physical plant resources than offering all psychosocial services on site. To conserve both psychosocial health services and the personnel and resources needed to make referrals, however, it is important for providers to implement approaches for doing so efficiently and effectively. This is an area that would benefit from further study.

Case Management[13]

Case management consists of a variety of activities necessary to coordinate some or all of the health-related care needed by patients (Zwarenstein et al., 2004). Although these activities often vary with the severity of the illness, the needs of the individual, and the specific model of case management employed (Gilbody et al., 2003; Marshall et al., 2004), case management services that address psychosocial health needs typically include assessment of the patient's need for supportive services; individual care planning, referral, and connection of the patient with other necessary services and supports; ongoing monitoring of the patient's care plan; advocacy and education; and monitoring of the patient's symptoms. These activities can be performed by an appointed individual or a group.

A review by the Cochrane Collaboration of the effectiveness of case management across various diseases and health conditions is under way; as of this writing, results are not yet available.[14] However, a qualitative review conducted for the Medicare program of coordinated care programs most effective in reducing hospital admission, total medical costs, or both across a variety of diagnoses identified case management as one of two effective interventions (Chen et al., 2000). Disease-specific systematic reviews and randomized controlled studies of case management in chronic conditions other than cancer, such as HIV/AIDS (Handford et al., 2006), mental illnesses (Ziguras et al., 2000, 2002), and diabetes (Norris et al., 2002), generally have shown that a variety of forms of case management have positive impacts on health outcomes. A meta-analysis of 37 randomized controlled trials of collaborative care for the treatment of depression in primary care found that case management is a key determinant of effective treatment of depression (Gilbody et al., 2006b). However, there have

---

[13]The discussion in this section distinguishes between case management provided by a resource *person* working with both the patient and the involved clinicians and disease management *programs*. The latter often involve transfer of the overall medical and related health care management of a patient's specific disease to a separate organization or program, often through a contract. Disease management programs can also offer case management services by an individual.

[14]Personal communication, Merrick Zwarenstein, February 7, 2007.

been few experimental studies of case management in cancer care, and their results vary widely.

McCorkle and colleagues (2000) studied the effect of case management by advanced practice nurses on older postsurgical patients with solid tumors. The intervention consisted of home visits and telephone calls over a 4-week period that involved assessment, information sharing, and skills training for patients and family caregivers. The nurse-managed patients experienced better 2-year survival rates, confined to the group with later-stage disease (67 vs. 40 percent 2-year survival). Another randomized trial examined the effect of nurse case management on women with breast cancer. The results suggest that case management by an oncology nurse for the 12 months following diagnosis increased the likelihood that patients participated in decision making and received evidence-based treatment (Goodwin et al., 2003). Results of other randomized trials in England and Australia, however, suggest that much remains to be learned about the effectiveness of the various activities of nurse case managers in cancer care (McLachlan et al., 2001). One study of the effects of a nurse coordinator intervention with terminally ill cancer patients found no significant differences in symptoms, psychiatric morbidity, or care satisfaction between nurse-managed and control patients and families (Addington-Hall et al., 1992). In an analysis of the health care utilization and cost impacts of the nurse coordinator intervention, however, Raftery and colleagues (1996) found significant reductions in use of hospital and home care with care management. The Australian investigators studied 450 Cancer Institute outpatients with multiple cancers and stages of disease. All patients completed a baseline computerized assessment that included informational, psychosocial, and physical needs; functioning, symptoms, and quality of life; and depressive symptoms. For patients in the intervention group, a nurse coordinator reviewed the assessment results and formulated an individualized care plan in accordance with preset psychosocial guidelines. In addition, a summary of the assessment was made available to the physician seeing the patient that day. The nurses linked patients with needed services, monitored patients and families for changing needs, and attempted to coordinate the activities of the clinical team in support of the management plan. Although counseling was frequently recommended, fewer than 30 percent of patients accepted this recommendation. No significant improvements in satisfaction of needs, psychosocial functioning, or quality of life were found.

In summary, case management has demonstrated effectiveness in the care of high-risk patients with major chronic illnesses, but its role in cancer care remains uncertain. Despite this uncertainty, a number of health plans have implemented case management activities for patients with cancer (AHIP, 2007). Case management directed at increasing adherence to evidence-based treatment (Goodwin et al., 2003) and increasing the self-management skills of patients and family caregivers (McCorkle et al., 2000) may well be effective.

On-site Collocation and Clinical Integration of Services

Multiple studies of mental health care have found that same-site delivery of mental health and primary care is effective in linking patients to the collocated services (Druss et al., 2001; Samet et al., 2001) and can improve treatment outcomes (Unutzer et al., 2001; Weisner et al., 2001). In a 1995 study of a nationally representative sample of outpatient drug use treatment units, same-site delivery of services was more effective than formal arrangements with external providers, referral agreements, or case management in ensuring that patients would utilize necessary services (a first step in collaborative care) (Friedmann et al., 2000).

Integrating psychosocial health care into medical care settings facilitates patient follow-through on referrals, allows for face-to-face verbal communication in addition to or as an alternative to communicating in writing, and allows for informal sharing of the views of different disciplines and easy exchange of expertise (Pincus, 2003). Studies of care collaboration also have shown that physical proximity of would-be collaborators facilitates collaboration (IOM, 2004).

The opportunities for face-to-face communication provided by collocated services are important because multiple studies have identified effective communication between providers as a key feature of care collaboration (Baggs and Schmitt, 1988; Shortell et al., 1994; Schmitt, 2001). "Effective" communication is described as frequent and timely (Shortell et al., 1994; Gittell et al., 2000),[15] and is characterized by discussion with contributions by all parties, active listening, openness, a willingness to consider other ideas and ask for opinions, questioning (Baggs and Schmitt, 1997; Shortell et al., 1994), and the free flow of information among participants. This type of communication is less easily achieved through electronic, mail, and telephone communications. Nonetheless, when physical collocation and integration of services is not feasible, other strategies for linking patients with needed services (e.g., through formal referral arrangements or use of case managers) can be used.

Care/System Navigators

Use of care/system navigators, as well as individual patient advocates, is similar to case management and may also help link patients to needed psychosocial services. Such programs in cancer care were developed initially

---

[15]As well as accurate, understandable, and satisfying.

to help low-income patients participate in screening for the detection of cancer and aid those with suspicious screening findings in gaining access to diagnostic and treatment services. Initially, patient navigators tended to be local community residents without professional credentials, but more recently some have proposed that nurses, social workers, and other health workers play a navigator role. This variation in the background of the navigator relates to differences in role expectations. While all navigator programs focus on helping patients overcome barriers to receiving effective services, some also include patient education and patient advocacy roles (Dohan and Schrag, 2005).

Evidence to date for the effectiveness of patient navigator programs is confined largely to their effectiveness in getting patients screened for the detection of cancer. One of the few randomized trials of this type of patient navigation (Jandorf et al., 2005) found that patient navigators increased the prevalence of screening for colorectal cancer. Results of other quasi- and nonexperimental evaluations suggest that such programs increase screening rates and may modestly increase the proportion of patients detected with early-stage disease (Dohan and Schrag, 2005). Some qualitative evidence suggests that navigators help patients overcome barriers, both logistical (e.g., transportation) and attitudinal, although their role in helping patients once diagnosed has received little study. However, a recent randomized trial evaluating the impact of a patient navigation program on follow-through with diagnosis among women with abnormal mammograms found that the intervention significantly increased the percentage of women achieving diagnostic resolution (Ell et al., 2007).

In summary, patient navigator programs appear to help low-income patients participate in cancer screening and perhaps diagnosis. Whether such programs can also be effective in linking a diverse patient population to appropriate psychosocial services and how they differ from case management functions described above remains uncertain, however. The American Cancer Society (ACS) and NCI have both launched major initiatives to implement and evaluate patient navigator programs. The ACS program involves placing trained ACS staff in strategically selected health care facilities with oncology treatment services to provide adult cancer patients and families with personalized and reliable information about the disease, referral to ACS resources, and timely follow-up. NCI has launched a Patient Navigation Research Program to address unequal access to standard oncology care by developing interventions designed to reduce the time to delivery of standard cancer services, cancer diagnosis, and treatment after an abnormal finding. Patient navigators in this program will assist patients and their families throughout the period of care by, for example, arranging various forms of financial support, scheduling transportation to appointments, and organizing child care during appointments. ACS is working with NCI on an evaluation of these patient navigator programs.[16] NCI's Community Cancer Centers Pilot Program includes patient navigators as one facet of these new centers (NCI, undated).

Supporting Patients in Managing Their Illness

Illness self-management is defined as an individual's "ability to manage the symptoms, treatment, physical and psychosocial consequences and lifestyle changes inherent in living with a chronic condition" (Barlow et al., 2002:178). Effective approaches for providing this support are reviewed in Chapter 3. Given the diverse physical, psychological, and social challenges posed by cancer, its treatment, and its sequelae, providing patients and their caregivers with knowledge, skills, abilities, and support in managing the psychosocial and biomedical dimensions of their illness and health is critical to effective health care and health outcomes for these patients.

Coordinating Psychosocial and Biomedical Health Care

A 2007 systematic review of systematic reviews of the effectiveness of care coordination, conducted by the Agency for Healthcare Research and Quality (AHRQ) (McDonald et al., 2007), found more than 40 definitions of care coordination and related terminology and 20 different coordination interventions.[17] The report provides the following working definition of care coordination:

> Care coordination is the deliberate organization of patient care activities between two or more participants (including the patient) involved in a patient's care to facilitate the appropriate delivery of health care services. Organizing care involves the marshalling of personnel and other resources needed to carry out all required patient care activities, and is often managed by the exchange of information among participants responsible for different aspects of care. (McDonald et al., 2007:v)

The AHRQ review found that the most common care coordination mechanisms addressed in the literature are multidisciplinary team care, case management, and disease management (the last of which is defined variably or not at all). The review found the strongest evidence for the effectiveness

---

[16]Personal communication, Nancy Single, PhD, ACS, September 11, 2006.

[17]Case management, collaborative care, disease management, geriatric assessment/evaluation and management, integrated programs, interprofessional education, key worker assigned coordination function, multidisciplinary clinic, multidisciplinary program (comprehensive), multidisciplinary teams, navigation program, nurse-doctor collaboration, organized specialty clinic, organized cooperation, shared care, specialist outreach clinic, assertive community treatment, team coordination, team coordination and delivery, and system-level interventions.

of coordination using a variety of strategies for individuals with congestive heart failure, diabetes, severe mental illness, a recent stroke, or depression, although the reviewers noted that it was not possible to identify the key component(s) of the care coordination interventions that were responsible for their effectiveness. Significantly, the review found that when systematic reviews addressed "other clinical areas such as rheumatoid arthritis, pain management, asthma, and *cancer* [emphasis added], there is insufficient evidence to draw firm conclusions" (McDonald et al., 2007:7). Nonetheless, until research provides better direction with respect to coordination within the context of cancer care, clinicians caring for these patients and their families will need to implement mechanisms for coordinating care based on the findings of care coordination studies for other diseases and for populations with varied conditions and on the limited studies addressing care coordination in cancer.

Cancer care typically requires multiple professional caregivers to provide accurate diagnosis and staging, surgical treatment, adjuvant or definitive chemotherapy and/or radiotherapy, and ongoing management of comorbid problems, as well as psychosocial support. The multiple handoffs involved in typical cancer care generate opportunities for confusion, redundancy, breakdowns in communication, and medical errors. Patients and families, with variable help from their clinicians, must often take the initiative to ensure that relevant information is shared across providers and that care is coordinated. The psychosocial problems described earlier, as well as the complexities of oncology care, can make it difficult if not impossible for patients and caregivers to carry out this role. This difficulty is exacerbated by the fact that care coordination as a psychosocial intervention must fulfill a dual function: coordination of psychosocial health services with biomedical services, and coordination of biomedical care provided by multiple clinicians.

Consistent with the findings of the AHRQ evidence review, both types of care coordination are likely to be achievable in various ways, including the activities described in the preceding section that are effective in linking patients to needed psychosocial health services, such as case management and collocated, clinically integrated services. A study of the efforts of hospitals and cancer centers to coordinate the care of patients with breast cancer also found the use of regularly scheduled multidisciplinary meetings and patient support personnel, such as patient educators and care navigators (Bickell and Young, 2001). In a randomized controlled trial of the integration of medical care with mental health services, same-site location, common charting, enhanced channels of communication (including joint meetings and e-mail), and in-person contact were found to facilitate the development of common goals and the sharing of information between medical and mental health providers (Druss et al., 2001). Other coordination mechanisms likely to impact psychosocial care and outcomes include the use of guidelines and protocols that incorporate attention to psychosocial issues; patient support, such as educational, navigation, or case management interventions, to assist patients in having their needs met; and use of information systems to help ensure that providers and patients have the information they need when they need it to facilitate care (Bickell and Young, 2001).

Consistent with these findings, Ouwens and colleagues' (2005) analysis of systematic reviews of programs for the chronically ill identified program components associated with positive effects on patient-reported outcomes, such as patients' functional health status, satisfaction with care, and hospitalization. These components included, among others, structured clinical follow-up, often supported by case management; multidisciplinary team care facilitated by regular communication and multidisciplinary care plans in accordance with evidence-based protocols or guidelines; and feedback, reminders, and education for health professionals.

The use of multidisciplinary teams has been found to be effective in reducing mortality and hospitalizations for individuals with heart failure (McAlister et al., 2004). Such teams have been promoted by the British National Health Service and are widely implemented in the United Kingdom. In a comprehensive assessment of the literature and the U.K. experience with multidisciplinary teams in cancer care, however, Fleissig and colleagues (2006:935) conclude that "research showing the effectiveness of MDT [multidisciplinary teams] working is scarce." Houssami and Sainsbury's (2006) review of the literature on multidisciplinary approaches for patients with breast cancer found 15 studies, none of which was experimental. While there was some suggestion of better survival, this was attributed to characteristics of the hospital and surgeons (especially patient volume) rather than to the functioning of teams. Psychosocial outcomes were not included in this review.

In addition to the low-tech approach of having on-site nursing staff or other personnel provide care coordination, the high-tech approach of using shared patient records can be used to coordinate patient care. Electronic health records (EHRs) are an important mechanism for sharing patient information among collaborating providers and have been highlighted as one of the essential components of the developing National Health Information Infrastructure (NHII). Although sharing of patient information maintained in paper-based records can take place, the electronic capture and storage of patient information is a more thorough and efficient mechanism for timely access to needed information by the many providers serving a patient. EHRs allow (1) the longitudinal collection of electronic information pertaining to an individual's health and health care, (2) immediate electronic access—by authorized users only—to person- and population-level information, (3) provision of knowledge and decision support to enhance the quality of patient care, and (4) support for efficient health care delivery (IOM, 2003). Given these advantages, NCI is requiring organizations participating in its Community Cancer Centers Program to be able to build information technology capability, including electronic patient records (Niederhuber, 2006). Indeed, although still a minority, hospitals and ambulatory practices are increasingly investing in EHRs; however, these investments typically are being made by larger facilities, creating what is referred to as the "adoption gap" between large and small organizations (Brailer and Terasawa, 2003).

Whereas EHRs function to serve the information needs of health care professionals, personal health records (PHRs) generally focus on the collection of information to help individual patients better manage their health care. Early forms of PHRs differed in size, format, and content and were paper-based, relying on manual collection of information from patients and clinicians. Patients' or caregivers' actual use of these PHRs varied depending on their intended use and perceived value. Although patient-reported levels of satisfaction with PHRs were consistently high (83–93 percent) in several studies involving patients with cancer and diabetes and women with children (Drury et al., 1996; Davis and Bridgford, 2001; Lecouturier et al., 2002; Hampshire et al., 2004), rates of actual use ranged from 37 to 97 percent (Drury et al., 1996, 2000; Davis and Bridgford, 2001; Williams et al., 2001; Lecouturier et al., 2002; Hampshire et al., 2004; Walton et al., 2006). Providers' level of satisfaction with using information from PHRs also varied (Drury et al., 2000; Davis and Bridgford, 2001; Williams et al., 2001; Lecouturier et al., 2002, Hampshire et al., 2004), and the few studies examining improvements in clinical status as a result of the use of PHRs found no significant differences (Drury et al., 2000; Williams et al., 2001).

Electronic versions of PHRs are becoming increasingly available as a feature offered by national health plans. These PHRs generally contain medical and pharmacy claims information and medical information libraries, and have areas for patients to record laboratory results and various health status findings (e.g., blood pressure, weight, height for children) and to collect health risk appraisal information. The committee could find no studies of the effectiveness of electronic PHRs. Research is needed to learn more about their potential value in linking cancer patients to psychosocial health services; informing their medical care; and perhaps most important, supporting them in managing their illness.

Consistent with the wide variation in the care coordination mechanisms reviewed above, the AHRQ review of care coordination concluded that the effectiveness of care coordination mechanisms will most likely depend upon appropriately matching the type(s) of care coordination mechanism(s) used with the needs of patients, although "more conceptual, empirical, and experimental research is required to explore this hypothesis" (McDonald et al., 2007:vi). In the interim, clinical practices should adopt approaches to care coordination that best address the needs of their patient population and fit their organizational and work design characteristics.

Following Up on Care Delivery

Patient follow-up is present in all of the models listed in Table 4-1 and has been cited in several reviews identifying effective interventions for improving health care processes and outcomes (Chen et al., 2000; Stuck et al., 2002). Follow-up can take place in a variety of ways, including telephone calls to patients to monitor their status (Brown et al., 2004b; Gilbody et al., 2006b; Kornblith et al., 2006), home visits by care managers or other personnel, as part of a scheduled outpatient visit, or through Internet or web-based technology.

Follow-up involves two discrete activities. First is the determination of which services, if any, the patient used, any problems encountered, and satisfaction with services provided. Second is rescreening and assessment to identify new or unmet needs that are then addressed.

A RECOMMENDED STANDARD FOR CARE

From the evidence presented above, the committee concludes that enough is now known to support the adoption of a standard of care for the delivery of psychosocial health services in cancer care. The committee recommends the following:

Recommendation: The standard of care. All parties establishing or using standards for the quality of cancer care should adopt the following as a standard:

All cancer care should ensure the provision of appropriate psychosocial health services by

- facilitating effective communication between patients and care providers;[18]
- identifying each patient's psychosocial health needs;
- designing and implementing a plan that
  - links the patient with needed psychosocial services,
  - coordinates biomedical and psychosocial care,

---

[18]Although the language of this standard refers only to patients, the standard should be taken as referring to both patients and families when the patient is a child, has family members involved in providing care, or simply desires the involvement of family members.

– engages and supports patients in managing their illness and health; and
• systematically following up on, reevaluating, and adjusting plans.

Multiple organizations could significantly influence adherence to this standard of care. NCI, as the nation's leader in cancer care, could include requirements for addressing psychosocial health needs in all of its protocols; standards for designating clinical or comprehensive cancer centers; and other programs, such as its Quality of Cancer Care Initiative. NCI also could work with other organizations in the public and private sectors to incorporate psychosocial health care into existing cancer care initiatives, such as the Centers for Disease Control and Prevention's National Comprehensive Cancer Control Program and the Veterans Health Administration's National Cancer Strategy. Private-sector leaders in cancer care could do the same. For example, standards-setting organizations such as NCCN and the American College of Surgeons' Commission on Cancer could incorporate the committee's recommended standard and its components into their own standards. Funders of leading initiatives to improve the quality of cancer care also could incorporate this standard into their programs.

Because individual clinical practices vary by their setting and patient population as well as by available resources in their practice and local community, *how* individual health care practices implement the standard of care and the level at which it is done will likely vary. Nevertheless, it is possible for all providers to meet this standard in some way. Examples of how some cancer care providers are doing so today and suggestions as to how others could do so, even with limited resources, are described in the next chapter. What organizations implementing this standard today have in common is attention to how care is delivered at their practice settings and a willingness to redesign care processes when needed—characteristics that require strong leadership, well known as a critical factor in the success of any major change initiative or quality improvement effort (Burns, 1978; Bodenheimer et al., 2004; National Institute of Standards and Technology, 2007).

ANNEX 4-1

EMPIRICALLY VALIDATED MODELS OF AND CLINICAL PRACTICE GUIDELINES FOR THE EFFECTIVE DELIVERY OF PSYCHOSOCIAL HEALTH SERVICES

Building Health Systems for People with Chronic Illnesses

Building Health Systems for People with Chronic Illnesses was a national initiative, funded by The Robert Wood Johnson Foundation from 1993 to 2002, aimed at improving the delivery of biomedical, mental health, and social support services for people with disabilities and chronic conditions requiring long-term care.[19] A qualitative analysis of the five programs most successful in integrating the delivery of all three types of care identified the following as key elements in achieving such outcomes as improved health, reduced use of the emergency room and hospital inpatient and residential mental health care, and reduced or contained costs: (1) screening, needs assessment, and care planning; (2) consumer participation, decision support, and self-determination in care planning; and (3) mechanisms for linking biomedical and psychosocial health services, such as use of interdisciplinary teams and case management (Palmer and Somers, 2005).

Chronic Care Model

The Chronic Care Model is intended to improve the health outcomes of people with chronic illness by creating informed, activated patients who can interact effectively with prepared, proactive health care teams (Bodenheimer et al., 2002). To this end, the model prescribes six key actions for health care organizations serving individuals with chronic illness: (1) supporting patients in learning about and managing their illnesses (illness self-management); (2) helping patients use community resources to manage their health; (3) redesigning patient care by, for example, redefining roles of care team members, offering case management services for complex cases, and providing regular follow-up of all patients; (4) using clinical information systems to support individual patient care planning and coordination of care and to otherwise facilitate efficient and effective care;

---

[19]"Long-term care" refers to the "wide range of medical, nursing, custodial, social, and community services provided over an extended period of time for the chronically ill," especially for individuals with developmental disabilities, traumatic injuries, or degenerative disease or older adults with declines in mobility and cognitive function (Palmer and Somers, 2005:4).

(5) using decision support (for patients as well as clinicians) to promote evidence-based care; and (6) creating overarching organizational mechanisms to promote safe, high-quality care (ICIC, 2007). These elements were developed from the findings of a review of the published literature on promising strategies for management of chronic illness. They were refined as a result of input from a large panel of national experts, and subsequently tested nationally across various health care settings through The Robert Wood Johnson Foundation's Improving Chronic Illness Care program.

Components of the Chronic Care Model have been associated with improved health outcomes in a number of studies (Bodenheimer et al., 2002). In conjunction with the Robert Wood Johnson program, the American Association of Medical Colleges launched an Academic Chronic Care Collaborative (ACCC) to improve care of persons with chronic conditions who receive their care in academic health systems and to ensure that clinical education occurs in an exemplary environment. Teams from 22 academic settings extensively redesigned their care strategies using the Chronic Care Model for persons with diabetes, asthma, and chronic obstructive pulmonary disease and achieved improvements in patient care and outcomes (AAMC, 2006). A RAND Corporation evaluation of the implementation of the Chronic Care Model in four quality improvement collaboratives sponsored by the Institute for Healthcare Improvement also found that implementation of the model for patients with diabetes, congestive heart failure, and asthma improved health care, as well as some dimensions of patients' illness self-management and health.[20] RAND's before-and-after study included 2,032 intervention patients and 1,837 control patients at 30 participating organizations. Improvements were seen in measures of technical quality of care, such as blood glucose control and use of appropriate heart disease medications. Improved patient outcomes included reductions in emergency room visits and hospital admissions for those with congestive heart failure, improvements in health-related quality of life for patients with asthma, and reductions in risk factors for heart disease (blood pressure, cholesterol, blood glucose levels) for individuals with diabetes.[21]

Clinical Practice Guidelines for Distress Management

The National Comprehensive Cancer Network (NCCN), an alliance of 21 leading cancer centers in the United States, offers a number of resources for improving health care provided to individuals with cancer (NCCN, 2007b). These resources include clinical practice guidelines, one set of

---

[20]Although improvements were not detected in all outcomes.
[21]Unpublished data from Emmett B. Keeler, PhD, RAND Corporation, February 20, 2007.

which addresses the management of distress (NCCN, 2007a). NCCN's consensus-based distress guidelines call for (1) screening of all patients at their initial visit, at appropriate intervals, and as clinically indicated to determine the level and nature of distress; (2) further evaluation, triage, and referral of patients with significant distress to appropriate resources for care; and (3) education of patients and their families about distress and its management (NCCN, 2006).

Clinical Practice Guidelines for the Psychosocial Care of Adults with Cancer

Australia's Clinical Practice Guidelines for the Psychosocial Care of Adults with Cancer were developed from a systematic review of research evidence. Although most of the guidelines address how to care for individual symptoms, such as anxiety, or practical problems, such as financial or work-related concerns, the guidelines also recommend certain cross-cutting activities to be carried out in treatment settings. These activities include providing patients with information to support their decision making, screening all patients for clinically significant anxiety and depression, ensuring continuity of care through the designation of a person responsible for care coordination, and developing referral pathways and networks (National Breast Cancer Centre and National Cancer Control Initiative, 2003).

Improving Supportive and Palliative Care for Adults with Cancer

The National Institute for Clinical Excellence (NICE) in the United Kingdom has promulgated guidance on improving supportive and palliative care for adults with cancer. The specific model of care delivery put forth in this guidance is difficult to generalize to the United States because it is based on an infrastructure for cancer care specific to the United Kingdom, such as designated Cancer Networks[22] for specific geographic areas charged with delivering components of a comprehensive National Cancer Plan. However, NICE's guidance recommends the performance of certain generic activities as part of its model for delivering supportive and palliative services, including assessment of patients' psychological, social, spiritual, and financial support needs alongside an assessment of physical needs; promotion of continuity and coordination of care through such mechanisms as multidisciplinary teams and interprofessional communication strategies; systems to support patients and their caregivers in participating in care; provision of

---

[22]Cancer Networks are explicit partnership arrangements among care providers in local health and social service organizations and the voluntary sector.

patient information; and explicit partnerships between various agencies to ensure access to and receipt of needed services (NICE, 2004).

Models for Treating Depression in Primary Care

An estimated 5–9 percent of patients in primary care settings meet criteria for having major depression (Pignone et al., 2002), and many people with depression are treated in primary care as opposed to mental health settings (Kessler et al., 2005). In addition to its direct effects on health and well-being, depression affects the utilization of and adherence to treatment for general medical conditions (discussed in Chapter 2). Although treatment of depression does not encompass all psychosocial health services, problems encountered in providing high-quality mental health care for depression in primary care settings are similar to problems encountered in detecting and managing the broader array of psychosocial health problems seen in oncology settings. Both situations involve an attempt to provide for specialty services in an environment not intended primarily for the delivery of those services. Models for ensuring care for depression in primary care settings have been developed and tested through research and a number of major initiatives. These models can inform strategies for delivering the broader array of psychosocial health services.

Collaborative Care Model

Although the term "collaborative care" is used to refer to a variety of types of interventions, one model of collaborative care developed by Katon and colleagues that has been tested in randomized controlled trials consists of a systematic approach to the structured involvement of mental health specialists in primary care. This approach employs (1) a negotiated definition of the clinical problem in terms that both patient and physician understand; (2) joint development of a care plan with goals, targets, and implementation strategies; (3) provision of support for self-management training and cognitive and behavioral change; and (4) active sustained follow-up using visits, phone calls, e-mail, and web-based monitoring and decision-support systems (Katon, 2003). In an initial randomized controlled trial of this intervention (supplemented by increased frequency of primary care visits in the first 6 weeks of treatment and scheduled visits with psychiatrists) involving 199 patients with depression seen at a primary care clinic over a 12-month period, intervention patients with major depression (but not those with minor depression) showed significantly greater improvement in symptoms than patients who received usual care (Katon et al., 1995). These findings were repeated in successive trials (Katon et al., 1996, 1999).

In a pilot study, collaborative care also has been found effective in treating low-income Latinas with cancer (Dwight-Johnson et al., 2005).

Three Component Model (3CM™) of the MacArthur Initiative on Depression and Primary Care

Based on a review of research findings, the John D. and Catherine T. MacArthur Foundation Initiative on Depression and Primary Care developed a Three Component Model (3CM™) in which the primary care clinician, a care manager, and a mental health specialist collaborate with the patient and with each other in providing care. Primary care processes also are reengineered to promote illness self-management, quantitative monitoring of the response to care, and modification of treatment as needed. Care processes include screening and assessment using standardized tools to identify the target population (patients with depression), patient education and engagement in shared decision making, use of a designated case manager to provide telephone support for the depressed patient and periodic feedback to the clinician on the patient's response to treatment, and formal linkages with mental health specialists (Anonymous, 2004, 2006). A randomized controlled trial of this model in three medical groups and two health plans in the United States involving 60 affiliated primary care practices and 405 patients demonstrated significantly reduced symptoms of depression and increased remission rates compared with usual treatment (Dietrich et al., 2004). 3CM™ has been recommended as an approach for ensuring comprehensive survivorship care to cancer patients through "shared care" collaborations between specialist and primary care clinicians (Oeffinger and McCabe, 2006).

Project IMPACT Collaborative Care Model

Another model of care for delivering psychosocial health services was developed by a national panel of experts for the Improving Mood—Promoting Access to Collaborative Treatment for Late-Life Depression (IMPACT) project. This model consists of systematic assessment to determine a diagnosis; collaboration among patients and primary care and specialty providers to define the problem, develop a therapeutic alliance, and formulate a personalized treatment plan; follow-up and monitoring of treatment outcomes by a case manager; and use of protocols for the involvement of consultation or greater involvement in care by specialists. In a randomized controlled trial of the IMPACT project at 18 primary care clinics associated with eight health care organizations in five states with ethnically and socioeconomically diverse patients, patients with depression treated according to the IMPACT model, compared with those receiving usual care, were significantly more likely to receive treatment for their depression at all follow-up periods; report greater satisfaction with their care; have significantly lower scores for depression; have a higher rate of complete remission of depression; experience less health-related impairment in work, family, and social functioning; and report better overall quality of life (Unutzer et al., 2001, 2002).

Partners in Care

Partners in Care was a quality improvement intervention for depression care conducted from 1995 to 2000 in 46 primary care clinics within six diverse, nonacademic managed care plans in the western, midwestern, and eastern United States. The study included two programs: one directed at improving depression care using medications and the other at resources to support psychotherapy. Along with quality improvement techniques for changing care delivery (e.g., education of clinical staff in evidence-based depression care), both programs included (1) proactive case detection and clinical assessment; (2) activation of patients to promote knowledge about their condition and motivation to follow treatment regimens; (3) care planning and case management; (4) formal mechanisms for ongoing, effective collaboration between primary care providers and mental health specialists; and (5) follow-up. The two programs proved to be about equally successful. A group-level, randomized controlled trial of the quality improvement interventions found increased rates of appropriate care, decreased symptoms of probable mental illness, and increased health-related quality of life in the intervention group compared with the group receiving usual care (Wells et al., 2000, 2004; RAND Corporation, 2007).

Promoting Excellence in End-of-Life Care Program

Between 1998 and 2004, The Robert Wood Johnson Foundation funded 22 demonstration projects aimed at developing innovative models for delivering palliative care to people with progressive, life-threatening conditions. Projects in the Promoting Excellence in End-of-Life Care Program varied greatly with respect to their target populations (e.g., pediatric patients, persons with serious mental illness, prison inmates, military veterans, renal dialysis patients, Native Americans, Native Alaskans, African Americans, and inner-city medically underserved populations), geographic areas and settings in which they were located (urban, rural, and frontier settings; integrated health systems; hospitals; outpatient clinics; cancer centers; nursing homes; renal dialysis clinics; inner-city public health and safety net systems; and prisons), and the ways in which the delivery of palliative care was organized.

Because each project conducted its own evaluation using different methods and metrics, it was not possible to report outcomes of the program as a whole. However, a qualitative review found that despite their differences, all projects had certain key processes in common: comprehensive assessment of physical, psychosocial, and spiritual domains; interdisciplinary care; care planning; regular communication among providers, patients, and families; care management to achieve coordinated care; ongoing monitoring; and patient and family education. The review also concluded that the projects in the aggregate demonstrated that by individualizing patient and family assessment, effectively employing existing resources, and aligning services with specific patient and family needs, it was possible to improve the quality of care in ways that were financially feasible and acceptable to patients/families, health care providers, and payers (Byock et al., 2006).

REFERENCES

AAMC (Association of American Medical Colleges). 2006. *Academic chronic care collaborative congress.* Seattle, WA. http://www.aamc.org/patientcare/iicc/congress.htm (accessed January 22, 2007).

Adams, R. J., B. J. Smith, and R. E. Ruffin. 2001. Impact of physician participatory style in asthma outcomes and patient satisfaction. *Annals of Allergy, Asthma and Immunology* 86(3):269–271.

Addington-Hall, J. M., L. D. MacDonald, H. R. Anderson, J. Chamberlain, P. Freeling, J. M. Bland, and J. Raftery. 1992. Randomised controlled trial of effects of coordinating care for terminally ill cancer patients. *British Medical Journal* 305(6865):1317–1322.

Adler, H. M. 2007. Toward a biopsychosocial understanding of the patient–physician relationship: An emerging dialogue. *Journal of General Internal Medicine* 22(2):280–285.

AHIP (America's Health Insurance Plans). 2007. *Innovations in chronic care.* http://www.ahipresearch.org/PDFs/Innovations_InCC_07.pdf (accessed April 3, 2007).

Akizuki, N., T. Akechi, T. Nakanishi, E. Yoshikawa, M. Okamura, T. Nakano, Y. Murakami, and Y. Uchitomi. 2003. Development of a brief screening interview for adjustment disorders and major depression in patients with cancer. *Cancer* 97(10):2605–2613.

Andrykowski, M. A., M. J. Cordova, J. L. Studts, and T. W. Miller. 1998. Posttraumatic stress disorder after treatment for breast cancer: Prevalence of diagnosis and use of the PTSD Checklist-Civilian version (PCL-C) as a screening instrument. *Journal of Consulting and Clinical Psychology* 66(3):586–590.

Anonymous. 2004. *Depression management tool kit. The MacArthur initiative on depression and primary care at Dartmouth and Duke June 7, 2004.* http://www.depression-primary care.org/imges/pdf/macarthur_toolkit.pdf (accessed June 7, 2004).

Anonymous. 2006. *MacArthur initiative on depression and primary care.* http://www.depression-primarycare.org/about/background/ (accessed January 18, 2007).

Arora, N. K. 2003. Interacting with cancer patients: The significance of physicians' communication behavior. *Social Science and Medicine* 57(5):791–806.

Asadi-Lari, M., and D. Gray. 2005. Health needs assessment tools: Progress and potential. *International Journal of Technology Assessment in Health Care* 21(3):288–297.

Baggs, J., and M. Schmitt. 1988. Collaboration between nurses and physicians. *IMAGE: Journal of Nursing Scholarship* 20(3):145–149.

Baggs, J., and M. Schmitt. 1997. Nurses' and resident physicians' perceptions of the process of collaboration in an MICU. *Research in Nursing and Health* 20(1):71–80.

Barlow, J., C. Wright, J. Sheasby, A. Turner, and J. Hainsworth. 2002. Self-management approaches for people with chronic conditions: A review. *Patient Education and Counseling* 48(2):177–187.

Barry, M. J., D. C. Cherkin, Y. Chang, F. J. Fowler, and S. Skates. 1997. A randomized trial of a multimedia shared decision-making program for men facing a treatment decision for benign prostatic hyperplasia. *Disease Management and Clinical Outcomes* 1(1):5–14.

Benbassat, J., D. Pilpel, and M. Tidhar. 1998. Patients' preferences for participation in clinical decision making: A review of published surveys. *Behavioral Medicine* 24(2):81–88.

Berrios-Rivera, J. P., R. L. Street Jr., M. G. Garcia Popa-Lisseanu, M. A. Kallen, M. N. Richardson, N. M. Janssen, D. M. Marcus, J. D. Reveille, N. B. Warner, and M. E. Suarez-Almazor. 2006. Trust in physicians and elements of the medical interaction in patients with rheumatoid arthritis and systemic lupus erythematosus. *Arthritis and Rheumatism* 55(3):385–393.

Bickell, N. A., and G. J. Young. 2001. Coordination of care for early-stage breast cancer patients. *Journal of General Internal Medicine* 16(11):737–742.

Bodenheimer, T., E. H. Wagner, and K. Grumbach. 2002. Improving primary care for patients with chronic illness. *Journal of the American Medical Association* 288(14):1775–1779.

Bodenheimer, T., M. C. Wang, T. G. Rundall, S. M. Shortell, R. R. Gillies, N. Oswald, L. Casalino, and J. C. Robinson. 2004. What are the facilitators and barriers in physician organizations' use of care management processes? *Joint Commission Journal on Quality and Safety* 30(9):505–514.

Boyes, A., S. Newell, A. Girgis, P. McElduff, and R. Sanson-Fisher. 2006. Does routine assessment and real-time feedback improve cancer patients' psychosocial well-being? *European Journal of Cancer Care* 15(2):163–171.

Brailer, D. J., and E. Terasawa. 2003. *Use and adoption of computer-based patient records in the United States*. Presentation to IOM Committee on Data Standards for Patient Safety on January 23, 2003. http://www.iom.edu/file.asp?id=10988 (accessed October 17, 2004).

Briss, P., B. Rimer, B. Reilley, R. C. Coates, N. C. Lee, P. Mullen, P. Corso, A. B. Hutchinson, R. Hiatt, J. Kerner, P. George, C. White, N. Gandhi, M. Saraiya, R. Breslow, G. Isham, S. M. Teutsch, A. R. Hinman, R. Lawrence, and Task Force on Community Preventive Services. 2004. Promoting informed decisions about cancer screening in communities and healthcare systems. *American Journal of Preventive Medicine* 26(1):67–80.

Brown, R., P. Butow, M. J. Boyer, and M. H. Tattersall. 1999. Promoting patient participation in the cancer consultation: Evaluation of a prompt sheet and coaching in question-asking. *British Journal of Cancer* 80(1/2):242–248.

Brown, R., P. Butow, S. Dunn, and M. H. Tattersall. 2001. Promoting patient participation and shortening cancer consultations: A randomised trial. *British Journal of Cancer* 85(9):1273–1279.

Brown, R. F., P. N. Butow, M. A. Sharrock, M. Henman, F. Boyle, D. Goldstein, and M. H. Tattersall. 2004a. Education and role modelling for clinical decisions with female cancer patients. *Health Expectations* 7(4):303–316.

Brown, R., J. Schore, N. Archibald, A. Chen, D. Peikes, K. Sautter, B. Lavin, S. Aliotta, and T. Ensor. 2004b. *Coordinating care for Medicare beneficiaries: Early experiences of 15 demonstration programs, their patients, and providers*. Princeton, NJ: Mathematica Policy Research, Inc.

Bruera, E., J. S. Wiley, J. L. Palmer, and M. Rosales. 2002. Treatment decisions for breast carcinoma. Patient preferences and physician perceptions. *American Cancer Society* 94(7):2076–2080.

Bruera, E., C. Sweeney, J. Willey, J. L. Palmer, S. Tolley, M. Rosales, and C. Ripamonti. 2003. Breast cancer patient perception of the helpfulness of a prompt sheet versus a general information sheet during outpatient consultation: A randomized, controlled trial. *Journal of Pain and Symptom Management* 25(5):412–419.

Burns, J. 1978. *Leadership*. New York: Harper and Row.

Butow, P. N., S. M. Dunn, M. H. Tattersall, and Q. J. Jones. 1994. Patient participation in the cancer consultation: Evaluation of a question prompt sheet. *Annals of Oncology* 5(3):199–204.

Butow, P. N., R. Brown, S. Cogar, M. H. Tattersall, and S. M. Dunn. 2002. Oncologists' reactions to cancer patients' verbal cues. *Psycho-Oncology* 11(1):47–58.

Butow, P. N., R. Devine, M. Boyer, S. Pendlebury, M. Jackson, and M. H. Tattersall. 2004. Cancer consultation preparation package: Changing patients but not physicians is not enough. *Journal of Clinical Oncology* 22(21):4401–4409.

Byock, I., J. S. Twohig, M. Merriman, and K. Collins. 2006. Promoting excellence in end-of-life care: A report on innovative models of palliative care. *Journal of Palliative Medicine* 9(1):137–151.

Cegala, D. J., L. McClure, T. M. Marinelli, and D. M. Post. 2000. The effects of communication skills training on patients' participation during medical interviews. *Patient and Education Counseling* 41(2):209–222.

Chen, A., R. Brown, N. Archibald, S. Aliotta, and P. D. Fox. 2000. *Best practices in coordinated care*. Princeton, NJ: Mathematica Policy Research.

Cooper-Patrick, L., J. Gallo, J. J. Gonzales, H. T. Vu, N. R. Powe, C. Nelson, and D. E. Ford. 1999. Race, gender, and partnership in the patient–physician relationship. *Journal of the American Medical Association* 282(6):583–589.

Curry, C., T. Cossich, J. P. Matthews, J. Beresford, and S. A. McLachlan. 2002. Uptake of psychosocial referrals in an outpatient cancer setting: Improving service accessibility via the referral process. *Supportive Care in Cancer* 10(7):549–555.

Davis, T. M. E., and A. Bridgford. 2001. A comprehensive patient-held record for diabetes. Part two: Large-scale assessment of the Diabetes Databank by patients and health care workers. *Practical Diabetes International* 18(9):311–314.

Davison, B. J., and S. L. Goldenberg. 2003. Decisional regret and quality of life after participating in medical decision-making for early-stage prostate cancer. *BJU International* 91(1):14–17.

Davison, B. J., M. E. Gleave, S. L. Goldenberg, L. F. Degner, D. Hoffart, and J. Berkowitz. 2002. Assessing information and decision preferences of men with prostate cancer and their partners. *Cancer Nursing* 25(1):42–49.

Davison, B. J., P. A. Parker, and S. L. Goldenberg. 2003. Patients' preferences for communicating a prostate cancer diagnosis and participating in medical decision-making. *BJU International* 93(1):47–51.

Del Piccolo, L., M. Mazzi, A. Saltini, and C. Zimmermann. 2002. Inter and intra individual variations in physicians' verbal behaviour during primary care consultation. *Social Science & Medicine* 55(10):1871–1885.

Derogatis, L. R. 2006. *BSI © 18 (brief symptom inventory 18)*. Pearson Education, Inc. http://www.pearsonassessments.com/tests/bsi18.htm#quickfacts (accessed January 3, 2007).

Dietrich, A. J., T. E. Oxman, J. W. W. Jr., H. C. Schulberg, M. L. Bruce, P. W. Lee, S. Barry, P. J. Raue, J. J. Lefever, M. Heo, K. Rost, K. Kroenke, M. Gerrity, and P. A. Nutting. 2004. Re-engineering systems for the treatment of depression in primary care: Cluster randomized controlled trial. *British Medical Journal* 329(7466):602.

Dohan, D., and D. Schrag. 2005. Using navigators to improve care of underserved patients: Current practices and approaches. *Cancer* 104(4):848–855.

Dowsett, S. M., J. L. Saul, P. N. Butow, S. M. Dunn, M. J. Boyer, R. Findlow, and J. Dunsmore. 2000. Communication styles in the cancer consultation: Preferences for a patient-centered approach. *Psycho-Oncology* 9(2):147–156.

Drury, M., J. Harcourt, and M. Minton. 1996. The acceptability of patients with cancer holding their own shared-care record. *Psycho-Oncology* 5(2):119–125.

Drury, M., P. Yudkin, J. Harcourt, R. Fitzpatrick, L. Jones, C. Alcock, and M. Minton. 2000. Patients with cancer holding their own records: A randomised controlled trial. *British Journal of General Practice* 50(451):105–110.

Druss, B., R. Rohrbaugh, C. Levinson, and R. Rosenheck. 2001. Integrated medical care for patients with serious psychiatric illness: A randomized trial. *Archives of General Psychiatry* 58(9):861–868.

Dwight-Johnson, M., K. Ell, and P. Lee. 2005. Can collaborative care address the needs of low-income Latinas with comorbid depression and cancer? Results from a randomized pilot study. *Psychosomatics* 46(3):224–232.

Eakin, E. G., and L. A. Strycker. 2001. Awareness and barriers to use of cancer support and information resources by HMO patients with breast, prostate, or colon cancer: Patient and provider perspectives. *Psycho-Oncology* 10(2):103–113.

Ell, K., B. Vourlekis, P. J. Lee, and B. Xie. 2007. Patient navigation and case management following an abnormal mammogram: A randomized clinical trial. *Preventive Medicine* 44(1):26–33.

Engel, J., and J. Kerr. 2003. Predictors of quality of life of breast cancer patients. *Taylor & Francis Health Sciences* 42(7):710–718.

Epstein, R. M., and R. L. Street. 2007. Patient-centered communication in cancer care: Promoting healing and reducing suffering. NIH Publ. No. 07-6225. Bethesda, MD: National Cancer Institute.

Fleissig, A., V. Jenkins, S. Catt, and L. Fallowfield. 2006. Multidisciplinary teams in cancer care: Are they effective in the UK? *Lancet Oncology* 7(11):935–943.

Flood, A. B., J. E. Wennberg, R. F. Nease, F. J. Fowler, J. Ding, and L. M. Hynes. 1996. The importance of patient preference in the decision to screen for prostate cancer. Prostate Patient Outcomes Research Team. *Journal of General Internal Medicine* 11(6):342–349.

Flynn, K. E., M. A. Smith, and D. Vanness. 2006. A typology of preferences for participation in healthcare decision making. *Social Science and Medicine* 63(5):1158–1169.

Fortner, B., T. Okon, L. Schwartzberg, K. Tauer, and A. C. Houts. 2003. The cancer care monitor: Psychometric content evaluation and pilot testing of a computer administered system for symptom screening and quality of life in adult cancer patients. *Journal of Pain and Symptom Management* 26(6):1077–1092.

Friedmann, P., T. D'Aunno, L. Jin, and J. Alexander. 2000. Medical and psychosocial services in drug abuse treatment: Do stronger linkages promote client utilization? *HSR: Health Services Research* 35(2):443–465.

Frosch, D. L., R. M. Kaplan, and V. Felitti. 2001. The evaluation of two methods to facilitate shared decision making for men considering the prostate-specific antigen test. *Journal of General Internal Medicine* 16(6):391–398.

Gaston, C. M., and G. Mitchell. 2005. Information giving and decision-making in patients with advanced cancer: A systematic review. *Social Science and Medicine* 61(10):2252–2264.

Gattellari, M., P. N. Butow, and M. H. Tattersall. 2001. Sharing decisions in cancer care. *Social Science and Medicine* 52(12):1865–1878.

Gilbody, S. M., A. O. House, and T. Sheldon. 2002. Routine administration of Health Related Quality of Life (HRQoL) and needs assessment instruments to improve psychological outcome—a systematic review. *Psychological Medicine* 32(8):1345–1356.

Gilbody, S. M., P. Whitty, J. Grimshaw, and R. Thomas. 2003. Educational and organizational interventions to improve the management of depression in primary care: A systematic review. *Journal of the American Medical Association* 289(23):3145–3151.

Gilbody, S. M., A. O. House, and T. A. Sheldon. 2006a. Outcome measures and needs assessment tools for schizophrenia and related disorders. The Cochrane Library 1.

Gilbody, S. M., P. Bower, J. Fletcher, D. Richards, and A. J. Sutton. 2006b. Collaborative care for depression: A cumulative meta-analysis and review of longer term outcomes. *Archives of Internal Medicine* 166(21):2314–2321.

Gittell, J., K. Fairfield, B. Bierbaum, W. Head, R. Jackson, M. Kelly, R. Laskin, S. Lipson, J. Siliski, T. Thornhill, and J. Zuckerman. 2000. Impact of relational coordination on quality of care, postoperative pain and functioning, and length of stay. *Medical Care* 38(8):807–819.

Goodwin, J. S., S. Satish, E. T. Anderson, A. B. Nattinger, and J. L. Freeman. 2003. Effect of nurse case management on the treatment of older women with breast cancer. *Journal of the American Geriatrics Society* 51(9):1252–1259.

Gordon, H., R. L. Street, P. A. Kelly, J. Souchek, and N. P. Wray. 2005. Physician–patient communication following invasive procedures: An analysis of post-angiogram consultations. *Social Science and Medicine* 61(5):1015–1025.

Gordon, H., R. L. Street, B. F. Sharf, P. A. Kelly, and J. Souchek. 2006a. Racial differences in trust and lung cancer patients' perceptions of physician communication. *Journal of Clinical Oncology* 24(6):904–909.

Gordon, H., R. L. Street, B. F. Sharf, and J. Souchek. 2006b. Racial differences in doctors' information-giving and patients' participation. *American Cancer Society* 107(6): 1313–1320.

Greenfield, S., S. Kaplan, J. E. Ware Jr., E. Yano, and H. Frank. 1988. Patients' participation in medical care: Effects on blood sugar control and quality of life in diabetes. *Journal of General Internal Medicine* 3(5):448–457.

Grimshaw, J., R. Winkeins, L. Shirran, C. Cunningham, A. Mayhew, R. Thomas, and C. Fraser. 2006. Interventions to improve outpatient referrals from primary care to secondary care. *Cochrane Database of Systematic Reviews* (4).

Guadagnoli, E., and P. Ward. 1998. Patient participation in decision-making. *Social Science and Medicine* 47(3):329–339.

Hack, T. F., L. F. Degner, P. Watson, and L. Sinha. 2006. Do patients benefit from participating in medical decision making? Longitudinal follow-up of women with breast cancer. *Psycho-Oncology* 15(1):9–19.

Hampshire, A. J., M. E. Blair, N. S. Crown, A. J. Avery, and E. I. Williams. 2004. Variation in how mothers, health visitors and general practitioners use the personal child health record. *Child: Care, Health & Development* 30(4):307–316.

Handford, C. D., A. M. Tynan, J. M. Rackal, R. H. Glazier. 2006. Setting and organization of care for persons living with HIV/AIDS. *Cochrane Database of Systematic Reviews* (3):CD004348.

Hegel, M. T., C. P. Moore, E. D. Collins, S. Kearing, K. L. Gillock, R. L. Riggs, K. F. Clay, and T. A. Ahles. 2006. Distress, psychiatric syndromes, and impairment of function in women with newly diagnosed breast cancer. *Cancer* 107(12):2924–2931.

Heisler, M., R. R. Bouknight, R. A. Hayward, D. M. Smith, and E. A. Kerr. 2002. The relative importance of physician communication, participatory decision making, and patient understanding in diabetes self-management. *Journal of General Internal Medicine* 17(4):243–252.

Hoffman, B. M., M. A. Zevon, M. C. D'Arrigo, and T. B. Cecchini. 2004. Screening for distress in cancer patients: The NCCN rapid-screening measure. *Psycho-Oncology* 13(11): 792–799.

Houssami, N., and R. Sainsbury. 2006. Breast cancer: Multidisciplinary care and clinical outcomes. *European Journal of Cancer* 42:2480–2491.

ICIC (Improving Chronic Illness Care). 2007. *Improving chronic illness care.* http://www. improvingchroniccare.org/index.html (accessed January 12, 2007).

IOM (Institute of Medicine). 2001. *Crossing the quality chasm: A new health system for the 21st century.* Washington, DC: National Academy Press.

IOM. 2003. *Health professions education: A bridge to quality.* A. Greiner and E. Knebel, eds. Washington, DC: The National Academies Press.

IOM. 2004. *Keeping patients safe: Transforming the work environment of nurses.* A. E. K. Page, ed. Washington, DC: The National Academies Press.

IOM. 2007. *Implementing cancer survivorship care planning.* Washington, DC: The National Academies Press.

Jacobsen, P. B., and S. Ransom. 2007. Implementation of NCCN distress management guidelines by member institutions. *Journal of the National Comprehensive Cancer Network* 5(1):93–103.

Jacobsen, P. B., K. A. Donovan, P. C. Trask, S. B. Fleishman, J. Zabora, F. Baker, and J. C. Holland. 2005. Screening for psychologic distress in ambulatory cancer patients. *Cancer* 103(7):1494–1502.

Jandorf, L., Y. Gutierrez, J. Lopez, J. Christie, and S. H. Itzkowitz. 2005. Use of a patient navigator to increase colorectal cancer screening in an urban neighborhood health clinic. *Journal of Urban Health* 82(2):216–224.

Janz, N. K., P. A. Wren, L. A. Copeland, J. C. Lowery, S. L. Goldfarb, and E. G. Wilkins. 2004. Patient–physician concordance: Preferences, perceptions, and factors influencing the breast cancer surgical decision. *Journal of Clinical Oncology* 22(15):3091–3098.

Kahán, Z., K. Varga, R. Dudás, T. Nyári, and L. Thurzó. 2006. Collaborative/active participation per se does not decrease anxiety in breast cancer. *Pathology Oncology Research* 12(2):93–101.

Kaplan, S., S. Greenfield, and J. Ware. 1989. Assessing the effects of physician-patient interactions on the outcomes of chronic disease. *Medical Care* 27(3 Supplement):S110–S127.

Kaplan, S. H., B. Gandek, S. Greenfield, W. Rogers, and J. E. Ware Jr. 1995. Patient and visit characteristics related to physician's participatory decision-making style: Results from the Medical Outcomes Study. *Medical Care* 33(12):1176–1187.

Kaplan, S., S. Greenfield, B. Gandek, W. H. Rogers, and J. E. Ware. 1996. Characteristics of physicians with participatory decision making styles. *Annals of Internal Medicine* 124(5):497–504.

Katon, W. J. 2003. The Institute of Medicine "Chasm" report: Implications for depression collaborative care models. *General Hospital Psychiatry* 25(4):222–229.

Katon, W. J., M. V. Korff, E. Lin, E. Walker, G. E. Simon, T. Bush, P. Robinson, and J. Russo. 1995. Collaborative management to achieve treatment guidelines: Impact on depression in primary care. *Journal of the American Medical Association* 273(13):1026–1031.

Katon, W. J., P. Robinson, M. V. Korff, E. Lin, T. Bush, E. Ludman, G. Simon, and G. Walker. 1996. A multifaceted intervention to improve treatment of depression in primary care. *Archives of General Psychiatry* 53(10):924–932.

Katon, W. J., M. V. Korff, E. Lin, G. Simon, E. Walker, J. Unutzer, T. Bush, J. Russo, and E. Ludman. 1999. Stepped collaborative care for primary care patients with persistent symptoms of depression. *Archives of General Psychiatry* 56(12):1109–1115.

Katz, S. J., P. M. Lantz, N. K. Janz, A. Fagerlin, K. Schwartz, L. Liu, D. Deapen, B. Salem, I. Lakhani, and M. Morrow. 2005. Patient involvement in surgery treatment decisions for breast cancer. *Journal of Clinical Oncology* 23(24):5526–5533.

Kazak, A. E., A. Prusak, M. McSherry, S. Simms, D. Beele, M. Rourke, M. Alderfer, and B. Lange. 2001. The Psychosocial Assessment Tool (PAT)©: Pilot data on a brief screening instrument for identifying high risk families in pediatric oncology. *Families, Systems and Health* 19(3):303–317.

Keating, N., E. Guadagnoli, M. B. Landrum, C. Borbas, and J. C. Weeks. 2002. Treatment decision making in early-stage breast cancer: Should surgeons match patients' desired level of involvement? *Journal of Clinical Oncology* 20(6):1473–1479.

Keeley, R.D., J. L. Smith, P. A. Nutting, L. Miriam Dickinson, W. Perry Dickinson, and K. M. Rost. 2004. Does a depression intervention result in improved outcomes for patients presenting with physical symptoms? *Journal of General Internal Medicine* 19(6): 615–623.

Kerr, J., J. Engel, A. Schlesinger-Raab, H. Sauer, and D. Hölzel. 2003a. Communication, quality of life and age: Results of a 5-year prospective study in breast cancer patients. *Annals of Oncology* 14(3):421–427.

Kerr, J., J. Engel, A. Schlesinger-Raab, H. Sauer, and D. Hölzel. 2003b. Doctor–patient communication: Results of a four-year prospective study in rectal cancer patients. *Diseases of the Colon and Rectum* 46(88):1038–1046.

Kessler, R. C., O. Demler, R. G. Frank, M. Olfson, H. A. Pincus, E. E. Walters, P. Wang, K. B. Wells, and A. M. Zaslavsky. 2005. Prevalence and treatment of mental disorders, 1990 to 2003. *The New England Journal of Medicine* 352(24):2515–2523.

Kiesler, D. J., and S. M. Auerbach. 2006. Optimal matches of patient preferences for information, decision-making and interpersonal behavior: Evidence, models and interventions. *Patient Education and Counseling* 61(3):319–341.

Kindler, C., L. Szirt, D. Sommer, R. Hausler, and W. Langewitz. 2005. A quantitative analysis of anaesthetist–patient communication during the pre-operative visit. *Anaesthesia* 60(1):53–59.

Kornblith, A., J. Dowell, and I. Herndon. 2006. Telephone monitoring of distress in patients aged 65 years or older with advanced stage cancer: A cancer and leukemia group b study. *Cancer* 107(11):2706–2714.

Kruijver, I. P. M., B. Garssen, A. P. Visser, and A. J. Kuiper. 2006. Signalising psychosocial problems in cancer care: The structural use of a short psychosocial checklist during medical or nursing visits. *Patient Education and Counseling* 62(2):163–177.

Lecouturier, J., L. Crack, K. Mannix, R. H. Hall, S. Bond. 2002. Evaluation of a patient-held record for patients with cancer. *European Journal of Cancer Care* 11(2):114–121.

Liao, L., J. G. Jollis, E. R. DeLong, E. D. Peterson, K. G. Morris, and D. B. Mark. 1996. Impact of an interactive video on decision making of patients with ischemic heart disease. *Journal of General Internal Medicine* 11(6):373–376.

Linden, W., D. Yi, M. C. Barroetavena, R. MacKenzie, and R. Doll. 2005. Development and validation of a psychosocial screening instrument for cancer. *Health and Quality of Life Outcomes* 3:54.

Lowe, B., J. Unutzer, C. M. Callahan, A. J. Perkins, and K. Kroenke. 2004. Monitoring depression treatment outcomes with the Patient Health Questionnaire-9. *Medical Care* 42(12):1194–1201.

Maliski, S. L., L. Kwan, T. Krupski, A. Fink, J. R. Orecklin, and M. S. Litwin. 2004. Confidence in the ability to communicate with physicians among low-income patients with prostate cancer. *Urology* 64(2):329–334.

Maly, R. C., B. Leake, and R. A. Silliman. 2004. Breast cancer treatment in older women: Impact of the patient-physician interaction. *Journal of the American Geriatrics Society* 52(7):1138–1145.

Marshall, M., A. Gray, A. Lockwood, and R. Green. 2004. *Case management for people with severe mental disorders* (Cochrane Review, Issue 4). Chichester, UK: John Wiley and Sons, Ltd.

Mazur, D. J., and D. H. Hickam. 1997. Patients' preferences for risk disclosure and role in decision making for invasive medical procedures. *Journal of General Internal Medicine* 12(2):114–117.

Mazur, D. J., and J. F. Merz. 1996. How older patients' treatment preferences are influenced by disclosures about therapeutic uncertainty: Surgery versus expectant management for localized prostate cancer. *Journal of the American Geriatric Society* 44(8):934–937.

Mazur, D. J., D. H. Hickam, and M. D. Mazur. 2005. The role of doctor's opinion in shared decision making: What does shared decision making really mean when considering invasive medical procedures? *Health Expectations* 8(2):97–102.

McAlister, F. A., S. Stewart, S. Ferrua, and J. V. McMurray. 2004. Multidisciplinary strategies for the management of heart failure patients at high risk for admission. A systematic review of randomized trials. *Journal of the American College of Cardiology* 44(4):810–819.

McCorkle, R., N. Strumpf, I. Nuamah, D. C. Adler, M. E. Cooley, C. Jepson, E. J. Lusk, and M. Torosian. 2000. A specialized home care intervention improves survival among older post-surgical cancer patients. *Journal of the American Geriatrics Society* 48(12):1707–1713.

McDonald, K., V. Sundaram, D. Bravata, R. Lewis, N. Lin, S. Kraft, M. McKinnon, H. Paguntalan, and D. Owens. 2007. Care coordination. AHRQ Publication No. 04(07)-0051-7, Vol. 7. In *Closing the quality gap: A critical analysis of quality improvement strategies*. Edited by K. G. Shojania, K. M. McDonald, R. M. Wachter, and D. K. Owens. Rockville, MD: Agency for Healthcare Research and Quality. http://www.ahrq.gov/downloads/pub/evidence/pdf/caregap/caregap.pdf (accessed August 17, 2007).

McDonald, M. V., S. D. Passik, W. Dugan, B. Rosenfeld, D. E. Theobald, and S. Edgerton. 1999. Nurses' recognition of depression in their patients with cancer. *Oncology Nursing Forum* 26(3):593–599.

McLachlan, S. A., A. Allenby, J. Matthews, A. Wirth, D. Kissane, M. Bishop, J. Beresford, and J. Zalcberg. 2001. Randomized trial of coordinated psychosocial interventions based on patient self-assessments versus standard care to improve the psychosocial functioning of patients with cancer. *Journal of Clinical Oncology* 19(21):4117–4125.

Mitchell, A., and J. Coyne. 2007. Do ultra-short screening instruments accurately detect depression in primary care? A pooled analysis and meta-analysis of 22 studies. *British Journal of General Practice* 57(535):144–151.

National Breast Cancer Centre and National Cancer Control Initiative. 2003. *Clinical practice guidelines for the psychosocial care of adults with cancer.* Camperdown, NSN, Australia: National Health and Medical Research Council.

National Institute of Standards and Technology. 2007. *Baldrige National Quality Program: Health care criteria for performance excellence.* Gaithersburg, MD: United States Department of Commerce.

NCCN (National Comprehensive Care Network). 2006. Distress management. In *NCCN clinical practice guidelines in oncology.* http://www.nccn.org/professionals/physician_gls/PDF/distress.pdf (accessed August 10, 2006).

NCCN. 2007a. *Distress management (V.I.2007), 08-10-06.* http://www.nccn.org/professionals/physician_gls/PDF/distress.pdf (accessed January 17, 2007).

NCCN. 2007b. *National Comprehensive Cancer Network.* http://www.nccn.org/default.asp (accessed November 16, 2007).

NCCS (National Coalition for Cancer Survivorship). 2007. *Cancer survival toolbox®.* http://www.cancersurvivaltoolbox.org (accessed March 23, 2007).

NCI (National Cancer Institute). undated. *NCI community cancer centers program—frequently asked questions.* http://ncccp.cancer.gov/Media/FactSheet.htm (accessed August 27, 2007).

NICE (National Institute for Clinical Evidence). 2004. *Guidance on cancer services: Improving supportive and palliative care for adults with cancer: The manual.* http://ww.nice.org. uk/page.aspx?0=csgspfullguideline (accessed July 12, 2006).

Niederhuber, J. E. 2006. NCCCP increases patient access to quality cancer care. *NCI Cancer Bulletin* 3(43).

Norris, S. L., P. J. Nichols, C. J. Caspersen, R. E. Glasgow, M. M. Engelgau, L. Jack, G. Isham, S. R. Snyder, V. G. Carande-Kulis, S. Garfield, P. Briss, and D. McCulloch. 2002. The effectiveness of disease and case management for people with diabetes. A systematic review. *American Journal of Preventive Medicine* 22(Supplement 4):15–38.

O'Connor, A. M., H. A. Llewellyn-Thomas, and E. R. Drake. 1995. *An annotated bibliography of research on shared decision making.* Toronto, Ontario: National Cancer Institute of Canada.

Oeffinger, K. C., and M. S. McCabe. 2006. Models for delivering survivorship care. *Journal of Clinical Oncology* 24(32):5117–5124.

Onel, E., C. Hamond, J. H. Wasson, B. B. Berlin, M. G. Ely, V. P. Laudone, A. E. Tarantino, and P. C. Albertsen. 1998. Assessment of the feasibility and impact of shared decision making in prostate cancer. *Urology* 51(1):63–66.

Ouwens, M., H. Wollersheim, R. Hermens, M. Hulscher, and R. Grol. 2005. Integrated care programmes for chronically ill patients: A review of systematic reviews. *International Journal for Quality in Health Care* 17(2):141–146.

Palmer, L., and S. Somers. 2005. *Integrating long-term care: Lessons from building health systems for people with chronic illnesses.* A national program of The Robert Wood Johnson Foundation. Center for Health Care Strategies, Inc. http://www.chcs.org/usr_doc/ CHCSBHSFINAL.pdf (accessed January 24, 2007).

Passik, S., W. Dugan, M. McDonald, and B. Rosenfeld. 1998. Oncologists' recognition of depression in their patients with cancer. *Journal of Clinical Oncology* 16(4):1594–1600.

Peele, P. B., L. A. Siminoff, Y. Xu, and P. M. Ravdin. 2005. Decreased use of adjuvant breast cancer therapy in a randomized controlled trial of a decision aid with individualized risk information. *Medical Decision Making* 25(3):301–307.

Piccolo, L. D., A. Saltini, C. Zimmermann, and G. Dunn. 2000. Differences in verbal behaviors of patients with and without emotional distress during primary care consultations. *Psychological Medicine* 30(3):629–643.

Pignone, M. P., B. N. Gaynes, J. L. Rushton, C. M. Burchell, C. T. Orleans, C. D. Mulrow, and K. N. Lohr. 2002. Screening for depression in adults: A summary of the evidence for the U.S. Preventive Services Task Force. *Annals of Internal Medicine* 136(10):765–776.

Pincus, H. A. 2003. The future of behavioral health and primary care: Drowning in the mainstream or left on the bank? *Psychosomatics* 44(1):1–11.

Pruyn, J. F. A., H. A. G. Heule-Dieleman, P. P. Knegt, F. R. Mosterd, M. A. G. van Hest, H. A. M. Sinnige, A. T. H. Pruyn, and M. F. de Boer. 2004. On the enhancement of efficiency in care for cancer patients in outpatient clinics: An instrument to accelerate psychosocial screening and referral. *Patient Education & Counseling* 53(2):135–140.

Raftery, J., J. Addington-Hall, L. MacDonald, H. Anderson, J. Bland, J. Chamberlain, and P. Freeling. 1996. A randomized controlled trial of the cost-effectiveness of a district coordinating service for terminally ill cancer patients. *Palliative Medicine* 10(2):151–161.

Ramfelt, E., K. Lutzen, and G. Nordström. 2005. Treatment decision-making in a group of patients with colo-rectal cancer before surgery and a one-year follow-up. *European Journal of Cancer Care* 14(4):327–335.

RAND Corporation. 2007. *Overview of the partners in care study.* http://www.rand.org/ health/projects/pic/overview.html (accessed February 26, 2007).

Recklitis, C. J., S. K. Parsons, M.-C. Shih, A. Mertens, and L. Robinson. 2006. Factor structure of the brief symptom inventory—18 in adult survivors of childhood cancer: Results from the childhood cancer survivor study. *Psychological Assessment* 18(1):22–32.

Richards, S., and J. Coast. 2003. Interventions to improve access to health and social care after discharge from hospital: A systematic review. *Journal of Health Services and Research Policy* 8(3):171–179.

Robinson, J. W., and D. L. Roter. 1999. Psychosocial problem disclosure by primary care patients. *Social Science and Medicine* 48(10):1353–1362.

Rost, K. M., K. S. Flavin, K. Cole, and J. B. McGill. 1991. Change in metabolic control and functional status after hospitalization impact of patient activation intervention in diabetic patients. *Diabetes Care* 14(10):881–889.

Roter, D., J. Hall, and Y. Aoki. 2002. Physician gender effects in medical communication. *Journal of the American Medical Association* 288(6):756–764.

Roth, A. J., A. B. Kornblith, L. Batel-Copel, E. Peabody, H. I. Scher, and J. C. Holland. 1998. Rapid screening for psychologic distress in men with prostate carcinoma: A pilot study. *Cancer* 82(10):1904–1908.

Samet, J. H., P. Friedmann, and R. Saitz. 2001. Benefits of linking primary medical care and substance abuse services: Patient, provider, and societal perspectives. *Archives of Internal Medicine* 161(1):85–91.

Schmitt, M. 2001. Collaboration improves the quality of care: Methodological challenges and evidence from U.S. health care research. *Journal of Interprofessional Care* 15(1):47–66.

Schofield, P., and P. N. Butow. 2003. Psychological responses of patients receiving a diagnosis of cancer. *Annals of Oncology* 14(1):48–56.

Schwartzberg, L., B. Fortner, and A. Houts. 2007. *Use of technology to enhance doctor-patient interactions*. American Society of Clinical Oncology Education Book. Alexandria, VA: American Society of Clinical Oncology. Pp. 686–791.

Shortell, S., J. Zimmerman, D. Rousseau, R. Gillies, D. Wagner, E. Draper, W. Knaus, and J. Duffy. 1994. The performance of intensive care units: Does good management make a difference? *Medical Care* 32(5):508–525.

Siminoff, L. A., J. H. Rose, A. Zhang, and S. J. Zyzanski. 2005. Measuring discord in treatment decision-making; progress toward development of a cancer communications and decision-making assessment tool. *Psycho-Oncology* 15(6):528–540.

Siminoff, L. A., G. C. Graham, and N. H. Gordon. 2006a. Cancer communication patterns and the influence of patient characteristics: Disparities in information-giving and affective behaviors. *Patient Education and Counseling* 62(3):355–360.

Siminoff, L. A., N. H. Gordon, P. Silverman, T. Budd, and P. M. Ravdin. 2006b. A decision aid to assist in adjuvant therapy choices for breast cancer. *Psycho-Oncology* 15(11):1001–1013.

Sleath, B., and R. Rubin. 2003. The influence of Hispanic ethnicity on patients' expression of complaints about and problems with adherence to antidepressant therapy. *Clinical Therapeutics* 25(6):1739–1749.

Sleath, B., D. Roter, B. Chewning, and B. Svarstad. 1999. Asking questions about medication: Analysis of physician–patient interactions and physician perceptions. *Medical Care* 37(11):1169–1173.

Stewart, M. 1995. Effective physician–patient communication and health outcomes: A review. *Canadian Medical Association* 152(9):1423–1433.

Street, R. L. Jr., and H. S. Gordon. 2006. The clinical context and patient participation in post-diagnostic consultations. *Patient Education and Counseling* 64(1–3):217–224.

Street, R. L. Jr., E. Krupat, R. A. Bell, R. L. Kravitz, and P. Haidet. 2003. Beliefs about control in the physician–patient relationship. Effect on communication in medical encounters. *Journal of General Internal Medicine* 18(8):609–616.

Street, R. L. Jr., H. S. Gordon, M. M. Ward, E. Krupat, and R. L. Kravitz. 2005. Patient participation in medical consultations. Why some patients are more involved than others. *Medical Care* 43(10):960–969.

Stuck, A. E., M. Egger, A. Hammer, C. E. Minder, and J. C. Beck. 2002. Home visits to prevent nursing home admission and functional decline in elderly people: Systematic review and meta-regression analysis. *Journal of the American Medical Association* 287(8):1022–1028.

Thind, A., and R. Maly. 2006. The surgeon–patient interaction in older women with breast cancer: What are the determinants of a helpful discussion? *Annals of Surgical Oncology* 13(6):778–793.

Thompson, C., and M. Briggs. 2000. Support for carers of people with Alzheimer's type dementia. *Cochrane Database of Systematic Reviews* (2):CD000454.

Timmermans, L., R. W. van der Maazen, K. P. van Spaendonck, J. W. Leer, and F. W. Kraaimaat. 2006. Enhancing patient participation by training radiation oncologists. *Patient Education and Counseling* 63(1–2):55–63.

Trask, P. C. 2004. Assessment of depression in cancer patients. *Journal of the National Cancer Institute Monographs* 2004(32):80–92.

Trask, P. C., A. Paterson, M. Riba, B. Brines, K. Griffith, P. Parker, J. Weick, P. Steele, K. Kyro, and J. Ferrara. 2002. Assessment of psychological distress in prospective bone marrow transplant patients. *Bone Marrow Transplantation* 29(11):917–925.

Unutzer, J., W. Katon, J. W. Williams, C. M. Callahan, L. Harpole, E. M. Hunkeler, M. Hoffing, P. Arean, M. T. Hegel, M. Schoenbaum, S. M. Oishi, and C. A. Langston. 2001. Improving primary care for depression in late life. *Medical Care* 39(8):785–799.

Unutzer, J., W. Katon, C. M. Callahan, J. W. Williams, E. Hunkeler, L. Harpole, M. Hoffing, R. D. D. Penna, P. H. Noel, E. H. B. Lin, P. A. Arean, M. T. Hegel, L. Tang, T. R. Belin, S. Oishi, and C. Langston. 2002. Collaborative care management of late-life depression in the primary care setting. *Journal of the American Medical Association* 288(22):2836–2845.

U.S. Preventive Services Task Force. 2002. *Screening for depression.* http://www.ahrq.gov/clinic/uspstf/uspsdepr.htm (accessed February 21, 2007).

van Roosmalen, M. S., P. F. Stalmeier, L. C. Verhoef, J. E. Hoekstra-Weebers, J. C. Oosterwijk, N. Hoogerbrugge, U. Moog, and W. A. van Daal. 2004. Randomized trial of a shared decision-making intervention consisting of trade-offs and individualized treatment information for BRCA1/2 mutation carriers. *Journal of Clinical Oncology* 22(16):3293–3301.

Walsh-Burke, K., and C. Marcusen. 1999. Self-advocacy training for cancer survivors. The Cancer Survival Toolbox. *Cancer Practice* 7(6):297–301.

Walton, S., H. Bedford, and C. Dezateux. 2006. Use of personal child health records in the UK: Findings from the millennium cohort study. *British Medical Journal* 332(7536):269–270.

Weisner, C., J. Mertens, S. Parthasarathy, C. Moore, and Y. Lu. 2001. Integrating primary medical care with addiction treatment: A randomized controlled trial. *Journal of the American Medical Association* 286(14):1715–1723.

Wells, K. B., C. Sherbourne, M. Schoenbaum, N. Duan, L. Meredith, J. Unutzer, J. Miranda, M. Carney, and L. Rubenstein. 2000. Impact of disseminating quality improvement programs for depression in managed primary care: A randomized controlled trial. *Journal of the American Medical Association* 283(12):212–220.

Wells, K., C. Sherbourne, M. Schoenbaum, S. Ettner, N. Duan, J. Miranda, J. Unutzer, and L. V. Rubenstein. 2004. Five-year impact of quality improvement for depression: Results of a group-level randomized controlled trial. *Archives of General Psychiatry* 61(4):378–386.

Wen, K.-Y., and D. H. Gustafson. 2004. Needs assessment for cancer patients and their families. *Health and Quality of Life Outcomes* 2:11.

Whelan, T., M. Levine, A. Willan, A. Gafni, K. Sanders, D. Mirsky, S. Chambers, M. A. O'Brien, S. Reid, and S. Dubois. 2004. Effect of a decision aid on knowledge and treatment decision making for breast cancer surgery. A randomized trial. *Journal of the American Medical Association* 292(4):435–441.

Williams, J. G., W. Y. Cheung, N. Chetwynd, D. R. Cohen, S. El-Sharkawi, I. Finlay, B. Lervy, M. Longo, and K. Malinovszky. 2001. Pragmatic randomised trial to evaluate the use of patient held records for the continuing care of patients with cancer. *Quality in Health Care* 10(3):159–165.

Wong, F., D. Stewart, J. Dancey, M. Meana, M. P. McAndrews, T. Bunston, and A. M. Cheung. 2000. Men with prostate cancer: Influence of psychological factors on information needs and decision-making. *Journal of Psychosomatic Research* 49(1):13–19.

Woods, V. D., S. B. Montgomery, R. P. Herring, R. W. Gardner, and D. Stokols. 2006. Social ecological predictors of prostate-specific antigen blood test and digital rectal examination in black American men. *Journal of the National Medical Association* 98(4):492–504.

Xu, K., T. F. Borders, and A. A. Arif. 2004. Ethnic differences in parents' perception of participatory decision-making style of their children's physicians. *Medical Care* 42(4):328–335.

Zabora, J., K. BrintzenhofeSzoc, P. Jacobsen, B. Curbow, S. Piantadosi, C. Hooker, A. Owens, and L. Derogatis. 2001. A new psychosocial screening instrument for use with cancer patients. *Psychosomatics* 42(3):241–246.

Zachariae, R., C. Pederson, A. B. Jensen, E. Ehrnrooth, P. B. Rossen, and H. von der Maase. 2003. Association of perceived physician communication style with patient satisfaction, distress, cancer-related self-efficacy, and perceived control over the disease. *British Journal of Cancer* 88(5):658–665.

Zigmond, A., and R. Snaith. 1983. The hospital anxiety and depression scale. *Acta Psychiatrica Scandinavica* 67(6):361–370.

Ziguras, S. J., and G. W. Stuart. 2000. A meta-analysis of the effectiveness of mental health case management over 20 years. *Psychiatric Services* 51(11):1410–1421.

Ziguras, S. J., G. W. Stuart, and A. C. Jackson. 2002. Assessing the evidence on case management. *British Journal of Psychiatry* 181(1):17–21.

Zwarenstein, M., B. Stephenson, and L. Johnston. 2004. Case management: Effects on professional practice and health care outcomes: Protocol. *Cochrane Database of Systematic Reviews* (1).

5

Implementing the Standard of Care

CHAPTER SUMMARY

Chapter 4 put forth a model (standard of care) for addressing psychosocial health needs. This chapter presents real-life illustrations of how this standard is already being implemented by some oncology practices and can be implemented by others, illustrating the feasibility of meeting the standard of care in situations with varying levels of resources.

Patients diagnosed with cancer are treated by many different types of clinicians across all phases of their cancer care. Some of these clinicians specialize in oncology; others, such as primary care physicians and general surgeons, have a patient population that is more heterogeneous with respect to diagnosis. The committee believes that all clinicians providing care for patients with cancer should attend to psychosocial health needs as part of their practice, but that oncologists can and should lead the way in addressing these needs. The committee therefore recommends that all providers of cancer care institute reliable processes to meet the standard of psychosocial health care. The National Cancer Institute (NCI), organizations setting standards for cancer care, and consumer advocacy organizations should promote these efforts by incorporating the recommended standard of care into their agendas, protocols, policies, and standards. NCI, the Centers for Medicare & Medicaid Services, and the Agency for Healthcare Research and Quality, individually or together, should conduct a program designed to demonstrate additional approaches to meeting the standard of care in different geographic areas and care settings, with more vulnerable populations, and in locations with varying resources.

Cancer treatment is delivered in a variety of settings, including, for example, the practices of medical oncologists; primary care providers;

surgeons; radiologists; and other specialists, such as hematologists and urologists (see Table 5-1).[1] As stated in Chapter 4, the committee believes that the delivery of psychosocial health services should occur from diagnosis through all stages of the illness, and therefore, the standard for delivering psychosocial health care articulated in Chapter 4 should guide the activities of all clinicians delivering cancer care. Nonetheless, as adult and pediatric oncologists are recognized specialists in the delivery of cancer care, they should lead the way in implementing this standard of care. This chapter focuses on how they can do so.

APPROACHES TO THE DELIVERY OF
PSYCHOSOCIAL HEALTH SERVICES

As of 2005, an estimated 12,000 oncologists practiced in the United States in a variety of practice settings and arrangements, including teaching hospitals (33 percent), group practices (46 percent), solo practices (9 percent), and other arrangements. The majority of oncologists (56 percent) worked with nurse practitioners and physician assistants who provided patient education and counseling, pain and symptom management, follow-up care for patients in remission, and other activities as part of patient care (AAMC Center for Workforce Studies, 2007).

Oncology practices can take two general approaches to the delivery of psychosocial health services in accordance with the model and standard for care set forth in Chapter 4: (1) providing the needed services and interventions directly themselves by offering collocated, integrated psychosocial and biomedical health care, or (2) establishing effective linkages and coordination of care with other providers.[2] This chapter describes and provides real-life examples of both approaches. Also described is a third approach, a potential variation on the second that involves the use of remote providers of psychosocial health services and can be employed in communities that lack substantial psychosocial health care resources.

Many organizations blend these approaches, collocating some psychosocial health services on site while coordinating and supplementing

---

[1]The committee located no data describing how cancer care differs across these different settings of care.

[2]The committee recognizes that there are cases in which another party (e.g., another health care provider treating a serious comorbid condition or a designated intermediary, such as a disease management entity) also has responsibility for securing appropriate psychosocial health services. However, the committee does not distinguish this as a separate approach to implementing the model because coordination of care requires effective linkages among *all* parties involved, and because at present and for the foreseeable future, the committee believes that the dangers of too little attention to psychosocial problems outweigh the dangers of duplicative attention to those problems.

TABLE 5-1 Distribution of Adult Ambulatory Cancer Care Visits by Site of Visit, Physician Specialty, and Clinic Type, United States, 2001–2002[a]

Visit Characteristic	Number/Percentage
Annual number of visits (in 1,000s)	20,574
Site of visit (%)	
Physician's office	89
Hospital outpatient department	11
Physician office visits[b] (%)	
Oncology	18
Primary care	32
General surgery	10
Specialty surgery	3
Dermatology	7
Urology	14
Other medical specialty	15
Hospital outpatient department[c] (%)	
General medicine	78
Surgery	14
Other	8

[a]Adults were categorized as being aged 25 and older. Visits for non-melanoma skin cancer were excluded.
[b]Radiologists were excluded from the sample of office-based physicians.
[c]Clinics providing chemotherapy, radiotherapy, physical medicine, and rehabilitation were excluded from the sample of hospital outpatient departments.
SOURCE: Analyses of the 2001 and 2002 National Ambulatory Medical Care Survey and the National Hospital Ambulatory Medical Care Survey, as presented in IOM and NRC, 2006.

their services with the delivery of other services from off-site providers. As discussed in Chapter 4, there is some evidence that collocated, integrated services are more effective than arrangements with off-site providers in ensuring that patients receive necessary care (Friedmann et al., 2000). Integrating psychosocial health care into medical care settings also facilitates patient follow-through on referrals, and allows for better communication between individuals caring for patients and easy exchange of expertise (Pincus, 2003). Studies of care collaboration also have shown that physical proximity facilitates collaboration among health care providers (IOM, 2004). However, when physical collocation of services is not possible, other strategies for linking patients with needed services are required.

Approach 1: Collocated, Integrated Psychosocial and Biomedical Health Care

In this approach, all components of the model described in Chapter 4 (identification of individuals with psychosocial health needs, care planning, linking of patients to providers of the needed services, support for patients in illness self-management, coordination of psychosocial with biomedical health care, and follow-up) take place at the same site where biomedical health care is provided, as well as some psychosocial health services. The physical plant and personnel requirements for implementing this approach are substantial. Examples are found in clinics attached to academic medical centers, but also in some leading community-based oncology practices.

Examples

The Rebecca and John Moores Cancer Center, University of California, San Diego   The Moores Cancer Center's Science of Caring Program provides comprehensive psychosocial health care integrated with biomedical treatment for all patients with cancer seen in its outpatient clinic. At each outpatient's initial visit, patient and family meet with a social worker who provides printed information about the psychosocial health services offered on site and an orientation to these services. At this first visit (and at regular intervals thereafter), every patient also uses a laptop computer to complete a simple touch-screen questionnaire—"How Can We Help You and Your Family?"—developed by the center. The questionnaire consists of a list of problems faced by patients with cancer. Patients are asked to identify the extent to which each problem affects them and whether they would like any help in dealing with it. Patients' responses (encrypted for privacy) are quickly disseminated by e-mail to their health care team of physicians, nurses, psychologists, and social workers. The data are also transmitted automatically to a software program that allows for their analysis.

Patients are linked to needed psychosocial health services in multiple ways. First, the computer-based screening program provides an automatic link. For some problems, such as those involving transportation, the program generates a printout of resources that is presented to patients by administrative staff[3] at the end of their appointment. For problems requiring a more complex intervention, the automated screening tool generates an e-mail to the team member with the expertise to address the problem. Full-time, on-site social workers also provide case management and refer patients to a wide variety of psychosocial health services available on site (e.g., support groups, educational seminars, psychotherapy, stress management) and from providers in the community.

Psychosocial care is coordinated with medical care by several means. The collocation of psychosocial and biomedical services facilitates timely

---

[3]Administrative staff also receive training and monthly updates on the value of the screening process.

and direct face-to-face communication among providers. Additional communication takes place during weekly team meetings and monthly meetings with community partners. A designated community health program manager creates linkages between the cancer center and community groups. The center has integrated, on-site relationships with The Wellness Community, the American Cancer Society (ACS), San Diego Hospice, and ACS's Cancer Navigator Program, among others. Patients and families receive help in illness self-management through an individualized orientation program designed to empower, inform, and guide them through treatment. A centrally located Patient and Family Education Center staffed by trained volunteers (most of whom are cancer survivors) offers computers with guided navigation to sources of information and services; information in print and video form; and donated items such as blankets, pillows, hats, and wigs. A Patient Advisory Council chaired by a family caregiver also meets monthly and makes specific recommendations to center leadership. For example, the council reviewed the center's physical plant before the center opened, and reviews all marketing materials, website designs, and patient education materials.

Follow-up on the receipt of needed services, their effectiveness, and the need for any changes occurs in multiple ways. Rescreening of each patient takes place whenever there is a change in treatment (unless the person was screened within the past 30 days) or every 2 months, whichever comes first. Program evaluation also takes place on a quarterly basis when a random chart audit is performed.

The program staff includes eight social workers, one psychologist, one psychology fellow, a part-time psychiatrist, one community outreach manager, and many students. Social workers are funded with "hard money" as part of the center's ongoing personnel budget. Although the psychologist bills for services provided, complete reimbursement often does not occur because of low payment rates and failure to receive any reimbursement when the provider is outside the network of some third-party insurers (see Chapter 6 for a discussion of this issue). Funding for the psychosocial program comes from philanthropy, the cancer center itself, clinical fees, shared programs with community groups, and grants. The director of the program spends substantial time fundraising for an endowed foundation to cover the costs of nonreimbursed services.

As a result of this year-and-a-half-old program, the center's scores on its annual Press-Ganey Oncology Outpatient patient satisfaction survey have tripled. The director identifies two characteristics of the program as key to its success: (1) the collocation and integration of its services with biomedical cancer care; and (2) its active alliances with community organizations (e.g., the center implements programs for The Wellness Community at the center and in the community, and The Wellness Community in turn pays in part for the services of a psychologist).[4]

The West Clinic, Memphis, Tennessee[5]   The West Clinic consists of three free-standing ambulatory oncology practices in metropolitan Memphis plus three satellite offices 60–90 minutes away from the main offices. Screening of patients for psychosocial health problems and quality-of-life assessment take place at every visit by means of the computer-based Patient Care Monitor (PCM) screening instrument (described in Chapter 4), which quickly collects information from individuals about their cancer-related symptoms while they are in the waiting room before meeting with the clinician. Validated instruments gauge pain levels, fatigue, and mental health status. Results are scored and attached to the patient's chart. More in-depth assessment of individuals experiencing significant distress is provided by psychologists located at the largest site (but able to travel to other sites as needed).

For some psychosocial health problems, patients receive the needed services directly on site; for others, they are referred to resources in the community by clinic nurses and social workers on an ad hoc basis. Some psychosocial services are offered at the three main ambulatory oncology clinics through on-site psychologists, social workers, nurses, palliative care specialists, other professional psychosocial staff, and volunteers, with dedicated space provided for nonclinical activities. A quality-of-life interview and information session with a psychologist are offered to every patient and family prior to the start of treatment. Many psychosocial services are also provided by West Clinic's approximately 200 trained[6] volunteers through a practice-based 501c3 foundation created by the clinic (Wings Cancer Foundation). Coordination of psychosocial and biomedical care is accomplished through collocated psychosocial and medical personnel.

The Wings Cancer Foundation offers support to patients and families in illness self-management through support groups, a lending library, nutritional counseling, exercise and strength building, yoga and relaxation classes, and crisis intervention. In addition, a separate patient education system provides wireless, notebook-sized computers (e-tablets) that patients use while waiting for their appointments or receiving treatment. The e-tablets deploy a proprietary intranet or Internet-based system called the Cancer Support Network, which provides patients with targeted educational

---

[4]Personal communication, Matthew J. Loscalzo, MSW, Director of Patient and Family Support Program, Rebecca and John Moores UCSD Cancer Center, March 12, 2007.

[5]Personal communication, Lee Schwartzberg, MD, Medical Director, April 13, 2007.

[6]Volunteers undergo formal training on such issues as patient safety, communication, and the Health Insurance Portability and Accountability Act.

information in text, graphic, video, and audio formats on a wide range of topics such as pain management, symptoms and treatment of psychological distress, and other matters relevant to cancer care.

The West Clinic credits the commitment of its leadership for its success in building the infrastructure and resources needed to deliver integrated psychosocial and biomedical health services in the context of a community-based practice.

Discussion

As discussed in Chapter 4, the benefits of collocated, integrated psychosocial and biomedical health care services include better access to needed services for patients and greater ease of communication and coordination between collocated providers. Moreover, some comprehensive programs, such as that of the Moore Center, offer their services to the community at large. The difficulties of this approach are that it requires a physical plant large enough to accommodate diverse personnel and a sufficiently large and varied labor pool in the community to staff interdisciplinary teams. Moreover, some experts in pediatric cancer care report that some cancer survivors do not want to receive services from the center in which they received their cancer care when it is no longer necessary because of negative emotions associated with the facility, a desire to "get on with their life," or the geographic inaccessibility of the facility (Friedman et al., 2006). When collocation of services is either infeasible or undesirable, psychosocial health services can be obtained through other community providers (Approach 2) or potentially through providers located remotely from the patient using telephone or Internet access (Approach 3).

Approach 2: Provision of Psychosocial Health Services Using Local Resources

Examples

Kansas City Cancer Center[7] (KCCC) is a full-service medical and radiation oncology practice that includes 29 medical oncologists, 8 radiation oncologists, and 11 oncology nurse practitioners (NPs) and oncology certified nurses. The center addresses patients' psychosocial health problems not by providing the needed services on site to the approximately 200–300 patients seen each day at its 11 urban/suburban locations, but by linking patients with community providers.

---

[7]Personal communication, John E. Hennessy, Nancy J. Washburn, and Barbara W. Adkins, Kansas City Cancer Center, March 13, 2007.

KCCC NPs screen patients at their initial and subsequent visits using a one-page screening tool to detect depression, pain, fatigue, and other problems. If the patient answers yes to either of the first two questions (a two-question depression screening tool), the Patient Health Questionnaire-9 (PHQ-9) screening tool for depression is administered to help determine whether the patient is in fact experiencing depression. Positive findings are addressed using a treatment algorithm standardized across clinical sites (Adkins et al., 2005).[8] If an intervention is established, the NP documents it in a note that the physician reviews so as to be able to follow up on the symptoms. The patient may also have a follow-up visit with the NP. NPs and physicians often alternate seeing patients in order to assess the physical, psychosocial, and spiritual needs of patients.

Based on the results of the screen and periodic psychosocial assessments, KCCC nurses link patients with multiple psychosocial services available in the Kansas City area. Cancer Action, for example, is a community-based nonprofit agency in Kansas City offering an array of programs and services that address the physical, social, emotional, financial, and spiritual needs of people with cancer and their families and friends. All Cancer Action programs and services are free of charge (see http://www.canceractionkc.org). For patients who are uninsured or underinsured, Swope Parkway Health Center, Catholic Charities, the Alliance for the Mentally Ill of Greater Kansas City, Samuel Rodgers Health Center, and Kansas City Free Health Clinic offer mental health counseling either free of charge or on a sliding scale. KCCC also has partnered with Metro CARE, WyJoCARE, and Northland CARE, organizations of specialists that have agreed to take a limited number of uninsured patients. For patients who are working, many employers have employee assistance programs that offer counseling free of charge. If the employees need further counseling, KCCC refers them to a counselor for continuation of care. If there is no employee assistance program where patients work, they are referred based on their insurance.

KCCC also partners with Turning Point: The Center for Hope and Healing, a 5-year-old 501c3 organization whose mission is to strengthen resilience in individuals living with cancer or other serious or chronic illnesses by providing education and other tools to help them manage their illness and live life to its fullest. Turning Point served approximately 3,400 people in the Kansas City area in 2006; approximately 85 percent of these were cancer patients, 55 percent of whom were referred by KCCC. The more than 50 different education and support programs provided by Turning Point to adults, children, families, and friends include counseling; exercise classes; nutrition classes; and specialized classes such as Surviving

---

[8]KCCC partnered with the Mid America Coalition for Health Care to create the treatment algorithm. The coalition also recommended the use of the PHQ-9 tool.

and Thriving, a comprehensive program for those having completed cancer treatment and having no signs of disease, as well as a program for people being treated for stage 3 or 4 cancer. Group programs are provided free of charge to participants as a result of extensive partnerships with area health care providers, employers, and others whose contributions pay for the services. Although individual counseling generally requires payment of a fee, Kansas City Turning Point provides up to five counseling visits free of charge to KCCC patients or family members if the patient has advanced disease. Turning Point is unique in that its services are not just for individuals dealing with cancer, an approach that may be more feasible in less densely populated areas that may have fewer patients with cancer and fewer community organizations dedicated to cancer care. The number of individuals being served by Turning Point is growing at an average rate of 64 percent annually.[9]

KCCC NPs also help patients manage their illness by providing them detailed, one-on-one education on treatment and management of the side effects of chemotherapy. Psychosocial health issues are addressed not only during but also after treatment. KCCC has a survivorship program that provides education about the adjustments required after treatment. Patients are given the *LiveStrong*® Survivorship Notebook, which contains information on the emotional effects of cancer. In addition, NPs meet with patients approximately 2 months after completion of treatment to address survivorship issues.

Care coordination and follow-up are provided by the NPs, who perform these activities as part of their regular patient care. KCCC bills and receives reimbursement for NP assessment, linkage, coordination, and follow-up activities from both government and nongovernment payors (this reimbursement approach is discussed in Chapter 6). No other foundation or special funding subsidizes these activities. KCCC does have a fund set up with the greater Kansas City Community Foundation, but is restricted from using these funds to subsidize the costs of operations; rather, this money is used to fund communitywide cancer education, awareness, and prevention activities. Another fund, created by one patient's family, provides oral chemotherapy drugs to patients who cannot afford them; this fund is administered by Cancer Action, which processes applications and determines eligibility.

Tahoe Forest Cancer Center (TFCC), located in Truckee, California (in the Lake Tahoe community), is another example of using community resources to deliver psychosocial health services to patients with cancer. In this case,

---

[9]Personal communication, Moira A. Mulhern, PhD, CEO of Turning Point, March 15, 2007.

a major source of resources is the community's 30-bed hospital, Tahoe Forest Hospital. A relocated oncologist and Tahoe Forest Hospital created a solo physician ambulatory oncology practice that routinely incorporates attention to psychosocial health needs as part of oncology care. The solo oncologist uses hospital personnel to help address psychosocial needs of patients.

TFCC's multidisciplinary staff of oncology nurses, social workers, physical therapists, and others are employees of the hospital (which also owns the free-standing ambulatory oncology office). Through these staff (who also work at the hospital), TFCC offers psychological services; social services; nutritional counseling; rehabilitation therapy; and support group meetings for cancer patients, family, and friends at the hospital's local Center for Health and Sports Performance. TFCC also offers the *Look Good . . . Feel Better Program*® and provides or links to a variety of other patient supports and resources on its website (http://www.tahoecancercenter. com).

Patients with psychosocial needs are identified during office visits or weekly meetings of the entire team. (The center does not yet use a standard screening tool.) Physicians link patients to psychosocial services by checking off "psychosocial evaluation" on a disposition sheet after patient visits. The staff schedules an appointment with the social worker, who then provides the necessary linkages to the psychosocial team. Coordination of biomedical and psychosocial care takes place at weekly team meetings. Follow-up is performed at these meetings and in the interim by TFCC nurses. Patients are supported in managing their cancer and its treatment in several ways. Each patient receiving chemotherapy spends 1 hour with a TFCC nurse for education about chemotherapy. In addition, patients receive customized printouts from the American Society of Clinical Oncology's (ASCO's) *People Living with Cancer* that provide specific details regarding their disease and planned treatments. TFCC also solicits volunteers from the community to provide assistance and companionship to patients receiving chemotherapy and help with other patient needs. TFCC's 250 patients are covered by a variety of insurers, including Medicare (18 percent), commercial insurance (61 percent), and Medicaid (19 percent); 2 percent pay out of pocket or are uninsured.[10]

Discussion

This approach is feasible for many oncology providers because of substantial growth in the number of providers of psychosocial health services

---

[10]Personal communication. Laurence J. Heifetz, MD, Medical Director, Tahoe Forest Cancer Center, August 10, 13, and 28, 2007.

in many communities. According to the report, *From Cancer Patient to Cancer Survivor: Lost in Transition,* "There is a wealth of cancer-related community support services available through voluntary organizations, many of them at no cost" (IOM and NRC, 2006:229). These services include, for example, nationwide programs of ACS, The Wellness Community, Gilda's Clubs, and other organizations that offer community-based services at many sites nationwide (some of these are summarized in Tables 3-2 and 3-3 in Chapter 3). These services also include regional, state, and local programs, such as Cancer Action in Kansas City and Sunstone Cancer Support Centers in southern Arizona (see http://www.sunstone healing.org/index.htm). This approach does not require physical space or a large staff. It does, however, require that organizations making referrals to other providers do so effectively, and that the referring organization have strong follow-up procedures in place.

Approach 3: Use of Remote Providers of Psychosocial Health Services

When a clinical practice has few staff and limited resources and/or is located where there are few or no psychosocial health care resources, such as in rural or remote areas, the only way to provide psychosocial health services on a frequent and timely basis may be to link patients with remote providers through telephone or Internet access. The NCI report *Patient Centered Communication in Cancer Care,* for example, notes that "telephone help lines can be a useful source of information and emotional support for patients with cancer" (Epstein and Street, 2007:138), and individuals with a recent cancer diagnosis, for example, often use NCI's Cancer Information Service to obtain information about cancer treatments in preparation for meeting with their clinician (Epstein and Street, 2007). Even practices that elect to deliver a wide variety of psychosocial health services directly may not by themselves be able to provide all of the services needed by every patient, and may still need to provide links to remote services. For example, despite the well-developed nature and breadth of services it provides, Moores Cancer Center refers many of its patients to CancerCare each month for educational programs and financial assistance.

This alternative may also be preferred by some individuals, even when psychosocial health services are available in their communities. Those with rare cancers may wish to connect with others who have their type of cancer, but find that the rarity of their condition means that this is impossible within their community. Others may simply desire the convenience or anonymity of receiving psychosocial services via the telephone or the Internet in their own homes. Adolescents and young adults who use the Internet routinely for multiple purposes also may prefer this mode of communicating.

Using remote resources to provide psychosocial health services to patients requires only that oncology providers have a mechanism for identifying patients with psychosocial needs; knowledge of a few key organizations providing a wide array of psychosocial health services to individuals with many different types of cancer (e.g., NCI's Cancer Information Service, ACS, CancerCare, the Lance Armstrong Foundation, and The Wellness Community); a way to support patients in accessing these resources by telephone or Internet; and a process for follow-up to ensure that patients accessed the services and that the services met their psychosocial health needs. Following is a discussion of how an organization with limited internal and local resources could address psychosocial needs following the model put forth in Chapter 4. This approach may not always be able to meet all psychosocial health needs; for example, some of the needed services, such as assistance with activities of daily living and chores, may not be available remotely. Nonetheless, this should not prevent providers from directing patients to remote resources that can meet as many of their needs as possible.

Implementation of the Use of Remote Resources

Clinical practices with limited resources can set the stage for effective patient–provider communication and delivery of psychosocial health services by communicating with patients about psychosocial health services at the outset of care. This could be accomplished, for example, through a short "Letter to My Patients" given to all patients at their first visit.[11] This letter could inform patients about the importance of communicating effectively and the relevance of psychological and social issues to their health and health care. Box 5-1 contains a sample letter that oncology practices could adapt to their own characteristics—for example, the extent to which a practice uses a team approach to care.

Practices could then use one of the low-tech approaches discussed in Chapter 4 that require few personnel and other resources to help identify patients with psychosocial health needs. The National Comprehensive Cancer Network's (NCCN's) Distress Thermometer, for example is a one-page screening tool, publicly available at no cost, that can be self-administered in less than a minute. This tool could be duplicated using an office copy machine and presented by clinical or administrative staff to all patients each time they come in for a visit along with other routine paperwork, such as insurance forms. When completed, the screening tool could be attached to the patient's chart and reviewed by the clinician together with the patient during the visit. To the extent that a clinician's evaluation of psychological

---

[11]This letter could also be used by clinical practices with greater internal and community resources.

**BOX 5-1
A Letter to My Patients**

Dear Partner in Care,

As we work together to treat your cancer, I will work very hard to give you the best health care for your cancer. As I do this, I will need your help in two important ways.

First, you and I will need to talk with each other as clearly as we can. Medical words can be hard to understand, and this office can be very busy, but you and the people important to you need to understand your illness, its treatment, and all their effects. If I or my staff don't explain things well enough or listen well enough, please tell us.

We also need you to tell us what is on your mind. For example, what questions do you have? How much information do you want to know? What is important to you as you decide about different treatments for your cancer?

COMMUNICATING WELL IS IMPORTANT TO YOUR CARE!

Second, emotional worries and problems that might not seem related to your health care actually are. Having worries, fears, or other emotional problems can make you feel more tired, have more pain, sleep more poorly, and get in the way of good health care—all of which affect your heath. Your health is also affected by problems such as not being able to pay for medications; not having a phone, transportation, or health insurance; or not being able to work.

At every visit, we will ask you to check off a list of any emotional or other problems you may be having. Although we may not be able to solve all of these problems ourselves, we know organizations that can help with many of them—and these are often just a toll-free phone call away.

PAYING ATTENTION TO YOUR EMOTIONAL AND SOCIAL
NEEDS IS PART OF HEALTH CARE TOO!

Please let me or other members of our health care team know if you have any questions. We want to give you the best health care possible!

---

and social problems added substantial time to the visit, the clinician could bill at a higher rate if reimbursed on a fee-for-service basis (see Chapter 6), although there is some evidence that use of a screening tool could reduce visit length (Pruyn et al., 2004).

All practices should be able to provide at least some of the psychosocial health services needed by patients—for example, information about the patient's diagnosis and treatment options, emotional support, and help in managing some of the symptoms of the illness and side effects of treatment.

For those psychosocial health service needs that exceed the practice's capabilities (e.g., material or logistical resources or peer support), the practice could have available a one-page handout listing organizations that can provide key psychosocial health services and can be accessed using a toll-free phone number. An example of such a patient handout is provided in Box 5-2. This handout could be adapted to include other resources, especially those locally available. The reverse side could include a broader list of resources for those who are comfortable with and have easy access to the Internet.

Follow-up with patients to check on their receipt of psychosocial health services and the effectiveness of the services could be accomplished either by checking with the patient at the next visit through the repeated use of the original screening tool, by monitoring between visits through telephone calls by office staff, or by asking patients or their caregivers to inform the practice if their psychosocial health care needs are not being met.

Remote Resources

As shown in Tables 3-2 and 3-3 in Chapter 3, a substantial number of nonprofit organizations provide psychosocial health services at no cost to patients via toll free phone lines, interactive Internet sites, or e-mail inquiry and response services. Virtual communities providing emotional support, information, and sometimes other psychosocial health services also are now commonplace. Their services are available to many cancer patients as a result of such Internet-based initiatives as those of PlanetCancer (http://www.planetcancer.org/html/index.php), which serves young adults, and The Wellness Community (http://www.thewellnesscommunity.org), which offers professionally led Internet support groups and educational programs to adults with all types of cancers via the Internet, in addition to its 21 Wellness Communities and 28 satellite centers at physical locations across the United States. As of June 30, 2006, 1,103 people were participating in the Wellness Community's 11 online support groups, 7 tumor-specific and mixed-diagnosis groups, 3 caregiver groups, 1 bereavement group, 1 teen group, and 1 Spanish-language group.

Another remote resource is the telephone education workshops provided by CancerCare for cancer patients, caregivers, and other interested persons. Approximately 2,000 people from the United States and countries such as Australia, Canada, China, Spain, and the United Kingdom attended each of three such workshops held in the first half of 2007. The utility of the workshops is indicated by the comments of those in attendance (see Box 5-3).

CHESS (Comprehensive Health Enhancement Support System) is another Internet-based resource that can provide remote information,

---

BOX 5-2
Example of Patient Handout on Sources of Help
in Managing Cancer and Its Treatment

If you need more information about your cancer and its treatment, you can call:

The National Cancer Institute. Information specialists can answer many questions about cancer, including most recent treatment advances.

By telephone Monday through Friday, 9:00 AM to 4:30 PM within all time zones across the United States: 1-800-4-CANCER (1-800-422-6237) and 1-800-332-8615 (TTY for the hearing impaired) (both toll free)
Service in English and Spanish

Questions can also be sent via e-mail to: cancergovstaff@mail.nih.gov

A "live" help service is available to answer general questions about cancer and provide help in navigating the NCI website at https://cissecure@nci.nih.gov/livehelp/welcome.asp#

The American Cancer Society

By telephone 24 hours a day, every day: 1-800-ACS-2345 and 1-866-228-4327 (TTY for the hearing impaired) (both toll free)
By the Internet at: http://www.cancer.org/asp/contactUs/cus_global.asp

If you need practical help, such as finding wigs or transportation or assistance with financial problems, you can call:

The American Cancer Society (same as above)

CancerCare

By telephone Monday through Thursday, 9:00 AM to 7:00 PM Eastern Standard Time, and Friday, 9:00 AM to 5:00 PM Eastern Standard Time (no weekend phone service): 1-800-813-HOPE (1-800-813-4673) (toll free)
By the Internet at: http://www.cancercare.org

If you would like to talk to someone about your concerns about having cancer or other concerns or talk with others who are living with cancer, you can call:

The American Cancer Society (same as above)

CancerCare (same as above)

---

emotional support, and decision-making and problem-solving assistance to people with cancer and other chronic illnesses (e.g., asthma, HIV, heart disease) and caregivers of persons with memory disorders and dementia. The design of the program is based on the results of literature reviews, needs assessment surveys typically involving several hundred patients and families,

BOX 5-3
Patient Comments on the Usefulness of
CancerCare's Telephone Education Workshops

My husband and I got a lot of good information from this workshop—very good advice at a difficult time for us. These programs are so helpful. Living in a rural area we don't always have the resources nearby.

Thank you for helping me to understand the aftermath of my treatment, what to look forward to and how to manage it.

What a fabulous way to reach people who, like me, are in remote areas and have limited access to support. This forum provides a much-needed service.

Thank you for your teleconferences. It keeps us in rural areas up on the latest.

I can't thank you enough for making these available via telephone for those of us in treatment or unable to travel.

Of course my own oncologist can't spend an hour talking with me. I feel so blessed that [these calls] provide me with top experts and up-to-the-minute information.

The topic was one I haven't seen presented anywhere else. It was very easy to call in and take part in the conference. I'm glad I did and I'm looking forward to the next one.

Thank you!!! When my aunt suffered breast cancer 20 years ago, she had to go it alone because she was too sick to get to support groups. I not only have email, but your teleconferences and the ability to refer to the podcast again to review points I may have missed. Thank you for taking advantage of technology for my benefit.

I actually listened via cell phone, while on vacation, sitting on the veranda of a grand old lodge, on one of Georgia's beautiful barrier islands, overlooking a wonderful marshy waterway that leads to the Atlantic. It was the best way I've ever found to deal with cancer issues!

The call-in portion was also very instructive given the fact that my wife and I have many of the same questions. After the discussion on "rocker" sole shoes, we found a location last Saturday and purchased a pair that is already giving me some needed comfort.

I can even participate in a conference during lunch or when I'm traveling. It's incredibly versatile and educational, useful and extremely helpful.

Keep these workshops coming. The more we know, the more able we are to judge if we are getting good and up-to-date care out here in rural areas.

I love these programs. They keep me up-to-date and I can go back to my doctor and we talk about all I have learned and I feel very in the know.

Thank you for offering these sessions and for offering them free of charge. They really do help survivors and offer a huge community service. Thank you for also offering the listening session after the workshop so those that miss the session can still hear the information.

SOURCE: CancerCare, 2007.

focus groups and interviews, and an ongoing demonstration. Because it addresses multiple conditions, the program can serve as a "one stop" resource for individuals who have other illnesses in addition to cancer.

CHESS services are accessed through home-based computers (organizations using the program often lend computers to patients who do not have them). As an example, information services for prostate cancer include brief answers to 400 frequently asked questions, links to more than 200 articles from the scientific and popular press, and WebLinks to connect users to other high-quality websites specific to the illness. A resource director also identifies local and national services and ways to connect with them. For emotional support, CHESS offers patients and families bulletin board–style discussion groups, each of which is limited to 50 participants and is professionally facilitated. *Ask an Expert* provides confidential responses to questions via NCI's cancer information service. Personal stories written by professional writers who interview people with cancer, as well as videos, show how individuals have managed problems frequently identified through needs assessments. Analysis, assessment, and decision-support services help patients think through issues important to them and make behavior changes. A health-tracking program collects data on an individual's health status every 2 weeks and charts change over time. The design of CHESS accommodates various coping and information-seeking styles by tailoring information and support to users' interests.

A team of decision, medical, information, and communication experts designs the decision-making and health-tracking tools. All CHESS modules are pilot-tested, then further refined on the basis of patient and clinician feedback before being released for dissemination. Modules are updated regularly to ensure that their content is accurate, relevant, and current and to improve their ease of use. All information is reviewed and updated (if needed) annually by advisory panels that include a range of professionals and patients. Intra-CHESS links and links to external websites also are checked biweekly. Patient feedback is actively solicited to identify voids in information and guide the development of system enhancements. Clinicians at participating research sites are encouraged to provide ideas for how CHESS can be adapted to better meet their needs. In addition, health care organizations are urged to review the content of modules before using them with their patients. Suggestions, questions, or feedback on the program content can be e-mailed to CHESS.

CHESS has been studied extensively across multiple illnesses, including cancer, and in a number of different ways, ranging from randomized trials and field tests designed to assess its impact on quality of life (Pingree et al., 1996; Gustafson et al., 1999; Shaw et al., 2006) to evaluation of the cost and effectiveness of different methods for disseminating the CHESS systems (Gustafson et al., 2005a,b). Results of these studies show positive effects on multiple dimensions, including emotional well-being, functional well-being, competence in dealing with health information, participation in health care, and quality of life. Other important findings are that underserved populations used CHESS more than socially advantaged populations and that they used it for different purposes. The former used the program more often to locate and analyze information and the latter more to participate in discussion groups (Gustafson et al., 2001, 2002).

Formerly a demonstration program, CHESS is now an ongoing program with continued operation and updating provided by the University of Wisconsin Comprehensive Cancer Center. Oncology practices and individual patients desiring to use it can do so.[12] The CHESS breast cancer program is available on the web in English and Spanish versions. The English version (Living with Breast Cancer) can be accessed at http://www.uwchessbc.org. The Spanish-language site, "Conviviendo con el Cancer de Seno," is a cultural and linguistic translation of the existing online Living with Breast Cancer program. The translation was performed by a multinational team from Mexico, Argentina, and Venezuela with guidance from the Dane County Latino Health Council. Partners, including the National Latino Cancer Research Network and the Center for Patient Partnerships, provided additional Latina-specific content. Conviviendo con el Cancer de Seno can be accessed at http://www.chess.wisc.edu/espanol/.[13]

Discussion

As useful as approaches such as The Wellness Community, CHESS, and other online and telephone services may be, there are some obstacles to their use. First, not all consumers may have access to the technology or the ability to use it in their homes, even if it is provided to them. Patients using entry-level computers with slow modems can be "timed out" by their Internet provider during a support session, causing an interruption in their participation. Second, it may not be possible to deliver all needed psychosocial health services on line. Delivery of mental health services over the Internet is still an evolving technology, and other services, such as cognitive testing, educational support, and support in performing activities of daily living, must still be provided directly. Nevertheless, telephone and Internet support can be used to provide some psychosocial health services, and clinicians should not let an inability to ensure the provision of all such services prevent their taking action to ensure the provision of as many as possible.

---

[12]By contacting 1-800-361-5481.
[13]Personal communication, David Gustafson, University of Wisconsin–Madison, July 10, 2007, and Fiona McTavish, Deputy Director of CHESS, July 16, 2007.

RECOMMENDATIONS

Based on the evidence presented in Chapters 3 and 4 and the additional evidence presented in this chapter on the feasibility of providing psychosocial health services in accordance with the standard recommended in Chapter 4, the committee makes the following recommendations.

Recommendation: Health care providers. All cancer care providers should ensure that every cancer patient within their practice receives care that meets the standard for psychosocial health care. The National Cancer Institute should help cancer care providers implement the standard of care by maintaining an up-to-date directory of psychosocial services available at no cost to individuals/families with cancer.

In making this recommendation, the committee appreciates that patients diagnosed with cancer are treated for their illness by many different types of providers—some specializing in oncology and others, such as primary care physicians and general surgeons, who have a patient population that is more heterogeneous with respect to diagnosis. Patients with cancer may make up a minority of patients seen by the latter clinicians. The committee believes that all providers should implement the above recommendation, but appreciates that those whose practices are not devoted to oncology may have other strategies, standards, and expectations placed on them by experts in the care of patients with other diseases. While the committee believes that the standard of psychosocial health care has applicability to all chronic diseases (as illustrated by the breadth of clinical conditions addressed by the models of care reviewed in Table 4-1 in Chapter 4), it calls upon oncology practices to lead the way in implementing this standard of care and providing cancer care "for the whole patient."

In making this recommendation, the committee also appreciates that there is not currently as ample a supply of psychosocial services as is necessary to meet all the needs of all patients, and some problems (such as a lack of health insurance and poverty) can be addressed only in a small way. Nevertheless, the committee urges all involved in the delivery of cancer care not to allow the perfect to be the enemy of the good. The inability to solve all psychosocial problems permanently should not preclude attempts to remedy as many as possible—a stance akin to treating cancer even when a successful outcome is not assured. Patient education and advocacy organizations can play a key role in bringing this about.

Recommendation: Patient and family education. Patient education and advocacy organizations should educate patients with cancer and their family caregivers to expect, and request when necessary, cancer care that meets the standard for psychosocial care. These organizations should also continue their work on strengthening the patient side of the patient–provider partnership. The goals should be to enable patients to participate actively in their care by providing tools and training in how to obtain information, make decisions, solve problems, and communicate more effectively with their health care providers.

Finally, the organizational, financial, and size differences among cancer care practices may influence the strategies providers use to implement the standard of care. For example, the economics of collocation and care coordination is affected by the volume of cases. Local resources also influence the way in which care is organized.

The committee concluded that evidence is sufficient to establish a standard for the delivery of psychosocial health care to patients with cancer. At the same time, as discussed in Chapter 4, much of the research underpinning this recommendation comes from populations with diseases other than cancer, and evidence in support of the individual components of the model is of variable strength. Thus a large-scale, systematic program demonstrating and evaluating the effects of the implementation of the standard of psychosocial health care at various oncology sites (e.g., comprehensive cancer centers attached to medical centers, freestanding oncology practices, and smaller oncology practices located outside of urban areas) would provide useful information about different ways to implement the standard as a whole and its individual components more efficiently in oncology practices and the impact of doing so. Demonstrating the model of care in general medical practices would provide additional valuable information. Patients with cancer may not constitute the majority of the patients of such practices, and a demonstration could address how these practices could implement the standard of psychosocial care. For example, would such a practice adopt the standard only for patients with cancer, for patients with other complex conditions as well, or for all patients? Such a demonstration program would allow the model to be honed over time and generate additional examples of how it can be implemented efficiently and effectively.

Moreover, measuring such outcomes as reductions in unmet needs and levels of distress, adherence to treatments, and cost-effectiveness would make it possible to compare different approaches to implementing the standard. A demonstration also could document effects of and approaches for successful implementation of the standard among vulnerable groups, such as those with low socioeconomic status, ethnic minorities, those with low health literacy, older adults, and the socially isolated. In addition, such a demonstration could examine different models of reimbursement, reveal additional ways of implementing the standard in resource-rich and non-resource-rich environments, and test the feasibility and soundness of performance measures for psychosocial health care. The demonstration could also examine how various types of personnel can be used to perform specific types of interventions and how those personnel can best be trained.

Recommendation: Support for dissemination and uptake. The National Cancer Institute, the Centers for Medicare & Medicaid Services (CMS), and the Agency for Healthcare Research and Quality (AHRQ) should, individually or collectively, conduct a large-scale demonstration and evaluation of various approaches to the efficient provision of psychosocial health care in accordance with the standard of care. This program should demonstrate how the standard can be implemented in different settings, with different populations, and with varying personnel and organizational arrangements.

REFERENCES

AAMC Center for Workforce Studies. 2007. *Forecasting the supply of and demand for oncologists: A report to the American Society of Clinical Oncology (ASCO) from the AAMC Center for Workforce Studies.* http://www.asco.org/ASCO/Downloads/ Cancer%20Research/Oncology%20Workforce%20Report%20FINAL.pdf (accessed August 15, 2007).

Adkins, B., T. Titus-Howard, V. Massey, N. Washburn, J. Molinaro, B. Lange, W. L. Bruning, S. Simmons, P. Gerken, V. Sommer, K. LaNoue, B. Rogers, and B. Wilson. 2005. Recognizing depression in cancer outpatients. *Community Oncology* 2(6):528–533.

CancerCare. 2007. *CancerCare Connect™ telephone education workshop: Report to the National Cancer Institute and Lance Armstrong Foundation unpublished data.* New York: CancerCare.

Epstein, R. M., and R. L. Street. 2007. *Patient-centered communication in cancer care: Promoting healing and reducing suffering.* Bethesda, MD: National Cancer Institute.

Friedman, D. L., D. R. Freyer, and G. A. Levitt. 2006. Models of care for survivors of childhood cancer. *Pediatric Blood & Cancer* 46(2):159–168.

Friedmann, P., T. D'Aunno, L. Jin, and J. Alexander. 2000. Medical and psychosocial services in drug abuse treatment: Do stronger linkages promote client utilization? *HSR: Health Services Research* 35(2):443–465.

Gustafson, D. H., R. Hawkins, E. Boberg, S. Pingree, R. E. Serlin, F. Graziano, and C. L. Chan. 1999. Impact of a patient-centered, computer-based health information/support system. *American Journal of Preventive Medicine* 16(1):1–9.

Gustafson, D. H., R. Hawkins, S. Pingree, F. McTavish, N. K. Arora, J. Mendenhall, D. F. Cella, R. C. Serlin, F. M. Apantaku, J. Stewart, and A. Sainer. 2001. Effect of computer support on younger women with breast cancer. *Journal of General Internal Medicine* 16(7):435–445.

Gustafson, D. H., R. P. Hawkins, E. W. Boberg, F. McTavish, B. Owens, M. Wise, H. Berhe, and S. Pingree. 2002. CHESS: 10 years of research and development in consumer health informatics for broad populations, including the underserved. *International Journal of Medical Informatics* 65(3):169–177.

Gustafson, D. H., F. McTavish, W. Stengle, D. Ballard, E. Jones, K. Julèsberg, H. McDowell, W. C. Chen, K. Volrathongchai, and G. Landucci. 2005a. Use and impact of ehealth system by low-income women with breast cancer. *Journal of Health Communication* 10(Supplement 1):157–172.

Gustafson, D. H., F. M. McTavish, W. Stengle, D. Ballard, E. Jones, K. Julèsberg, H. McDowell, G. Landucci, and R. Hawkins. 2005b. Reducing the digital divide for low-income women with breast cancer: A feasibility study of a population based intervention. *Journal of Health Communication* 10(Supplement 1):173–193.

IOM (Institute of Medicine). 2004. *Keeping patients safe: Transforming the work environment of nurses.* A. E. K. Page, ed. Washington, DC: The National Academies Press.

IOM and NRC (National Research Council). 2006. *From cancer patient to cancer survivor: Lost in transition.* M. Hewitt, S. Greenfield, and E. Stovall, eds. Washington, DC: The National Academies Press.

Pincus, H. A. 2003. The future of behavioral health and primary care: Drowning in the mainstream or left on the bank? *Psychosomatics* 44(1):1–11.

Pingree, S., R. Hawkins, D. Gustafson, E. Boberg, and E. Bricker. 1996. Can the disadvantaged ride the information highway? Hopeful lessons from a computer assisted crisis support system. *Journal of Broadcasting and Electronic Media* 40:331–353.

Pruyn, J. F. A., H. A. G. Heule-Dieleman, P. P. Knegt, F. R. Mosterd, M. A. G. van Hest, H. A. M. Sinnige, A. T. H. Pruyn, and M. F. de Boer. 2004. On the enhancement of efficiency in care for cancer patients in outpatient clinics: An instrument to accelerate psychosocial screening and referral. *Patient Education and Counseling* 53(2):135–140.

Shaw, B., D. Gustafson, R. Hawkins, F. McTavish, H. McDowell, S. Pingree, and D. Ballard. 2006. How underserved breast cancer patients use and benefit from ehealth programs: Implications for closing the digital divide. *American Behavioral Scientist* 49(6): 823–834.

6

Public- and Private-Sector Policy Support

CHAPTER SUMMARY

Policies set by public and private purchasers, oversight bodies, and other health care leaders shape how health care is accessed, what services are delivered, and the manner in which they are delivered. Many of these policies already support the provision of some psychosocial health care. The decision by Medicare and leading purchasers in the private sector to pay for behavioral health assessments and interventions is a strong example of these policies, as is Medicare's recent decision to increase payment levels for patient evaluation and management services. However, other reimbursement policies have not kept pace with the evidence for the strong influence of psychological and social problems on health care and outcomes set forth in Chapter 2. Reimbursement approaches for care coordination for individuals with complex needs are not well articulated. Restrictions on which clinicians can be paid can make it difficult to access those with special expertise and present a barrier to the collocation of clinical oncology and mental health services—a situation that is problematic since collocation is an effective approach for increasing access to mental health services and coordination of those services with biomedical care. Moreover, the results of many studies finding that poor-quality health care is widespread show that reimbursement by itself does not ensure the provision of needed health care services. Reimbursement and other incentives need to be aligned with quality measurement and improvement activities, which currently are inadequate in addressing psychosocial health services.

To overcome these obstacles, the committee recommends that group purchasers of health care coverage, health plans, and quality oversight

organizations take a number of actions to fully support the interventions
necessary to deliver effective psychosocial health services. The National
Cancer Institute, the Agency for Healthcare Research and Quality, and
the Centers for Medicare & Medicaid Services also should spearhead the
development and use of performance measures to improve the delivery of
these services.

SUPPORTS FOR AND CONSTRAINTS ON INTERVENTIONS TO DELIVER PSYCHOSOCIAL SERVICES

Chapter 4 delineates the processes that all oncology providers need
to have in place to ensure that the psychosocial problems affecting their
patients' health care and outcomes are effectively addressed. These include processes that (1) support effective patient–provider communication;
(2) identify individuals with psychosocial health needs; (3) link patients
with service providers; (4) coordinate psychosocial and biomedical care;
(5) help patients manage their illness; and (6) follow up to ensure the effectiveness of services. The need for these processes is already recognized
by many group purchasers, insurers, and other policy makers, as reflected
in their policies (see Table 6-1 and the discussion that follows). Other policies, however, do not reflect existing evidence on the need for and methods
of delivering psychosocial health care.

Medicare policies are of particular interest for several reasons. Because
60 percent of new cancer cases occur among people aged 65 and older,
Medicare is the principal payer for cancer care (IOM, 1999). Moreover,
Medicare typically pays about 83 percent of what private insurers pay
(MEDPAC, 2007); therefore, to the extent that Medicare payment rates
allow for reimbursement of practice expenses related to the processes enu-
merated above, reimbursement by private payers should do so to a greater
extent. Medicare also is a leader in technology assessment and coverage
determinations; its decisions are often followed by private-sector insurers.
Finally, Medicare's policies on coverage determination and rate setting are
more visible to the public than those of the private sector, enabling their
study. This section reviews key Medicare reimbursement policies and their
effects on the provision of psychosocial health services to individuals with
cancer. The discussion encompasses both "traditional" Medicare payments
to physicians—payments made to individual health care clinicians on a fee-
for-service (FFS) basis *after* an individual patient has made an outpatient
visit or undergone a procedure—and Medicare's *advance* (prospective,
capitated) payments to managed care and other health plans for the delivery
of an array of inpatient and outpatient services that a Medicare beneficiary
may need over a specified period of time (the Medicare Advantage [MA]

program).[1] Policies of private insurers and of Medicaid, the State Children's Health Insurance Program (SCHIP), and other government programs also are discussed as data are available.

Policies Addressing Effective Patient–Provider Communication

As indicated in Table 6-1, a few large-scale policy initiatives are under way to promote more effective patient–provider communication in general.[2] The Cancer Survival Toolbox (available free of charge) teaches people living with cancer how to obtain information, make decisions, solve problems, and generally communicate more effectively with health care providers (NCCS, 2007). The *Questions Are the Answer* Campaign (AHRQ, 2007b) and *Ask Me 3*™ initiative (Partnership for Clear Health Communication, undated) also encourage all patients to ask questions of their providers.

Policy support for the provider side of the patient–provider partnership is illustrated by the efforts of the Veterans Health Administration, whose Employee Education System provides mandatory and optional classes on such topics as clinician–patient communication to enhance health outcomes, communication to affect behavior change, and disclosure of unanticipated outcomes and medical errors. Other initiatives to improve patient–provider communication by organizations such as Kaiser Permanente, Geisinger Health System, the American Academy of Orthopedic Surgeons, Affinity Health System, and Washington State University are chronicled by the Institute for Healthcare Communication (2005), which has conducted more than 9,000 workshops for more than 120,000 clinicians and health care workers on improving communications between clinician and patient. Further support is provided by the Agency for Healthcare Research and Quality's (AHRQ's) Consumer Assessment of Healthcare Providers and Systems (CAHPS) Clinician and Group Survey Instruments. This ambulatory care survey tool has separate versions for adult specialty care and adult and child primary care, each containing multiple questions specifically asking patients about how their physician communicated and shared decision making with them (AHRQ, 2007a). In addition to these instruments' potential use as performance measures, the American Board of Medical Specialties (ABMS) is pursuing use of the specialty version to help determine physician competency in effective communication as part of its Maintenance

---

[1]MA plans serve approximately 17 percent of Medicare beneficiaries (MEDPAC, 2007).

[2]Many more initiatives are in place to improve provider communication with members of cultural and ethnic minorities and other vulnerable populations.

TABLE 6-1 Examples of Policy Support for Interventions to Deliver
Psychosocial Health Care

Interventions (from Figure 4-1 in Chapter 4)	Medicare	Medicaid/SCHIP
Support for Effective Patient–Provider Communication (excluding initiatives providing information on services only and those focused solely on cross-cultural communication)		

Private Insurance	Other Government Programs	Other Private Sector
• Some health plans and providers make patient–provider communication a priority throughout their organization. See examples at Institute for Healthcare Communication: http://www.healthcarecomm.org/index.php	Support is provided by: • Agency for Healthcare Research and Quality's (AHRQ) *Questions Are the Answer* campaign • AHRQ's Consumer Assessment of Healthcare Providers and Systems (CAHPS) Clinician and Group Survey questions on effective provider communication and shared decision making • Veterans Health Administration's mandatory and optional courses on effective communication for all employees and National Symposium on Clinician-Patient Communication • National Cancer Institute's (NCI): –Research Symposium on Consumer–Provider Communication in 2002 –Synthesis of literature on physicians' communication behaviors in cancer care and generally –State-of-the-science report *Patient-Centered Communication in Cancer Care* puts forth a comprehensive research agenda addressing patient-provider communication (Epstein and Street, 2007)	Support is provided by: • Accreditation Council for Graduate Medical Education (ACGME) Outcome Project competencies on residents' interpersonal and communication skills • American Board of Medical Specialties' Maintenance of Certification initiative • Cancer Survival Toolbox • Joint Commission *Speak Up*™ initiatives • Partnership for Clear Health Communication's *Ask Me 3*™ Initiative

continued

TABLE 6-1 Continued

Interventions (from Figure 4-1 in Chapter 4)	Medicare	Medicaid/SCHIP
Identification of Psychosocial Needs	• Medicare law generally proscribes fee-for-service (FFS) reimbursement for "screening," but screening still occurs in FFS and Medicare Advantage plans in several ways • Medicare FFS also provides full coverage for health and behavior assessment	Coverage and reimbursement vary by state, but generally: • Some screening covered for children under age 21 through the Medicaid Early Periodic Screening, Diagnosis, and Treatment (EPSDT) benefit • Coverage of Health and Behavior Current Procedural Terminology (CPT) codes varies by state
Care Planning; Linking of Patients with Psychosocial Services; Coordination of Psychosocial and Biomedical Care; Follow-up	• Some reimbursement is provided as part of FFS payments for medical Evaluation and Management (E/M) services, and payments for some E/M services increased in 2007 • Medicare Advantage plans' more flexible reimbursement also allows for these services • Multiple demonstration projects are ongoing to test models of care coordination	• Medicaid payments are generally low, but states' Primary Care Case Management (PCCM) programs offer some financial support, as do state Medicaid agency contracts with managed care plans; as of 2005, 25 states offered PCCM services with some limits • Most states also offer "targeted case management" to certain beneficiaries to enable access to and coordination of necessary medical, social, and educational care and other service needs (CMS, 2005a)

Private Insurance	Other Government Programs	Other Private Sector
• Coverage of mental health screening varies by health plan • Coverage for health and behavior assessment CPT codes is provided by many insurers	Other government programs reimburse or provide services to identify psychosocial needs, e.g., • Department of Veterans Affairs Medical Centers annually screen all patients for depression and alcohol misuse prompted by patients' computerized medical records • Older Americans Act programs also perform needs assessments	Voluntary organizations offer mental health screenings
• Some support is provided through nurse support systems for patients established by some private insurers • Some support also provided through the E/M billing codes reimbursed by private insurers • Managed care plans' more flexible reimbursement also facilitates these services (see, e.g., AHIP, 2007)	Support is provided by Maternal and Child Health Programs for Children with Special Health Care Needs	Support is provided by American Cancer Society's Patient Navigator program

continued

TABLE 6-1 Continued

Interventions (from Figure 4-1 in Chapter 4)	Medicare	Medicaid/SCHIP
Support for Illness Self-Management	• Full coverage is provided for Health and Behavior Intervention CPT codes • Patient and family instruction/education in managing illness is provided for in E/M codes • Multiple care coordination demonstrations are teaching illness management practices	• Patient and family instruction/education in managing illness is provided for in E/M codes, but Medicaid payment rates are lower than those of private insurance and Medicare, which may be a disincentive to provide these services

of Certification initiative.[3] A CAHPS specialty version could be used in oncology practices as a way to systematically measure and help improve patient–provider communication.

Despite the above initiatives to help patients and providers communicate more effectively, the limited number and scope of such initiatives constrains improvement in this area. The new CAHPS Clinician and Group Survey instruments can provide a vehicle to help educate both patients and providers and facilitate clinicians' adoption of new communication behaviors, but mechanisms need to be in place to collect the data from patients and relay them back to providers in ways that will improve communication. These mechanisms (discussed later in this chapter) are not yet in place. In addition, although ineffective patient–provider communication is not typically identified as resulting from a failure to reimburse for effective communication, financial incentives to see greater numbers of patients (and thereby limit providers' time with each patient) are sometimes cited as

---

[3]The ABMS Member Boards helped develop the three versions of the survey—one for adult primary care, one for proceduralists/surgeons, and one for pediatricians. The impetus for these efforts was the need for instruments to measure patient care experiences and physician–patient communication as an aspect of physician competence in the ABMS Maintenance of Competence Program. Personal communication, Stephen Miller, MD, President, ABMS, March 23, 2007.

Private Insurance	Other Government Programs	Other Private Sector
• Some coverage is provided for Health and Behavior Intervention CPT codes • Managed care plans' more flexible reimbursement also facilitates these services (see, e.g., AHIP, 2007) • Patient and family instruction/education in managing illness is provided for in E/M codes • Some telephonic case management or nurse support systems offered by some private insurers offer support	• Administration on Aging grant program to states and local communities, *Empowering Older People to Take More Control of Their Health through Evidence-Based Prevention*, requires use of illness self-management	• Large number of programs offered in the voluntary sector (see Chapter 3) • Employer programs and policies such as Employee Assistance Programs and leave policies, e.g., availability of extended leave of absence, flex time work hours, and unscheduled leave

a barrier to addressing psychosocial issues (Astin et al., 2006). Reimbursement policies could be structured in ways that would reward providers with the best performance in communicating with patients.

Policies Addressing the Identification of Psychosocial Needs

As discussed in Chapter 4, two general means are used to identify patients' psychosocial needs reliably: screening for problems, followed by an assessment, or bypassing screening and conducting a more comprehensive assessment by itself. Given the brevity of several reliable and valid screening instruments (as discussed in Chapter 4) and the fact that many of these instruments can be self-administered by the patient (often in the waiting room prior to contact with the physician, also as discussed in Chapter 4), the resources required to administer such instruments may not be substantial, although following up on numerous, complex needs thus identified may be, as discussed below.

Screening

Although FFS Medicare generally does not pay explicitly and separately for screening services (except when coverage for a specific screening

procedure is explicitly added to the Medicare statute by congressional action), this may not be a major barrier to the performance of psychosocial
screening by itself. First, the exemplar organizations described in Chapter
5 (and others identified by the committee but not discussed in this report)
all perform screening and more in-depth assessment under a variety of scenarios. These practices provide some evidence of the feasibility of screening
under current policies. Second, MA private plans are not restricted to offering services explicitly allowed under Medicare's FFS statutory provisions.
MA plans (especially health maintenance organization [HMO]–type plans,
as opposed to preferred provider organizations [PPOs] and private FFS
plans) often offer benefits beyond those in FFS Medicare, such as routine
health exams, some care coordination, and eyeglasses. Managed care plans
in the private sector also often offer additional services. For example, in
2005 *Aetna* began an initiative offering financial incentives to primary care
physicians to identify and care for certain health plan enrollees with depression. Primary care physicians who serve *Aetna* enrollees are trained in the
use of the Patient Health Questionnaire-9 (PHQ-9) depression screening
tool, are supplied with care management resources designed to support
patients and primary care providers, and have access to mental health
specialists for collaborative consultation (Moran, 2006). For every patient
identified though screening as positive for symptoms of depression, *Aetna*
pays the physician $15.00.[4]

Moreover, brief screening for some conditions takes place and is reimbursed as part of Medicare's FFS payment for office visits. For example,
when a nurse takes a patient's blood pressure at each routine visit, this is
essentially screening for hypertension. Similarly, if a primary care provider
incorporates depression screening or screening for alcohol misuse into a
visit for evaluation or management of physical symptoms or an already
documented medical condition, these screening services are included in
Medicare's payment for Evaluation and Management (E/M) services—one
of the most commonly delivered health services. Such screening is explicitly identified as a component of E/M services in the Current Procedural
Terminology (CPT) codes[5] reimbursed by all payers (public and private)
(Beebe et al., 2006).

---

[4]Personal communication, Hyong Un, MD, National Medical Director for Behavioral
Health, Aetna, March 29, 2007.

[5]CPT, maintained by the American Medical Association, is a listing of medical services and
procedures (and an accompanying numerical code for each) used by physicians and certain
other clinicians (e.g., physician assistants, nurse practitioners, and nurse midwives) to report
the services and procedures they perform as part of their claims to insurers for reimbursement.
CPT codes are designated by the federal government as the national standard for coding such
services.

Assessment of Psychosocial Needs

Assessing and following up on psychosocial problems takes more time than screening; as a result, payment becomes more of an issue. In 2002, new Health and Behavior Assessment and Intervention (H/B) codes were incorporated into the CPT coding set generally used by all ambulatory health care providers when submitting a claim for reimbursement.[6] At the time, these codes were described as a "paradigm shift" (Foxhall, 2000) because they allowed direct billing—by nonphysicians such as clinical psychologists—for psychosocial services for general medical illnesses such as diabetes or heart disease as opposed to mental illnesses. The new codes were intended to allow behavioral health specialists to address psychological, behavioral, emotional, cognitive, and social problems interfering with patients' ability to manage their physical illnesses. Prior to the new codes, the only way to deliver such services was to submit a bill for a mental health intervention, which required a diagnosis of mental illness.

Of note, when the American Psychological Association put forth its proposal for the adoption of these codes, the following pediatric oncology case study was used as one example of the range of interventions the codes were intended to capture:

> A 5-year-old boy undergoing treatment for acute lymphoblastic leukemia is referred for assessment of pain and severe behavioral distress and combativeness associated with repeated lumbar punctures and intrathecal chemotherapy administration. Previously unsuccessful approaches had included pharmacologic treatment of anxiety (Ativan), conscious sedation using Versed, and finally, chlorohydrate, which only exacerbated the child's distress as a result of partial sedation. General anesthesia was ruled out because the child's asthma increased respiratory risk to unacceptable levels.
>
> Intervention: The patient was assessed using standard questionnaires (e.g., the Information-Seeking scale, Pediatric Pain Questionnaire, Coping Strategies Inventory), which, in view of the child's age, were administered in a structured format. The medical staff and child's parents were also interviewed. On the day of a scheduled medical procedure, the child completed a self-report distress questionnaire. Behavioral observations were also made during the procedure using the CAMPIS-R, a structured observation scale that quantifies child, parent, and medical staff behavior.[7]

As defined in the 2007 CPT coding manual (Beebe et al., 2006:410–411),

---

[6]Reimbursement generally does not take place without a code to describe accurately the service delivered.

[7]Personal communication, Diane Pedulla, JD, American Psychological Association, January 5, 2007.

Health and behavior assessment procedures are used to identify the psychological, behavioral, emotional, cognitive, and social factors important to the prevention, treatment, or management of physical health problems.

The focus of the assessment is not on mental health but on the biopsychosocial factors important to physical health problems and treatments. The focus of the intervention is to improve the patient's health and well-being utilizing cognitive, behavioral, social, and/or psychophysiological procedures designed to ameliorate specific disease-related problems.

Codes 96150-96155 describe services offered to patients who present with primary physical illnesses, diagnoses, or symptoms and may benefit from assessments and interventions that focus on the biopsychosocial factors related to the patient's health status . . .

96150 health and behavior assessment (e.g., health-focused clinical interview, behavioral observations, psychophysiological monitoring, health-oriented questionnaires), each 15 minutes face-to-face with the patient, initial assessment
96151 re-assessment
96152 health and behavior intervention, each 15 minutes, face-to-face; individual
96153 group (2 or more patients)
96154 family (with the patient present)
96155 family (without the patient present).

Each of the H/B codes refers to a 15-minute intervention; interventions requiring more time are billed by reporting multiple units of service. For example, a 30-minute assessment would be billed as two units of 96150. Currently, these codes are used most often by clinical psychologists.

The use of these codes and the delivery of the behavioral health services they represent are growing. Table 6-2 shows Medicare trend data for reimbursement of these services during 2003–2005 as reported by the American Psychological Association. All Medicare carriers now reimburse claims for services using these codes (except 96155, which Medicare does not cover). Although the extent to which private insurers and state Medicaid programs reimburse for these codes is not comprehensively tracked, in early 2007 an American Psychological Association list serve contained anecdotal reports of denial of reimbursement for these services by Medicaid, and coverage by private-sector health plans is not yet uniform.[8]

---

[8]Personal communication, Alan Nessman, American Psychological Association, March 27, 2007.

TABLE 6-2 Psychologist Claims Paid by Medicare, 2003–2005, by Type of Intervention, and Comparison 2005 Claims Paid for All Provider Types

Code	Description	2003 Psychologist Claims	2004 Psychologist Claims	2005 Psychologist Claims	2005 All Provider Claims
96150	H/B Assessment	50,660	74,371	78,008	90,016
96151	H/B Reassessment	51,888	47,599	18,421	21,913
96152	H/B Intervention—face-to-face, individual	136,904	245,088	291,103	300,463
96153	H/B Intervention—group (two or more patients)	9,252	16,431	17,873	34,052
96154	H/B Intervention—family (with patient present)	6,129	7,003	7,508	7,942
96155	H/B Intervention—family (without patient present)	Medicare does not reimburse for this type of intervention			
Total		254,833	390,492	412,913	454,386

SOURCE: American Psychological Association analysis of data from the Centers for Medicare & Medicaid Services' Physician/Supplier Procedure Summary Master File.

Policies Addressing Care Planning, Linking of Patients to Psychosocial Services, Care Coordination, and Follow-Up

Current Support in Fee-for-Service Reimbursement

Addressing patients' identified psychosocial needs by planning, linking patients to service providers, coordinating psychosocial with biomedical care, and following up on the receipt and effectiveness of services is provided for to some extent in existing FFS reimbursement policy. Although perhaps not always recognized (Adiga et al., 2006), the CPT codes for E/M services (reimbursed by all public- and private-sector insurers) explicitly (1) provide for physicians' need to take patients' "social history" and "relevant social factors" into account in evaluating and managing their symptom(s), condition, or illness; (2) provide for clinicians' review of mental health status; and (3) include "coordination of care with other providers or agencies . . . consistent with the nature of the problem(s) and the patient's and/or family's needs" as part of their definition. These codes also acknowledge that sometimes coordination of care may be the predominant purpose of an E/M visit: "When counseling and/or coordination of care dominates (more than 50%) of the physician/patient and/or family encounter . . . , then **time** [emphasis in original] may be considered the key or controlling factor to qualify for a particular level of E/M services" (Beebe et al., 2006:8). Further, the different levels of E/M services (and concomitant increasing payment levels) incorporate the time physicians spend before and after their face-to-face contact with patients performing such tasks as "arranging for further services, and communicating further with other professionals and the patient through written reports and telephone contact" (Beebe et al., 2006:5). This is one reason why Medicare does not reimburse separately for telephone contacts on a patient's behalf. Although there are separate CPT codes for telephone calls of varying length, Medicare considers this service to be bundled into the E/M CPT codes (CMS, 2006a).[9] Medicare's 2007 Payment Schedule, which went into effect on January 1, increased payments for some E/M services (e.g., code 99213, office visit for an established patient) (CMS, 2006a,b), but reduced payments for others (e.g., code 99203, office visit for a new patient) (Ginsburg and Berenson, 2007).

Thus, just as Medicare does not reimburse clinicians separately for the individual steps of performing a physical exam, taking a patient's history, making a diagnosis, and developing a treatment plan, it also does not pay separately for planning for meeting nonmedical service needs, making referrals and otherwise linking patients with other service providers, and coordinating care. In the past, when most health care was dominated by acute conditions, this payment strategy may not have attracted much attention, but as the conditions addressed by health care providers are increasingly those of older adults and those with chronic illnesses, these aspects of providing high-quality health care and the way clinicians are reimbursed for them are undergoing more scrutiny.

Further, although E/M codes typically can be used only by physicians and other practitioners licensed to practice independently (e.g., nurse practitioners and physician assistants), reimbursement for E/M services could also support the costs of nurses, social workers, or other personnel (e.g., patient navigators) employed by medical practices to assist in coordinating the care of their patients (MEDPAC, 2006). This potential exists by virtue of the way in which Medicare determines the rates it pays for E/M services.

---

[9]Reimbursement for telephone calls is problematic for other reasons. First, for both provider and payer, the costs of submitting, paying, and collecting on claims for reimbursement of calls would in many cases likely be greater than the reimbursement itself. Second, major difficulties are involved in ensuring financial integrity (i.e., auditing the number and length of calls). Third is the risk of "moral hazard"—an insurance concept denoting the phenomenon that occurs when an event is in the control of the insured, and the insured may wish the event (e.g., telephone calls) to occur. In such cases, the event does not well lend itself to the statistical principles that govern insurance (Berenson and Horvath, 2003).

The amount Medicare pays for a specific physician service is based in part on the relative value units (RVUs) Medicare assigns to that service compared with other types of physician services. (There are more than 7,000 Medicare-covered services, each with its own assigned RVUs.) Each service's RVUs are a composite of three factors: (1) the time and intensity of the direct work performed by physicians (or other practitioners licensed to practice independently) to provide the service (Work RVUs); (2) the practice expenses (PEs) associated with the service, such as costs of office space, supplies, equipment, and other clinical and administrative staff (PE RVUs); and (3) professional liability insurance RVUs.[10] To the extent that all physicians' clinical practices in the aggregate include nurses, medical assistants, social workers, or other support personnel who aid in planning, linking, coordinating, and following up on psychosocial service needs, this is reflected in physician PEs. Thus, to the extent that physicians typically employ such staff in their practices, Medicare indirectly reimburses for the services provided by these support personnel whenever it pays a claim for E/M services. Medicare payments then reflect what *is* current typical care, rather than what *should be.* The result is a situation in which clinicians may not want to invest in advanced work systems and personnel to provide better care because Medicare payments do not fully reimburse for them, while at the same time, Medicare payments do not well reimburse for these expenditures in part because physicians are not typically making them.

Limitations of Fee-for-Service Reimbursement

Despite the inclusion of care coordination functions in the definition of E/M codes, the potential to capture the costs of care coordination activities performed by other clinical and administrative personnel as part of physicians' PEs, the increase in Medicare reimbursement for some E/M services that took place in January 2007, and the adequacy of Medicare payment rates for physician services overall (MEDPAC, 2007), FFS payments may reimburse inadequately for the costs of planning, linking, coordination, and follow-up for several reasons. First, the care coordination work included in the definition of each E/M code refers only to the work performed by the physician or other licensed clinician with independent billing privileges (e.g., nurse practitioner). The time spent on this work by other support personnel may not be used to determine clinicians' billing for E/M services. Moreover, for Medicare, the practice expense portion of reimbursement

---

[10]Medicare's actual payment rate for each E/M CPT code is then determined by an equation that assigns a dollar amount to the individual RVU (a monetary "conversion factor"), multiplied by a geographic adjustment factor to account for cost variations in different geographic areas.

is based on survey data, with the aim of identifying the current typical practice expenses of physicians in general. To the extent that assistance with planning, linking, coordination, and follow-up on needed psychosocial services is currently limited in physician practices in general, estimates of the associated physician practice expenses will be limited as well. This situation financially penalizes practices that have in place mechanisms and personnel to help address patients' psychosocial needs; these practices will be reimbursed the same amount as those that have not taken such steps or have done so to a lesser degree.[11] Perhaps most important, experts have identified some fundamental limitations in the data sources and approaches used to calculate Medicare payment rates that have resulted in erosion of payment rates for E/M services over time (Ginsburg and Berenson, 2007).

Because of the above limitations of indirect reimbursement for planning, linking, coordination, and follow-up activities, some advocate that Medicare and other private insurers reimburse directly for explicit case management or care coordination services. Medicare FFS does not do so at present, and clinical practices participating in The Robert Wood Johnson Foundation's Depression in Primary Care Initiative found that likewise, "Few, if any explicit care management billing codes are recognized by third party payers, especially private insurers" (Bachman et al., 2006:280). Moreover, it is not clear to what extent insurers that do reimburse for case management services do so for the full array of psychosocial health services, rather than paying for a benefit that includes only coordination of biomedical care from multiple providers or a more limited array of services.

Several fundamental issues would need to be resolved if explicit reimbursement for case management/care coordination were to be implemented. First, the subset of patients for whom such services would be reimbursed would need to be identified. All patients with psychosocial health care needs require some degree of planning, linking, coordination, and follow-up, and this level of service is provided for in the construct of E/M services as described above. Most case management/care coordination initiatives target individuals with higher-than-average needs, sometimes with the expectation that the added services will generate lower costs. How should the subset of individuals for whom additional reimbursement is required be identified? Moreover, the entity that is to assume responsibility for coordinating care would need to be identified. This entity might vary by the characteristics of

---

[11]Conversely, if tomorrow all physicians identified attention to patients' psychosocial health needs as integral to the provision of medical care and put in place mechanisms to address these needs, the practice expenses associated with doing so could be captured in the data sources Medicare uses to estimate practice expenses, and this could lead to an increase in payment rates. However, since Medicare payments are based on the value of each service "relative" to another, when relative values (and payments) increase for some services, they decrease for others.

the physician group providing care, such as the size of its patient population and the degree to which information technology is present in the practice to support care coordination. Finally, the extent to which case management payment should be placed at risk would have to be addressed. Otherwise, Medicare would need to define the specific set of care coordination activities to be reimbursed, how they could be delivered, and who would be eligible for payment (MEDPAC, 2006).

Support from Capitated Payment

Capitated payment is a more flexible mode of reimbursement than FFS that may better promote planning, linking, coordination, and follow-up activities (Berenson and Horvath, 2003; Bodenheimer et al., 2004; MEDPAC, 2006). This is because payment is made not for an isolated visit or procedure, but for the care of each health plan member for the entire period in which he or she is enrolled in the plan. Although payment is made for the provision of a defined benefit package, capitated health plans frequently offer extra services and benefits (often tailored to members' level of risk) to better manage the care of their enrollees and improve health outcomes, which also may result in cost savings. Although there is no database that comprehensively documents the prevalence of these practices, America's Health Insurance Plans (AHIP) reports that health plans are increasingly using administrative data and predictive modeling to identify individuals most in need of additional support services, and then planning, linking to, coordinating, and following up on services through such mechanisms as health advocacy, social work, case management, and disease management services. Some of these services specifically target individuals with cancer (AHIP, 2007).

Other Policy Support

Public- and private-sector group purchasers and insurers are continuing to implement and test better ways to plan, link, coordinate, and follow up on needed care (although attention to psychosocial care is not always as evident in these initiatives as is the coordination of biomedical care delivered by different clinicians) (see, e.g., MEDPAC, 2006; AHIP, 2007). In 2006, for example, 26 percent of U.S. employers with three or more employees who offered health benefits to their workers included one or more disease management programs in their health plan with the largest enrollment (Claxton et al., 2006). A 2002 survey of the nation's managed care plans found that nearly all health plans offered some type of disease management program for some members (AHIP, 2004). The voluntary sector is also implementing programs to help fill this gap, such as the patient navigator program described in Chapter 4. Medicare in particular is implementing several care coordination demonstration projects to inform efforts to develop better support for planning, linking, coordinating, and following up on the delivery of necessary psychosocial health services (see Box 6-1). However, many of these initiatives assume that better care coordination will result in lower costs, and it is not clear whether better health care and health outcomes will do so. Many of these programs also target conditions other than cancer.

Policies Addressing Support for Illness Self-Management

Some support for illness self-management is provided for in the H/B codes discussed earlier in this chapter. Some support also is found in the E/M codes, which define "counseling" as part of an E/M visit. "Counseling" is defined as "discussion with a patient and/or family concerning one or more of the following areas: . . . instructions for management (treatment) and/or follow up, importance of compliance with chosen management (treatment options), risk factor reduction, patient and family education" (Beebe et al., 2006:1). Other separate CPT codes (98960, 98961, and 98962) are established for more focused "Education and Training for Patient Self-Management" on a one-to-one basis and for group programs. These codes are intended to report "educational and training services prescribed by a physician and provided by a qualified nonphysician health care professional using a standardized curriculum. . . . The qualifications of the nonphysician healthcare professionals and the content of the educational training programs must be consistent with guidelines or standards established or recognized by a physician society, nonphysician health care professional society/association, or other appropriate source" (Beebe et al., 2006:418). It is not known how many private insurers reimburse for this code, although, as with the provision of planning, linking, coordination, and follow-up on services, many health plans offer other forms of support to their enrollees in managing some aspects of some illnesses (AHIP, 2004, 2007). Medicare pays for separate illness self-management programs for diabetes only.

As discussed in Chapters 3 and 4, illness self-management programs that have been tested empirically generally have not focused on cancer. Instead, they have addressed other illnesses more traditionally viewed as chronic and involving uniform patient interventions that must be performed on a regular basis, such as monitoring blood glucose levels (diabetes) or measuring peak flow volume (asthma). Many programs designed to help cancer patients adopt healthful behaviors, manage the side effects of their illness and treatment, and improve their health also are offered in the voluntary sector (see Chapter 3).

BOX 6-1
Medicare Care Coordination Demonstration Projects

Medicare Health Support Demonstration. In this ongoing demonstration (authorized in 2003), the Centers for Medicare & Medicaid Services (CMS) entered into agreements with eight organizations to test disease management and other approaches to care coordination to see whether they could improve the quality of care and life for people who have heart failure and/or complex diabetes among their chronic conditions. This demonstration represents the first time a large-scale initiative of this type has been tried in fee-for-service (FFS) Medicare. Its design randomizes participants into intervention and control groups. Each participating organization offers self-care guidance and support to beneficiaries to help them manage their health, adhere to their physicians' plans of care, and ensure they know when to seek medical care. Organizations also are required to assist participants in managing their health holistically, including all comorbidities and relevant health care services, in a manner that is responsive to any unique individual needs (CMS, undated). Each organization is paid a prospective fee for the care coordination that is at partial risk if targeted savings are not achieved (MEDPAC, 2006).

Physician Group Practice Demonstration. This first pay-for-performance initiative for physicians under the Medicare program is testing whether performance-based payments would result in better care. During the 3-year project, CMS will reward physician groups that improve patient outcomes by coordinating care for chronically ill and high-cost beneficiaries. Because they will share in any financial savings that result, the groups have incentives to use care management strategies that, based on clinical evidence and patient data, can improve patient outcomes and lower total medical costs. Performance payments will be derived from savings expected through improvements in care coordination for an assigned beneficiary population; by law the demonstration is required to be budget neutral. Approaches to be used for better care coordination include disease management and case management services, improved access to care and providers, and use of electronic medical records and disease registries (CMS, 2007).

Care Management for High-Cost Beneficiaries. This 3-year demonstration, begun in 2005, is designed to test approaches to helping Medicare beneficiaries with complex medical needs achieve better health outcomes through improved care coordination. In addition to providing traditional FFS Medicare benefits, participating health care organizations offer a variety of additional services to coordinate care, including home visits, in-home monitoring devices, electronic medical records, self-care and caregiver support, education and outreach, tracking and reminders of individuals' preventive care needs, 24-hour nurse telephone lines, behavioral health care management, and transportation services. Organizations receive a monthly fee for each beneficiary to cover their administrative and care management costs; however, they are at financial risk if they do not meet established performance standards for achieving cost savings. Participating organizations also have the flexibility to stratify targeted beneficiaries according to risk and need and to customize interventions to meet individuals' personal needs (CMS, 2005b).

SUPPORTS FOR AND CONSTRAINTS ON SERVICE AVAILABILITY

In addition to the policy support for interventions aimed at delivering psychosocial services described above, policies need to support the availability and accessibility of the various services patients require. Multiple health and human services sectors of the U.S. economy are involved in either directly delivering or providing for these services. They include government purchasing and insuring programs, such as Medicare and Medicaid; private-sector purchasers and insurers; the large voluntary sector, including voluntary services provided by health care organizations, such as hospitals, that otherwise require reimbursement for their services; programs offered by federal and state government agencies, such as the National Cancer Institute (NCI), the Centers for Disease Control and Prevention (CDC), and state health departments; and the informal support system of family, friends, and other social networks that provide supportive services. Additionally, many services are available for purchase in the marketplace.

Policies Supporting Service Availability

Table 6-3 lists some of the psychosocial services available from the various sectors cited above, which together form a comprehensive array of such services. Several features of this array are particularly noteworthy. First is the complexity of the providers and the services they offer, which underscores the need for policy support for care coordination and care navigator services, as discussed in Chapter 4 and above. The large role of the voluntary sector also is clear, highlighting the invaluable role played by this sector in cancer care (see also Tables 3-2 and 3-3 in Chapter 3). This partial listing of available services also counters the potential concern that "there is no point in identifying individuals who need psychosocial services because there is nothing to offer them." The voluntary sector has striven to ensure the availability of substantial psychosocial services for patients with cancer and their families, and the committee concurs with an earlier IOM report that found a "wealth of cancer-related community support services" (IOM and NRC, 2006:229).

The important role of family and other informal supports in providing critically needed services such as transportation and assistance with activities of daily living also is visible, especially in light of the limited availability of these services from other sources. Policies need to support these informal supports for several reasons. First, informal caregivers often know the patient best, and can tailor their support to the patient's unique needs and preferences. Their service to the patient often comes from their personal love or affection, which a business or regulatory model of care cannot match. Further, informal supports are a major source of emotional and other support. A nationally representative study of individuals aged 70 or older found that those treated for cancer received an average of 10 hours of help in activities of daily living from informal caregivers per week, at an estimated annual cost (in 1998 dollars) of $1,200 per patient and just over one $1 billion nationally. The economic worth of caregiving is actually likely higher, as these estimates do not include costs of caring for patients younger than 70, those residing in a nursing home, and those not being treated for their cancer. Estimates also do not include a number of other costs, including those of addressing limitations not experienced by individuals "most of the time" (Hayman et al., 2001). If informal supports were unable to continue providing these services, the costs to patients and to the health care system would be sizable. Yet despite the widely accepted importance of supporting caregivers in carrying out this role, as discussed in Chapter 3, how best to accomplish this is a question not yet well answered by research.

Policies Constraining Service Accessibility

A final observation on the availability of services as illustrated in Table 6-3 is the extent to which "with limits" or "coverage depends on policy" describes the availability of mental health care. The lack of health insurance generally, greater limits placed on mental health benefits, and restrictions on access to some mental health providers can be a serious impediment to receipt of mental health services.

Absent or Inadequate Insurance Coverage

An estimated 44.8 million Americans (15.3 percent of the population) were without health insurance in 2005 (U.S. Census Bureau, 2007), and many more have only modest insurance coverage, coupled with an income level that limits their ability to pay health care costs out of pocket. The adverse effects of no or inadequate insurance are well documented and include poorer health, delayed treatment, and worse outcomes of medical treatment for people with cancer as well as other diseases (IOM, 2002). Even for those who are fully insured, coverage for mental health services is frequently more limited than that for other medical conditions. In 2002, 2 percent of workers with employer-sponsored health insurance did not have a mental health benefit. Of the 98 percent that had coverage, 74 percent had limits on the number of outpatient visits they could make in a year, and 22 percent had to pay a higher copayment for a mental health visit than for a general medical visit (Barry et al., 2003). Medicare similarly requires higher

TABLE 6-3 Some Availability of Psychosocial Services in Health and Human Services Sectors and from Informal Supports

Service	Medicare	Medicaid/ SCHIP	Private Insurance
Provision of Information (e.g., on cancer-related treatments, health, and psychosocial services)			
Peer Support for People with a Cancer Diagnosis			
Counseling/ Psychotherapy	Covered benefit with limits	Covered benefit with limits	Coverage depends on policy
Pharmacological Management of Mental Symptoms	Covered benefit with limits	Covered benefit with limits	Coverage depends on policy
Health Behavior Interventions	Included as part of Evaluation and Management (E/M) services, Health and Behavior (H/B) Interventions, and additional services from managed care plans		
Medical Supplies	Some coverage	Some coverage	Coverage depends on policy
Transportation		Some coverage in almost all states	
Family and Caregiver Support	Family education included as part of E/M services, services from managed care plans		
Assistance with Activities of Daily Living (ADLs)	Part-time or intermittent assistance reimbursed under certain circumstances	Some reimbursement under Medicaid's "personal care" benefit and state-specific waivers of federal law	Not typically covered unless insured has long-term care insurance

Voluntary Sector	Health Care Providers (nonreimbursed)	Out-of-Pocket Purchase	Other Government Programs	Informal Supports
Widely available from many voluntary organizations (see Table 3-2 in Chapter 3)	Varies by provider		National Cancer Institute and other federal programs, e.g., Administration on Aging, Veterans Health Administration	
Widely available	Some availability			Some availability
Some counseling available		Can be purchased	Veterans Health Administration	
		Can be purchased	Veterans Health Administration	
Much support	Varies by provider	Can be purchased	Centers for Disease Control and Prevention initiatives	
Some supplies provided at no charge		Can be purchased		A source of financial resources for purchase
Some support		Can be purchased	Area Agencies on Aging	Available
Much support		Can be purchased		
		Can be purchased	Area Agencies on Aging	A substantial resource for these services

continued

TABLE 6-3 Continued

Service	Medicare	Medicaid/SCHIP	Private Insurance
Legal Services (e.g., regarding the Americans with Disabilities Act, the Family and Medical Leave Act, wills, power of attorney, disposition of assets)			
Cognitive and Educational Assistance		Covered as needed for persons under age 21 under the Early Periodic Screening, Diagnosis, and Treatment (EPSDT) benefit	Reports of inconsistent coverage of pediatric neurocognitive evaluations
Financial Planning, Counseling, and Management of Day-to-Day Activities (e.g., bill paying)			
Insurance Counseling (e.g., health, disability)			
Eligibility Assessment/ Counseling for Other Benefits (e.g., Supplemental Security Income [SSI]/Social Security Disability Insurance [SSDI])			

Voluntary Sector	Health Care Providers (nonreimbursed)	Out-of-Pocket Purchase	Other Government Programs	Informal Supports
Some availability (e.g., Cancer Legal Resource Center); some in defined geographic areas (e.g., Legal Information Network for Cancer in Virginia)		Can be purchased	Some Area Agencies on Aging	
			An Individual Education Program (IEP) and services available to children with disabilities under the Individuals with Disabilities Education Act (IDEA)	
Limited availability		Can be purchased	Some Area Agencies on Aging	Day-to-day financial management assistance available, depending on individual's informal supports
Limited availability				
			Eligibility assessment as part of the specific government programs	

continued

TABLE 6-3 Continued

Service	Medicare	Medicaid/ SCHIP	Private Insurance
Financial Assistance	Pays for some health care for those over age 65 or with disabilities who have made social security payments	Pays for some health care for certain categories of persons with low income	Approximately 85% of Americans have some health insurance to help pay certain acute health care costs; far fewer have short- and long-term disability insurance

cost sharing for outpatient mental health care (50 percent)[12] compared with general medical visits (20 percent).

This situation has substantial implications for the receipt of psycho-social services. When people without insurance need treatment for cancer, they must begin a search to locate health care providers in their community who will treat them at no or reduced cost, are willing to work out a payment plan, or some combination of these.[13] Once they are successful in locating such a provider, they may be unlikely to have the energy, time, or other resources to repeat the search to locate another provider who will provide mental health services on a similar basis—services they may not even anticipate needing at the outset of their illness. Grateful to the provider of their biomedical treatment, they may be unwilling to ask the facilitator of those services to subsidize as well the cost of any mental health services. Heavy out-of-pocket costs for the biomedical treatment of their cancer may also make them less willing to seek out mental health services, which they may view as of lower priority than the treatment of their life-threatening cancer. As a consequence, they are at risk of foregoing those services. Members of the American Psychosocial Oncology Society (APOS) report the frequent failure of patients with cancer to pursue or continue mental health care because of limited insurance coverage (APOS, 2007).

---

[12]However, visits for medication management require only a 20 percent copayment.

[13]See, for example, http://www.natlbcc.org/nbccf/access/affordable.html or http://www.breastcancer.org/faq_insurance.html.

Voluntary Sector	Health Care Providers (nonreimbursed)	Out-of-Pocket Purchase	Other Government Programs	Informal Supports
Very limited availability from voluntary organizations (e.g., American Cancer Society, CancerCare, The Leukemia and Lymphoma Society, Patient Advocate Foundation)	Limited free and reduced-cost health care at some hospitals under Hill-Burton Act		Federal SSI and SSDI programs provide limited funds to certain disabled persons	Some provided by informal supports

The committee notes that in the first half of 2007 (when this report was being written) there was renewed interest in Congress in expanding health insurance to all Americans, and legislation had been introduced in both houses of Congress to achieve comparable coverage of mental and general health care by health insurance (S 558, Mental Health Parity Act of 2007, and HR 1424, Paul Wellstone Mental Health and Addiction Equity Act of 2007). The committee strongly endorses action on this issue.

Restricted Access to Mental Health Clinicians with Special Expertise or Those Located at the Site of Cancer Care

Even when insurance covers mental health services, the ability of a patient to access appropriate mental health care conveniently can sometimes be hindered. Insurance for mental health services is often provided by a health plan that limits the clinicians included as part of the network of providers available to those it insures. When this happens, individual mental health care clinicians, such as psychiatrists and psychologists, who do not belong to and cannot gain admission to that network may not be able to be reimbursed for services to patients insured by the plan (APOS, 2007). This can thwart appropriate mental health care in two ways.

First, individuals with complex comorbid mental health and general medical conditions (such as cancer) sometimes require mental health clinicians with expertise in the management of these complex conditions. In the case of cancer care, for example, a high level of knowledge of cancer-induced cytokine production and its relationship to depression (Raison and Miller, 2003), as well as the pharmacological treatment of such depression in the presence of a complex drug regimen for the treatment of cancer and other comorbid conditions, is required. For such situations, in 2003 ABMS approved a new subspecialty in psychosomatic medicine to address "the high prevalence of psychiatric disorders in patients with medical, surgical, obstetrical and neurological conditions, particularly for patients with complex and/or chronic conditions ('the complex medically ill')" (Lyketsos et al., 2001:5). Although there were only 583 psychiatrists in the United States with certification in this subspecialty as of 2007,[14] to the extent that these specialists are available in the community and the oncologist believes this expertise is needed to address the patient's depression, failure of the patient's health plan to allow these clinicians admittance to its network or otherwise provide reimbursement for their services can effectively deny the patient access to this care.

Additionally, some oncology providers wish to locate mental health care clinicians within their practices. Doing so facilitates collocated, integrated care—one of the recommended approaches for coordination of health care described in Chapters 4 and 5. However, if these practices' mental health clinicians cannot receive reimbursement because they are not admitted to the insuring health plan's network, this prevents integrated care and decreases access to mental health services for the patient. The Moffitt Cancer Center in Florida, for example, reports that some managed behavioral health plans will not reimburse staff mental health clinicians because they are not part of the plan's network, but also will not allow them to become part of the network.[15,16]

Such problems with health plan networks are not explicitly addressed in leading accreditation standards for behavioral health plans.[17] However, health plans need to consider expertise in the mental health treatment of patients with complex chronic diseases as an important competency of their provider panels. This is consistent with the findings and recommendations of other health care quality improvement initiatives (President's Advisory Commission on Consumer Protection and Quality in the Health Care Industry, 1998; Shalala, 2000).

---

[14]Personal communication, Jennifer Vollmer, American Board of Psychiatry and Neurology, September 4, 2007.

[15]Personal communication, Paul B. Jacobsen, PhD, Clinical Program Leader, Psychosocial and Palliative Care Program, Moffitt Cancer Center, April 6, 2007.

[16]The Rebecca and John Moores Cancer Center, University of California, San Diego, reports similar experiences, as described in Chapter 5.

[17]Personal communication, Kathleen C. Mudd, MBA, RN, Vice President, National Committee for Quality Assurance, April 4, 2007.

USE OF PERFORMANCE MEASUREMENT TO IMPROVE
THE QUALITY OF PSYCHOSOCIAL HEALTH CARE

Even if reimbursement policies were to fully support the provision of all the psychosocial services described above, individuals being treated for cancer might still be unlikely to receive the psychosocial health services they need to manage their illness effectively. The many studies of health care quality conducted in the United States in recent years that have found widespread deficiencies in care, including underprovision of needed services (Fisher et al., 2003; McGlynn et al., 2003; Hussey et al., 2004; AHRQ, 2006), clearly show that the availability of reimbursement by itself does not ensure the provision of needed health care. Accordingly, many professional associations, payers, regulators, accrediting bodies, consumer groups, and other organizations have undertaken initiatives to report publicly on the performance of health care providers in delivering quality health care, use payments to create incentives for higher-quality care, and/or directly implement quality improvement programs at the provider level. Two mechanisms are common to all three of these pathways to better health care: (1) measuring the attainment of certain aims of quality health care by health care providers and the health care system overall (performance measurement), and (2) using the results of performance measurement to leverage changes in the way health care is delivered (IOM, 2006b).

Use of these two mechanisms to improve the delivery of psychosocial services to cancer patients and their families is hindered in part by the same overall problem that afflicts all of U.S. health care: the nation's lack of "a coherent, goal oriented, consistent, and efficient system for assessing and reporting on the performance of the health care system" (IOM, 2006b:2). Certain health care organizations, group purchasers, communities, and others have nonetheless used performance measurement to achieve improvements in the segment of the health care system they can influence. However, there are two additional obstacles to similar efforts to improve the psychosocial health care provided to patients with cancer: less well-developed measures of the delivery of psychosocial health services, and a less well-developed network of organizations and partnerships to ensure the application of such measures.

Measurement of Psychosocial Health Care

As experts have noted, some areas of health care have better-developed performance measures than others (IOM, 2006b). Mental health care, for example, historically has been less well addressed in national performance measurement and quality improvement initiatives (IOM, 2006a), although this gap is narrowing. Performance measures for the delivery of a more comprehensive array of psychosocial health services in general and for patients with cancer in particular also are not very visible in major national performance measurement initiatives (see Table 6-4).

Table 6-4 reveals that psychosocial health services are not typically addressed in the limited number of measures of the quality of cancer care. Although components of the model for delivering psychosocial health care described in Chapter 4 (e.g., effective patient–provider communication) and specific psychosocial health services (e.g., treatment for depression) are addressed for health care overall, a well-thought-out, efficient, and strategic set of performance measures addressing psychosocial health care in general or for patients with cancer in particular is not evident. For example, there is no performance measure of the extent to which patients with cancer (or those with other chronic illnesses) have undergone screening or assessment to identify psychosocial problems. Neither are there measures of the extent to which these patients have been linked to needed services.

Measurement of the quality of care does not take place only in the context of performance measurement initiatives; programs that accredit certain types of health care providers are another venue for ensuring that organizations have in place the structures and processes necessary to deliver good-quality health care. The American College of Surgeons' multidisciplinary Commission on Cancer, for example, sets standards for cancer care delivered primarily in hospital settings, surveys hospitals to assess compliance with those standards, and uses the resulting data to evaluate hospital performance and develop effective educational interventions to improve cancer care at the national and local levels (American College of Surgeons, 2007). However, no organization targets the accreditation of organizations providing ambulatory cancer care. This is problematic as most patients with cancer receive treatment on an ambulatory rather than an inpatient basis.

Performance measurement is well recognized as essential to performance improvement. Measuring specific aspects of the quality of care and reporting the results back to providers is linked both conceptually and empirically to reductions in variations in care and increases in the delivery of effective care (Berwick et al., 2003; Jha et al., 2003). A number of organizations could help develop and test measures of psychosocial health care (e.g., the National Quality Forum, the AHRQ CAHPS team), but the existence of measures alone will not be sufficient to achieve change. Structures and processes to enable use of the measures and leadership with influence over how cancer care is delivered are needed to spearhead the development and use of such measures.

Means of Ensuring the Use of Performance Measures

Effective performance measurement requires mechanisms for conceptualizing the measures, translating these concepts into technical specifications,

TABLE 6-4 Performance Measures of Psychosocial Health Care Adopted/ Endorsed by Leading Performance Measurement Initiatives as of July 2007

Initiative	Number of Performance Measures Adopted/Endorsed	Number and Description of Adopted/ Endorsed Performance Measures Addressing Psychosocial Health Care in Community Settings
AQA Alliance (formerly Ambulatory Care Quality Alliance)	100 as of January 2007; 4 addressing cancer care (AQA, 2007)	• None among the 4 cancer care measures • Primary care measures include 4: advising smokers to quit and asking about tobacco use, and two addressing depression medication management • Dermatology measures include 1: counseling those with new or a history of melanoma to perform a skin self-exam
ASCO Quality Oncology Practice Initiative (QOPI)	52 measures as of Spring 2007 (ASCO, 2007)	• 2 address discussion of chemotherapy with patient • 6 address assessment of pain • 2 address smoking cessation • 4 address enrollment in hospice
Consumer Assessment of Healthcare Providers and Systems (CAHPS) Clinician and Group Adult Specialty Care Questionnaire	37 basic items and additional supplemental questions	• 6 supplemental questions address how well the physician communicated with the patient • 3 address shared decision making
Healthplan Employer Data and Information Set (HEDIS)	73 for 2007, 3 of which are survey instruments asking about satisfaction with the experience of care (NCQA, 2007)	• Follow-up after hospitalization for mental illness • Antidepressant medication management • Medical assistance with smoking cessation • Initiation and engagement of treatment for alcohol and other drug dependence • Mental health utilization: inpatient discharges and average length of stay (ALOS), percentage of health plan members receiving inpatient and intermediate care and ambulatory services • Chemical dependency utilization: inpatient discharges and ALOS • Identification of alcohol and other drug services • Medicare Health Outcomes Survey

continued

TABLE 6-4 Continued

Initiative	Number of Performance Measures Adopted/Endorsed	Number and Description of Adopted/Endorsed Performance Measures Addressing Psychosocial Health Care in Community Settings
2006 National Health Care Quality Report	211 measures, including 15 addressing effectiveness of cancer care	• Cancer-specific measures do not address psychosocial health services • 8 address effectiveness of mental health and substance abuse care • 15 address timeliness of care • 24 address patient–provider communication across conditions
National Quality Forum	• 6 measures for breast cancer; 4 for colorectal cancer (NQF, 2007a)	• No psychosocial measures among the breast and colorectal cancer measures
	• 9 measures of symptom management and end-of-life care for patients with cancer (NQF, 2006)	• Symptom management and end-of-life measures predominantly (8 or 9 of 9) address hospice, death, and last 30 days of life
	• 112 ambulatory care measures endorsed as of July 2007 for treatment of 9 noncancer conditions (e.g., asthma, diabetes), plus emergency care, geriatrics, medication management, patient experience with care, screening, and preventive care (NQF, 2007b)	• Ambulatory measures for mental health address major depressive disorders, new episodes of depression, attention-deficit hyperactivity disorder, bipolar disorder, alcohol and other drug treatment • Other ambulatory care measures address tobacco cessation, physical activity, and cancer screening • Patient experience of care measures include CAHPS survey of adult specialty care and survey for children with chronic conditions

pilot testing the measures, ensuring calculation and submission of the measures, auditing to ensure their accuracy, analyzing and displaying measurement results in a format suitable for the intended audiences, and maintaining the measures' accuracy and reliability over time (IOM, 2006a). Structures and processes for performing many of these functions already exist within the health care system. However, marshaling these resources, especially with respect to ensuring the calculation and submission of the measures, will require leadership.

Leadership

Leadership is a critical factor in the success of any major change initiative or quality improvement effort (Burns, 1978; Bodenheimer et al., 2004; National Institute of Standards and Technology, 2007). Fortunately, a number of organizations that already play a leadership role in oncology have the ability to influence quality through their certifying activities, financial support, and ability to inform consumers in the marketplace. Such organizations, working together, could constitute a critical mass of leadership creating substantial incentives for oncology providers to improve the delivery of psychosocial health care for patients with cancer and their families by supporting the development of a small, strategic set of performance measures addressing psychosocial health care and then incorporating these measures into their organizational policies and practices.

As the nation's leader in cancer care, NCI has a number of venues through which performance measures could be used to improve psychosocial health care. NCI's 61 designated cancer centers and comprehensive cancer centers together constitute the "centerpiece of the nation's effort to reduce morbidity and mortality from cancer" (NCI, 2004:2) and are "characterized by strong organizational capabilities, institutional commitment, and trans-disciplinary, cancer-focused science; experienced scientific and administrative leadership, and *state-of-the-art* cancer research and *patient care facilities* [emphasis added]" (NCI, undated-a). NCI could encourage these facilities to set the benchmark for performance in meeting standards for psychosocial health care incorporated in the performance measures, and to measure and report their performance in providing such care.

NCI's Outcomes Research Branch also coordinates and sponsors research aimed at improving cancer outcomes; reducing health disparities; and reducing the cancer burden on patients, families, and society. In doing so, it coordinates and funds research and applications designed to assess, monitor, and improve the quality of cancer care, and translates research findings into products and strategies for use by public and private policy makers who provide, pay for, regulate, and set standards for cancer care (NCI, undated-b). Incorporating the development and application of performance- measures of psychosocial health care into this agenda also could help advance the use of such measures.

Leading private-sector funders of cancer research and demonstrations, such as the American Cancer Society, Lance Armstrong Foundation, and Susan G. Komen for the Cure Foundation, also could incentivize the calculation and public reporting of performance measures of psychosocial health care by including questions about how organizations deliver such care in their requests for proposals, making awards based on applicants' performance in these areas, and requiring the calculation and reporting of the measures as a condition of their financial support. For example, the Lance Armstrong Foundation could require participants in its LIVE**STRONG** Survivorship Center of Excellence Network (Lance Armstrong Foundation, 2007) to calculate and submit the measures to a performance measures repository as part of membership in the network.

Organizations supporting patients with cancer and their families as consumers in the marketplace could also use performance measures to create strong incentives for improved performance in psychosocial health care. Approved performance measures constitute de facto standards of performance. Publicizing the measures (even before there are any measurement results) can help educate consumers about what services to expect and ask about when they begin their cancer care. Publicizing the measures can also filter up to employers (and other group purchasers), who want the best possible care for their employees facing treatment, and thereby to the insurers with whom they contract to provide coverage for health care.

An Infrastructure to Support Performance Measurement

As discussed above, successful performance measurement requires more than the creation of measures and an entity that will require their calculation. Structures and processes are needed to transform the concepts to be measured into sets of technical specifications, pilot test the measures, audit a sample of measures to ensure their accuracy, analyze and display measurement results, and maintain the accuracy of measurement specifications over time. Structures and processes for performing many of these functions already exist within the health care system. The National Quality Forum, for example, working in collaboration with many of its members, has developed or endorsed technical specifications for many measures across a wide variety of conditions. Accrediting bodies such as the Joint Commission and the National Committee for Quality Assurance (NCQA) serve as repositories of submitted data and convert the data to formats useful to consumers and others. Consolidating a combination of organizations and resources to carry out the various performance measurement–related activities will require planning, collaboration, and perhaps financial support. This, too, will require leadership across many sectors of cancer care.

CONCLUSIONS AND RECOMMENDATIONS

The committee concludes that, although the policies and practices of many organizations support the delivery of several components of psychosocial health care, such is not always the case. Available mechanisms to compensate providers for assessments and interventions to help patients manage their illness are not fully utilized by all insurers. While FFS reimbursement codes take into consideration the basic need to coordinate care, FFS reimbursement does not well support processes for care coordination that require additional resources. Although capitated payments to managed care plans allow better for the provision of linking services, care coordination, follow-up, and illness self-management support, these examples are still considered noteworthy, rather than "usual and customary" practice. Lack of health insurance, high cost sharing for patients, and health plan policies that hinder collocated services and access to certain providers also can keep patients from receiving needed services. Solutions exist that are feasible for group purchasers of health care coverage and health plans to implement.

Recommendation: Support from payers. Group purchasers of health care coverage and health plans should fully support the evidence-based interventions necessary to deliver effective psychosocial health services:

- Group purchasers should include provisions in their contracts and agreements with health plans that ensure coverage and reimbursement of mechanisms for identifying the psychosocial needs of cancer patients, linking patients with appropriate providers who can meet those needs, and coordinating psychosocial services with patients' biomedical care.
- Group purchasers should review cost-sharing provisions that affect mental health services and revise those that impede cancer patients' access to such services.
- Group purchasers and health plans should ensure that their coverage policies do not impede cancer patients' access to providers with expertise in the treatment of mental health conditions in individuals undergoing complex medical regimens such as those used to treat cancer. Health plans whose networks lack this expertise should reimburse for mental health services provided by out-of-network practitioners with this expertise who meet the plan's quality and other standards (at rates paid to similar providers within the plan's network).
- Group purchasers and health plans should include incentives for the effective delivery of psychosocial care in payment reform programs—such as pay-for-performance and pay-for-reporting initiatives—in which they participate.

In the above recommendation, "group purchasers" include purchasers in the public sector (e.g., Medicare and Medicaid), as well as group purchasers in the private sector (e.g., employer purchasers). In recommending that group purchasers include in their contracts and agreements with health plans provisions to ensure the coverage and reimbursement of mechanisms to identify psychosocial needs, link patients to psychosocial health services, and coordinate these services with biomedical care, the committee is not necessarily calling for these interventions to be reimbursed separately by group purchasers and health plans. Rather, these parties should assess the extent to which these processes are explicitly addressed in their agreements with each other and with health care providers, make these expectations explicit if they are not already so, and assess the adequacy of their payment rates for these processes. Purchasers and health plans may find, for example, that these interventions are currently provided for in their capitated payments or included to some extent in FFS reimbursements. In contrast, mechanisms may need to be developed for reimbursing higher-than-average levels of care coordination. The predictive modeling techniques now being used by some health plans can help identify when special reimbursement of or arrangements for care coordination may be called for.

With respect to reimbursement of out-of-network providers when necessary, mental health care providers "with expertise in the treatment of mental health conditions in individuals undergoing complex medical regimens such as those used to treat cancer" include mental health care providers who possess this expertise through formal education (such as specialists in psychosomatic medicine), as well as mental health care providers who have gained expertise though their clinical experiences, such as mental health clinicians collocated with and part of an interdisciplinary oncology practice.

The recommended approach of guaranteeing access to such expertise through the use of out-of-network providers is consistent with similar recommendations of other health care quality initiatives (Shalala, 2000), including the President's Advisory Commission on Consumer Protection and Quality in the Health Care Industry (1998), whose patient Bill of Rights states: "All health plan networks should provide access to sufficient numbers and types of providers to assure that all covered services will be accessible without unreasonable delay. . . . If a health plan has an insufficient number or type of providers to provide a covered benefit with the appropriate degree of specialization, the plan should ensure that the consumer obtains the benefit outside the network at no greater cost than if the benefit were obtained from participating providers. Plans also should establish and maintain adequate arrangements to ensure reasonable proximity of providers to the business or personal residence of their members" (p. A-31).

Further, ensuring access to such providers means more than just allowing them to receive reimbursement; a health care provider possessing this expertise must be accessible to the cancer patient. If, for example, an individual with such expertise is collocated with the patient's other oncology providers, this individual should be allowed to receive reimbursement provided that (as specified in the recommendation above) he or she meets the plan's quality and other standards. The provider should also accept reimbursement at rates paid to similar providers within the plan's network.

In recognition that full implementation of the above recommendation will not by itself ensure the provision of appropriate psychosocial health services, the committee also makes the following recommendation.

Recommendation: Quality oversight. The National Cancer Institute, CMS, and AHRQ should fund research focused on the development of performance measures for psychosocial cancer care. Organizations setting standards for cancer care (e.g., National Comprehensive Cancer Network, American Society of Clinical Oncology, American College of Surgeons' Commission on Cancer, Oncology Nursing Society, American Psychosocial Oncology Society) and other standards-setting organizations (e.g., National Quality Forum, National Committee for Quality Assurance, URAC, Joint Commission) should

- Create oversight mechanisms that can be used to measure and report on the quality of ambulatory oncology care (including psychosocial health care).
- Incorporate requirements for identifying and responding to psychosocial health care needs into their protocols, policies, and standards.
- Develop and use performance measures for psychosocial health care in their quality oversight activities.

The research to be funded will need to transform concepts to be measured into technical specifications, pilot test the measures, audit a sample of measures to ensure their accuracy, analyze and display measurement results, and address how the accuracy and reliability of the measures will be maintained over time. The committee expects that these activities will make use of already established mechanisms and organizations that currently perform these functions, but that some funding may be needed to support certain other activities, such as the initial development of the measure specifications.

The committee also believes that a small number of measures (five or fewer) should be targeted for development, and that these could consist of structural as well as process and outcome-of-care measures. Structural measures are typically addressed in accreditation processes and could be used to deal with such areas of concern as whether a health plan or clinical practice requires or uses a validated instrument or approach to identify systematically all cancer patients with psychosocial needs. Patient report instruments, such as AHRQ's CAHPS Clinician and Group Survey questions, could also be used to obtain information from patients about the extent to which they were linked to needed psychosocial services and received education and training in managing their illness. Thus, the expert organizations to be encompassed by and consulted in this planning process would be diverse, including government agencies such as AHRQ; private-sector accreditation bodies such as the Commission on Cancer, NCQA, and the Joint Commission; and performance measurement bodies such as the National Quality Forum.

REFERENCES

Adiga, K., M. Buss, and B. W. Beasley. 2006. Perceived, actual, and desired knowledge regarding Medicare billing and reimbursement: A national needs assessment survey of internal medicine residents. *Journal of General Internal Medicine* 21(5):466–470.

AHIP (America's Health Insurance Plans). 2004. *2002 AHIP survey of health insurance plans: Chart book of findings.* Washington, DC: AHIP.

AHIP. 2007. *Innovations in chronic care.* Washington, DC: AHIP.

AHRQ (Agency for Healthcare Research and Quality). 2006. *National health care quality report.* Rockville, MD: U.S. Department of Health and Human Services, and AHRQ.

AHRQ. 2007a. *CAHPS clinician and group survey AHRQ, 3/22/2007.* https://www.cahps.ahrq.gov/content/products/CG/PROD_CG_CG40Products.asp?p=1021&s=213 (accessed March 23, 2007).

AHRQ. 2007b. *Questions are the answer.* http://www.ahrq.gov/questionsaretheanswer/ (accessed April 4 2007).

American College of Surgeons. 2007. *What is the Commission on Cancer?* http://www.facs.org/cancer/coc/cocar.html (accessed April 11, 2007).

APOS (American Psychosocial Oncology Society). 2007 (unpublished). *APOS reimbursement survey.*

AQA (Ambulatory Care Quality Alliance). 2007. *AQA approved quality measures, January 2007.* http://www.aqaalliance.org/files/ApprovedPerformanceMeasures.xls (accessed April 9, 2007).

ASCO (American Society of Clinical Oncology). 2007. *Summary of QOPI measures, Spring 2007.* http://www.asco.org/portal/site/ASCO/menuitem.c543a013502b2a89de91231032 0041a0/?vgnextoid=cdb7dd224254c010VgnVCM100000ed730ad1RCRD&cpsextcurr channel=1/ (accessed August 20, 2007).

Astin, J. A., K. Soeken, V. Sierpina, and B. Clarridge. 2006. Barriers to the integration of psychosocial factors in medicine: Results of a national survey of physicians. *Journal of the American Board of Family Medicine* 19(6):557–565.

Bachman, J., H. A. Pincus, J. K. Houtsinger, and J. Unutzer. 2006. Funding mechanisms for depression care management: Opportunities and challenges. *General Hospital Psychiatry* 28(4):278–288.

Barry, C. L., J. R. Gabel, R. G. Frank, S. Hawkins, H. H. Whitmore, and J. Pickreign. 2003. Design of mental health benefits: Still unequal after all these years. *Health Affairs* 22(5):127–137.

Beebe, M., J. A. Dalton, M. Espronceda, D. D. Evans, R. L. Glenn, G. Green, D. Hayden, A. Majerowicz, J. Meggs, M. L. Mindeman, K. E. O'Hara, M. R. O'Heron, D. Pavlovski, D. Rozell, L. Stancik, P. Thompson, S. Tracy, J. Trajkovski, and A. Walker. 2006. *Current Procedural Terminology*. CPT 2007 Professional Edition. Chicago, IL: American Medical Association.

Berenson, R. A., and J. Horvath. 2003. Confronting the barriers to chronic care management in Medicare. *Health Affairs* (Suppl. web exclusive):W3-37–W3-53.

Berwick, D. M., B. James, and M. J. Coye. 2003. Connections between quality measurement and improvement. *Medical Care* 41(1):Supplement I-30–I-38.

Bodenheimer, T., M. C. Wang, T. G. Rundall, S. M. Shortell, R. R. Gillies, N. Oswald, L. Casalino, and J. C. Robinson. 2004. What are the facilitators and barriers in physician organizations' use of care management processes? *Joint Commission Journal on Quality and Safety* 30(9):505–514.

Burns, J. 1978. *Leadership*. New York: Harper and Row.

Claxton, G., I. Gil, B. Finder, B. DiJulio, S. Hawkins, J. Pickreign, H. Whitmore, and J. Gabel. 2006. *Employer health benefits: 2006 annual survey*. Menlo Park, CA, and Chicago, IL: Henry J. Kaiser Foundation and Health Research and Educational Trust.

CMS (Centers for Medicare and Medicaid Services). Undated. *Medicare Health Support. Highlights of the program*. http://www.cms.hhs.gov/CCIP/02_Highlights.asp#TopOfPage (accessed November 18, 2007).

CMS. 2005a. *Medicaid at-a-glance*. CMS-11024-05. Washington, DC: Department of Health and Human Services.

CMS. 2005b. *Medicare to award contracts for demonstration projects to improve care for beneficiaries with high medical costs*. http://www.cms.hhs.gov/DemoProjectsEvalRpts/downloads/CMHCB_Press_Release.pdf (accessed April 4, 2007).

CMS. 2006a. Medicare program; revisions to payment policies, five-year review of work relative value units, changes to the practice expense methodology under the physician fee schedule, and other changes to payment under part B; revisions to the payment policies of ambulance services under the fee schedule for ambulance services; and ambulance inflation factor update for CY 2007. *Federal Register* 71(231):69623–70251.

CMS. 2006b. *CMS announces proposed changes to physician fee schedule methodology*. http://www.cms.hhs.gov/apps/media/press/release.asp?Counter=1887 (accessed March 19, 2007).

CMS. 2007. *Medicare physician group practice demonstration*. http://www.cms.hhs.gov/DemoProjectsEvalRpts/downloads/PGP_Fact_Sheet.pdf (accessed April 4, 2007).

Epstein, R. M., and R. L. Street. 2007. *Patient-centered communication in cancer care: Promoting healing and reducing suffering*. NIH Publication No. 07-6225. Bethesda, MD: National Cancer Institute.

Fisher, E., D. Wennberg, T. Stukel, D. Gottlieb, F. Lucas, and E. Pinder. 2003. The implications of regional variations in Medicare spending. Part 1: The content, quality, and accessibility of care. *Annals of Internal Medicine* 138(4):273–287.

Foxhall, K. 2000. New CPT codes will recognize psychologists' work with physical health problems. *Monitor on Psychology* 31(10):46–47.

Ginsburg, P. B., and R. A. Berenson. 2007. Revising Medicare's physician fee schedule: Much activity, little change. *New England Journal of Medicine* 356(12):1201–1203.

Hayman, J. A., K. M. Langa, M. U. Kabeto, S. J. Katz, S. M. DeMonner, M. E. Chernew, M. B. Slavin, and A. M. Fendrick. 2001. Estimating the cost of informal caregiving for elderly patients with cancer. *Journal of Clinical Oncology* 19(13):3219–3225.

Hussey, P., G. Anderson, R. Osborn, C. Feek, V. McLaughlin, J. Millar, and A. Epstein. 2004. How does the quality of care compare in five countries? *Health Affairs* 23(3):89–99.

Institute for Healthcare Communication. 2005. *Case studies.* http://www.healthcarecomm.
    org/index.php?sec=case (accessed April 13, 2007).
IOM (Institute of Medicine). 1999. *Ensuring quality cancer care.* M. Hewitt and J. V. Simone,
    eds. Washington, DC: National Academy Press.
IOM. 2002. *Care without coverage: Too little, too late.* Washington, DC: National Academy
    Press.
IOM. 2006a. *Improving the quality of health care for mental and substance-use conditions.*
    Washington, DC: The National Academies Press.
IOM. 2006b. *Performance measurement: Accelerating improvement.* Washington, DC: The
    National Academies Press.
IOM and NRC (National Research Council). 2006. *From cancer patient to cancer survivor:
    Lost in transition.* M. Hewitt, S. Greenfield, and E. Stovall, eds. Washington, DC: The
    National Academies Press.
Jha, A. K., J. B. Perlin, K. W. Kizer, and R. A. Dudley. 2003. Effect of the transformation of
    the Veterans Affairs health care system on the quality of care. *The New England Journal
    of Medicine* 348(22):2218–2227.
Lance Armstrong Foundation. 2007. *How network members are selected and funded.* http://
    www.livestrong.org/site/c.jvKZLbMRIsG/b.1537979/k.739/How_Network_Members_
    are_Selected_and_Funded.htm (accessed April 11, 2007).
Lyketsos, C., J. Levenson, and Academy of Psychosomatic Medicine Task Force for Subspe-
    cialization. 2001. *Proposal for recognition of "psychosomatic medicine" as a psychiatric
    subspecialty.* Academy of Psychosomatic Medicine. http://www.apm.org/subspecialty/
    ABPNsubspecialtyproposal.pdf (accessed April 6, 2007).
McGlynn, E., S. Asch, J. Adams, J. Keesey, J. Hicks, A. DeCristofaro, and E. Kerr. 2003. The
    quality of health care delivered to adults in the United States. *New England Journal of
    Medicine* 348(26):2635–2645.
MEDPAC (Medicare Payment Advisory Commission). 2006. Care coordination in fee-for-
    service Medicare. In *Report to the Congress: Medicare payment policy.* Washington,
    DC: MEDPAC.
MEDPAC. 2007. *Report to the Congress: Medicare payment policy, March 2007.* Washington,
    DC: MEDPAC.
Moran, M. 2006. Aetna to pay for depression screening by primary care physicians. *Psychi-
    atric News* 41(2):5.
National Institute of Standards and Technology. 2007. *Baldrige National Quality Program:
    Health care criteria for performance excellence.* Gaithersburg, MD: United States Depart-
    ment of Commerce.
NCCS (National Coalition for Cancer Survivorship). 2007. *Cancer survival toolbox®.* http://
    www.cancersurvivaltoolbox.org (accessed March 23, 2007).
NCI (National Cancer Institute). Undated-a. *Cancer centers program.* DHHS. http://cancer-
    centers.cancer.gov/about/index.html (accessed April 11, 2007).
NCI. Undated-b. *Outcomes research: Mission of the outcomes research branch.* http://
    outcomes.cancer.gov/about/ (accessed April 11, 2007).
NCI. 2004. *Policies and guidelines relating to the cancer center support grant.* http://
    cancercenters.cancer.gov/documents/CCSG_Guide12_04.pdf (accessed April 11, 2007).
NCQA (National Committee for Quality Assurance). 2007. *HEDIS® 2007 summary table
    of measures and product lines.* http://web.ncqa.org/Portals/0/HEDISQM/HEDIS2007/
    MeasuresList.pdf (accessed April 9, 2007).
NQF (National Quality Forum). 2006. *National quality forum endorses consensus standards for
    symptom management and end-of-life care for patients with cancer.* http://216.122.138.39/
    pdf/news/prCancerSxEOL10-12-06.pdf (accessed April 10, 2007).

NQF. 2007a. *National Quality Forum endorses consensus standards for diagnosis and treatment of breast & colorectal cancer.* http://www.qualityforum.org/pdf/news/prbreastcolon03-12-07.pdf (accessed April 10, 2007).

NQF. 2007b. *National voluntary consensus standards for ambulatory care.* http://www.qualityforum.org/pdf/ambulatory/tbAMBALLMeasuresendorsed%2007-27-07.pdf (accessed September 4, 2007).

Partnership for Clear Health Communication. Undated. *Ask me 3™.* http://www.askme3.org/for_patients.asp (accessed April 4, 2007).

President's Advisory Commission on Consumer Protection and Quality in the Health Care Industry. 1998. *Quality first: Better health care for all Americans.* Final report to the President of the United States. Washington, DC: U.S. Government Printing Office.

Raison, C. L., and A. H. Miller. 2003. Depression in cancer: New developments regarding diagnosis and treatment. *Biological Psychiatry* 54(3):283–294.

Shalala, D. 2000. *Report to Congress: Safeguards for individuals with special health care needs enrolled in Medicaid managed care.* Washington, DC: U.S. Department of Health and Human Services.

U.S. Census Bureau. 2007. *Census Bureau revises 2004 and 2005 health insurance coverage estimates.* Washington, DC: U.S. Department of Commerce.

7

Preparing the Workforce[1]

CHAPTER SUMMARY

Psychosocial health services are delivered by a wide variety of providers, including specialists in medical, nursing, and social work oncology; other physicians, nurses, and social workers; and a range of additional mental health professionals, such as psychologists and counselors. Although it is not possible to estimate the optimal supply of this workforce (individually or in the aggregate) to meet the nation's need for psychosocial health services for people diagnosed with cancer, it is clear that there currently exists a large health care workforce that routinely encounters and cares for this population and can deliver these services.

Institutions concerned with the preparation of this workforce address psychosocial issues in their standards for educational accreditation and licensure. However, many of these standards are brief and general, and there are limited systems in place to collect data on how these educational standards are translated into hours, methods, or content of such instruction or the resulting skills of the workforce. Consequently, it is not possible to know with certainty the characteristics of the education on psychosocial issues these health care providers receive, or their resulting competency in assessing and addressing psychosocial health needs.

To remedy educational contributions to inadequate provision of psychosocial health care, the committee recommends that educational accrediting organizations, licensing bodies, and professional societies examine their standards and licensing and certification criteria, and develop them as fully as possible in accordance with a model that integrates biomedical and psychosocial care. The education of the health care workforce

---

[1]Although (as discussed in Chapters 2 and 6) families and other informal caregivers provide substantial amounts of psychosocial health services, this chapter addresses the paid, professional workforce.

in psychosocial health needs and services could also be improved by a public–private collaboration aimed at (1) identifying and supporting the implementation of strategies for collecting better information about curricular content and methods addressing psychosocial health care; (2) identifying, refining, and broadly disseminating information to health care educators about workforce competency models and curricula relevant to providing psychosocial health services; (3) further developing faculty skills to teach psychosocial health care using evidence-based teaching strategies; and (4) strengthening accreditation standards pertaining to psychosocial health care in education programs and health care organizations.

A LARGE AND DIVERSE WORKFORCE

Currently, a large and diverse workforce either comes into contact with cancer patients and their families through the provision of cancer care or exists as a potential resource for these individuals. This considerably diverse workforce comprises distinct, although at times overlapping, sectors, including (1) clinicians who are involved principally in the provision of biomedical health care services; (2) mental health and counseling professionals; and (3) providers of other psychosocial services, such as information, logistical or material support, and financial assistance. This latter sector includes a large volunteer and peer support component.

A wide variety of licensed providers deliver some psychosocial health services: allopathic physicians (such as those practicing oncology, internal medicine, family medicine, pediatric hematology-oncology, and pediatrics), nurses, mental health professionals (such as psychiatrists, clinical psychologists, counselors, social workers, and pastoral counselors), and other social workers. Some of these providers deliver care exclusively to people diagnosed with cancer on the basis of their specialization in oncology or employment in programs devoted to serving these individuals. Others provide care to people diagnosed with cancer as just one segment of their total patient populations. For example, a previous Institute of Medicine (IOM) report, *From Cancer Patient to Cancer Survivor: Lost in Transition*, notes that primary care physicians provide the greatest amount of ambulatory cancer care in the United States (IOM and NRC, 2005).

Tables 7-1 and 7-2 provide estimates of the numbers of selected providers of various types who serve cancer patients and can play a role in either providing or ensuring the provision of psychosocial health services. Table 7-1 shows the number of physicians in various specialties certified by the American Board of Medical Specialties (ABMS)[2] or with membership in

---

[2]Initial certification, a process that evaluates the training, qualifications, and competence of physician specialists at the outset of their careers, is a major focus of ABMS and its Member Boards (Horowitz et al., 2004). Nearly 85 percent of licensed U.S. doctors are certified by at least one ABMS member board (ABMS, 2007).

TABLE 7-1 Estimates of the Supply of Selected Physician Types Available to Provide or Ensure the Provision of Psychosocial Health Services

Type of Physician Specialty	Credential or Membership Status	Amount
Internal Medicine	Board certified[a] (2006)	186,868
	Member of American College of Physicians[b] (2006)	120,000
Family Medicine	Board certified[c] (2006)	66,421
	Member of American Academy of Family Physicians[d] (2006)	94,000
Pediatrics	Board certified[e] (2005)	84,826
	Member of American Academy of Pediatrics[f] (2006)	60,000
Psychiatry	Board certified[g] (2005)	43,850
	Member of American Psychiatric Association[h] (2006)	35,000
Medical Oncology	Board certified[a] (2006)	10,016
	Member of American Society of Clinical Oncology[i] (2006)	20,000
Pediatric Hematology-Oncology	Board certified[e] (2006)	1,884
	Member of American Society of Pediatric Hematology/Oncology[j] (2006)	1,000

NOTE: Estimates of board-certified physicians are based on the number of valid certificates issued, and may not accurately reflect the number of currently practicing physicians in the United States. Also, because provider types may be credentialed as well as licensed or hold more than one credential, the numbers in each category are not mutually exclusive.
SOURCE: Numbers of board-certified physicians come from the [a]American Board of Internal Medicine (ABIM, 2006a); [c]American Board of Family Medicine (ABFM, 2006c); [e]American Board of Pediatrics (ABP, 2006b); and [g]American Board of Psychiatry and Neurology, Inc. (ABPN, 2006b). Professional organization membership comes from the [b]American College of Physicians (ACP, 2006); [d]American Academy of Family Physicians (AAFP, 2006); [f]American Academy of Pediatrics (AAP, 2006); [h]Personal communication, Lisa Corchado, American Psychiatric Association, September 4, 2007; [i]American Society of Clinical Oncology (ASCO, 2006); and [j]American Society of Pediatric Hematology/Oncology (ASPHO, 2006).

related professional societies. Table 7-2 shows the numbers of other health care personnel—generally those licensed and credentialed by relevant professional societies.

In addition to these licensed professionals, there are a host of other employed providers of psychosocial services that constitute a large and critical sector of the health care workforce. This sector includes individuals with bachelor's degrees, high school diplomas, or lesser education who are involved in diverse caregiver roles. They may provide information, transportation, financial advice, or case management, or may function as navigators in systems of care. They may also provide in-home support for activities of daily living and other services. Virtually no data or information is available about the numbers of these individuals or their characteristics, training, or performance. Finally, complementing the employed workforce

TABLE 7-2 Estimates of the U.S. Supply of Selected Nonphysician Providers Available to Provide or Ensure the Provision of Psychosocial Health Services

Type of Provider	Licensure or Credential Status	Number
Registered nurses (RNs)	Licensed[a] (as of 2004)	2,909,357
	RN with advance practice preparation and credentials in oncology[a] (2004)	2,573
	Member of Oncology Nursing Society[b] (2006)	33,000
	Oncology Certified Nurse (OCNs)[c] (2006)	21,195
	Advanced Oncology Certified Nurse (AOCN)[c] (2006)	1,381
	Certified Pediatric Oncology Nurse (CPONs)[c] (2006)	1,261
	Advanced Oncology Certified Nurse Practitioner (AOCNP)[c] (2006)	313
	Advanced Oncology Certified Clinical Nurse Specialist (AOCNS)[c] (2006)	128
	RN with advance practice preparation and credentials in psychiatry/mental health[a] (2004)	19,693
	Clinical nurse specialists in adult psychiatric and mental health[d] (2007)	6,851
	Clinical nurse specialist in child and adolescent mental health[d] (2007)	988
	Family psychiatric and mental health nurse practitioner[d] (2007)	635
	Adult psychiatric and mental health nurse practitioner[d] (2007)	1,750
Social workers	Employed social worker[e] (2004)	562,000
	Social worker employed in mental health and substance abuse services[e] (2004)	116,000
	Social worker employed in medical and public health[e] (2004)	110,000
	Social worker employed in child, family, and school social services[e]	272,000
	Licensed social worker[f] (2004)	310,000
	Member of National Association of Social Workers[g] (2006)	149,621
	Member of Association of Oncology Social Work[h] (2007)	1,000
	Member of Association of Pediatric Oncology Social Workers[i] (2006)	303
	Certified by the Board of Oncology Social Work Certification[j] (2007)	236
Psychologists	Licensed[k] (2004)	179,000
	Member (worldwide) of American Psychological Association (APA)[l] (2006)	148,000
	Member of APA Health Division[m] (2006)	532
Mental health counselors	Licensed[n] (2004)	96,000
Pastoral counselors	Certified[o] (2006)	3,000

NOTE: Estimates are based on the number of valid licenses or certificates issued, and may not accurately reflect the number of currently practicing providers in the United States. Because

TABLE 7-2 Continued

provider types may be credentialed as well as licensed or hold more than one credential, the numbers in each category are not mutually exclusive.

SOURCES: Number of providers and professional organization membership comes from the [a]Health Resources and Service Administration (HRSA, 2006); [b]Oncology Nursing Society (ONS, 2006); [c]Oncology Nursing Certification Corporation (ONCC, 2006); [d]Personal communication, Todd Peterson, American Nurse Credentialing Center, September 10, 2007; [e]U.S. Department of Labor (BLS, 2006d); [f]Center for Health Workforce Studies and NASW Center for Workforce Studies (2006); [g]National Association of Social Workers (NASW, 2006); [h]Personal communication, Ethan Gray, Association of Oncology Social Work, September 4, 2007; [i]Association of Pediatric Oncology Social Workers (Personal communication, D. Donelson, APOSW, November 15, 2006); [j]Personal communication, Kim Day, Board of Oncology Social Work Certification, September 5, 2007; [k]U.S. Department of Labor (BLS, 2006c); [l]American Psychological Association (APA, 2006a); [m]Personal communication, Wendy Williams, American Psychological Association, September 5, 2007; [n]U.S. Department of Labor (BLS, 2006a); and [o]American Association of Pastoral Counselors (AAPC, 2006).

are numerous volunteers who also provide information, support, and other forms of assistance. Again, there is little information available about the size, nature, preparation, and functioning of this important sector of the health care workforce.

This mix of different disciplines and licensed, unlicensed, and informal caregivers contributes to the difficulty of determining whether the number of workers is adequate to provide psychosocial health services. Ideally, one might want to estimate carefully the level of need for these services and then attempt to predict accurately the necessary workforce supply to meet that need. However, experts in health care workforce issues note decades of failure of efforts to estimate the size, composition, and distribution of the nation's health care workforce (Grumbach, 2002; Snyderman et al., 2002). Even in countries with centrally managed, universal health care systems, progress in medical technology and changes in the organization of care can create large forecasting errors. Predicting workforce supply in the United States is further complicated by the fact that demand for services is not tightly controlled, and the distribution of the workforce is neither controlled nor actively shaped through reimbursement mechanisms (Reinhardt, 2002). To complicate the matter, data on health professions are not collected in a routine, standardized fashion across the multiple disciplines (Hoge et al., 2007), and the dramatic growth in selected disciplines, such as clinical psychology and counseling, has reshaped the composition of the health care workforce. Another limitation on a forecasting effort is that the same function (e.g., care coordination, case management, or patient navigation) may be carried out by different types of professionals, paraprofessionals, or volunteers in different organizations or systems. Thus, workforce needs are heavily influenced at the local level by the assignment of functions to providers. For these and other reasons discussed in Appendix B, the development of estimates of the overall workforce capacity required to meet psychosocial health needs through modeling or other methods was not a feasible activity for this study.

Nonetheless, shortages and maldistribution of a variety of psychosocial health care providers, such as nurses and mental health clinicians is a long-recognized problem. In 1999, the Surgeon General's report on mental health stated: "The supply of well-trained mental health professionals is inadequate in many areas of the country, especially in rural areas. Particularly keen shortages are found in the numbers of mental health professionals serving children and adolescents with serious mental disorders, and older people" (DHHS, 1999:455). Echoing this statement, in 2003 the President's New Freedom Commission on Mental Health reported: "In rural and other geographically remote areas, many people with mental illnesses have inadequate access to care [and] limited availability of skilled care providers . . ." (New Freedom Commission on Mental Health, 2003:51). Shortages in the nursing workforce also have been well documented (HRSA, 2004). And the American Association of Medical Colleges estimates that the growing need for cancer care will soon outstrip the supply of oncologists, and predicts a shortage by 2020 (Erikson et al., 2007).

WORKFORCE EDUCATION IN BIOPSYCHOSOCIAL APPROACHES TO CARE

In addition to its numbers, the capacity of the health care workforce is determined by its knowledge, skill, and overall ability to deliver psychosocial health services. As described in previous chapters, this ability is influenced in part by how work in clinical practices is designed (Chapters 4 and 5) and how incentives from payers and oversight organizations operate (Chapter 6). However, the content and methods of professional education and training also affect the workforce's understanding and appreciation of the interrelatedness of biological, psychological, and social factors in influencing health, as well as its knowledge and skill in detecting and responding to adverse psychosocial stressors. Although most professions have developed educational standards addressing psychosocial issues, it is unclear how these standards have been translated into educational curricula and more important, whether they create the competencies needed in the health care workforce to meet psychosocial health needs effectively.

Professional education should prepare licensed clinicians to recognize and address psychosocial health needs just as they do biomedical needs. The education of mental health and social service professionals should also impart knowledge of and skills in addressing the effects of general medical illnesses on mental health and comorbid mental illnesses and on social needs. While the biopsychosocial model of health care has long been advocated (Engel, 1977), the extent to which this model is adequately implemented in educational curricula is unclear. Licensing and continuing education requirements and credentialing standards pertaining to psychosocial factors also are unclear and appear to be limited, with variations across professions.

Physicians

Education, training, and licensing requirements to practice medicine in the United States typically include graduating from college with an undergraduate degree; receiving an additional 4 years of undergraduate education at a medical school; passing a licensing examination; and completing up to 8 years of residency training, depending on a physician's chosen specialty (BLS, 2006b).

Undergraduate Medical Education

The IOM committee that authored the 2004 IOM report *Improving Medical Education: Enhancing the Behavioral and Social Science Content of Medical School Curricula* found that "existing national databases provide inadequate information on behavioral and social science content, teaching techniques, and assessment methodologies. This lack of data impedes the ability to reach conclusions about the current state and adequacy of behavioral and social science instruction in U.S. medical schools." The committee recommended that the "National Institutes of Health's Office of Behavioral and Social Sciences Research should contract with the Association of American Medical Colleges to develop and maintain a database on behavioral and social science curricular content, teaching techniques, and assessment methodologies in U.S. medical schools. This database should be updated on a regular basis" (IOM, 2004a:7). This recommendation has not been implemented.[3]

Accreditation of medical schools is conducted by the Liaison Committee on Medical Education (LCME), sponsored jointly by the Association of American Medical Colleges (AAMC) and the American Medical Association. Although LCME accreditation is "voluntary," it is required for "schools to receive federal grants for medical education and to participate in federal loan programs" (LCME, 2006b). Box 7-1 displays LCME accreditation standards that address psychosocial health services. The stan-

---

[3]Personal communication, M. Brownell Anderson, AAMC, November 9, 2006.

BOX 7-1
LCME Undergraduate Medical Education Accreditation
Standards That Address Psychosocial Health Services

- **ED-7.** It [the curriculum] must include current concepts in the basic and clinical sciences, including therapy and technology, changes in the understanding of disease, and the **effect of social needs and demands on care.**
- **ED-10.** The curriculum **must include behavioral and socioeconomic subjects**, in addition to basic science and clinical disciplines.
- **ED-13.** Clinical instruction must cover all organ systems, and include the important aspects of preventive, acute, chronic, continuing, rehabilitative, and end-of-life care.
- **ED-19.** There must be **specific instruction in communication skills** as they relate to physician responsibilities, **including communication with patients, families,** colleagues, and other health professionals [emphasis added].

SOURCE: LCME, 2006a.

---

dards intentionally are broad in scope to afford schools flexibility in the way they meet them.[4]

Each medical school defines its own curricular objectives (LCME, 2006a). In 1996, however, AAMC initiated the Medical School Objectives Project (MSOP) (AAMC, 1998) "to reach general consensus within the medical education community on the skills, attitudes, and knowledge that graduating medical students should possess" (AAMC, undated). The MSOP guidelines state, in part, that graduates must demonstrate "knowledge of the important non-biological determinants of poor health and of the economic, psychological, social, and cultural factors" that contribute to the development or continuation of ill health (AAMC, 1998:8). Yet neither the LCME standards nor the MSOP guidelines specify explicitly how to teach these subjects, how many hours should be devoted to their study, or what topics related to psychosocial health services should be covered. The extent to which the MSOP guidelines are being fulfilled is unclear.

A national survey of U.S. medical schools[5] conducted between 1997 and 1999 found that the concepts and measurement of such psychosocial factors as stress and social support were taught by 80 to 93 percent of schools (most often in required courses), but that psychosocial topics represented on average 14 percent of curricula (range from 1 to 60 percent), and

---

[4]Personal communication, Robert Eaglen, PhD, LCME/AAMC, October 10, 2006.
[5]46 percent response rate.

only 37 percent had a written curriculum on these topics. Student interest in and appreciation of the subject was mixed. About 50 percent of medical schools endorsed less than 40 hours of total instruction in psychosomatic/ behavioral medicine out of the 7,000–8,000 hours in the average medical school curriculum. The researchers concluded that the degree of coverage of the subject in undergraduate medical education appeared variable, but generally was unknown and difficult to assess (Waldstein et al., 2001). AAMC's online Curriculum Management and Information Tool (CurrMIT) currently serves as the database for tracking teaching techniques and assessment methodologies for these topics.[6] Although CurrMIT aids in analyzing curricular content, it is a voluntary system. About one-third of accredited U.S. medical schools are not actively entering data into the system. Further, medical schools that participate have flexibility in data entry, and as a result, the data submitted vary in detail from school to school.[7] As reported above, a 2004 IOM report found that existing national databases provide inadequate information on behavioral and social science content, teaching techniques, and assessment methodologies in U.S. medical schools.

Medical students' clerkship experiences and opinions reflect some satisfaction with current education and training in psychosocial health services (Yuen et al., 2006). In the 2006 Medical School Graduation Questionnaire, 86.5 percent of students reported receiving "appropriate" instruction in behavioral sciences (AAMC, 2006b).[8] Yet some medical students, residents, and practicing physicians have reported inadequate medical education on the role of psychosocial factors in health (Astin et al., 2005, 2006), which is related to clinicians' attention to psychosocial issues in their practices (Astin et al., 2006).

Medical Licensure

To practice legally as a physician, medical students must pass the three-step U.S. Medical Licensing Examination (USMLE). Step 1 of the exam (usually taken after the second year in medical school) assesses basic science knowledge according to general principles and individual organ systems. Approximately 10–20 percent of Step 1 addresses "behavioral considerations affecting disease treatment and prevention, including psychosocial, cultural, occupational and environmental" (USMLE, 2006:7). Box 7-2 shows the subtopics in the Step 1 exam that address psychosocial

---

[6]Personal communication, M. Brownell Anderson, AAMC, November 9, 2006.

[7]Personal communication, Robby Reynolds, AAMC, October, 23, 2006.

[8]In the *2006 All Schools Report*, the question was, "Do you believe that the time devoted to your instruction in the following areas was inadequate, appropriate, or excessive?" (*n*= 11,417); 9.2 and 4.4 percent, respectively, rated the time as "inadequate" or "excessive" (AAMC, 2006b).

BOX 7-2
General Principles of Gender, Ethnic, and
Behavioral Considerations for USMLE Step 1

Psychologic and social factors influencing patient behavior:

- personality traits or coping style, including coping mechanisms
- psychodynamic and behavioral factors, related past experience
- family and cultural factors, including socioeconomic status, ethnicity, and gender
- adaptive and maladaptive behavioral responses to stress and illness
- interactions between the patient and the physician or the health care system
- patient adherence, including general and adolescent

SOURCE: FSMB and NBME, undated-a.

health services. However, such test questions would most likely be woven together with questions dealing with chronic diseases instead of making up a separate section devoted to psychological and social factors.[9]

Similarly, Step 2 of the exam (usually taken after the fourth year of medical school) does not explicitly cover psychosocial health services, but a "broad spectrum of cases reflecting common and important symptoms and diagnoses" (USMLE, 2006:9). It tests clinical knowledge and communication and interpersonal skills using standardized patients.[10] Approximately 15–20 percent of the exam addresses "promoting preventive medicine and health maintenance," as in the assessment of risk factors and application of preventive measures, and approximately 15–25 percent addresses "applying principles of management," as in the care of people with chronic and acute conditions in ambulatory and inpatient settings (USMLE, 2006:8). Step 3 of the exam *may* cover psychosocial health services since "test items and cases reflect the clinical situations that a general, as yet undifferentiated, physician might encounter within the context of a specific setting" (FSMB and NBME, undated-b).

---

[9]Personal communication, G. Dillon, National Board of Medical Examiners, October 10, 2006.

[10]USMLE Step 2 assesses whether candidates can "apply medical knowledge, skills, and understanding of clinical science essential for the provision of patient care under supervision and includes emphasis on health promotion and disease prevention" (USMLE, 2006:2).

Graduate Medical Education

Medical school graduates seeking to receive board certification or enter independent practice must complete graduate medical education (GME, or residency training programs) of up to 8 years in length, depending on their specialty. Recognizing that the current teaching models focus more on accommodating biomedical content than on improving patient care (Leach, 2001), the Accreditation Council for Graduate Medical Education (ACGME), which accredits residency programs and sets their curricular standards, developed the Outcome Project (ACGME, 2007a)—a long-term effort to enhance the effectiveness of residency education and accreditation by increasing the emphasis on outcomes. The desired outcomes are focused on demonstrated competencies among physicians in training. Box 7-3 shows the "minimum language" version of the six general competencies endorsed by ACGME in 1999.

Internal Medicine Residency and Medical Oncology Subspecialty The American Board of Internal Medicine (ABIM) requires candidates for

---

BOX 7-3
General Competencies of the ACGME Outcome Project

1. Patient care that is compassionate, appropriate, and effective for the treatment of health problems and the promotion of health
2. Medical knowledge about established and evolving biomedical, clinical, and cognate (e.g., epidemiological and **social-behavioral) sciences and the application of this knowledge to patient care**
3. Practice-based learning and improvement that involves investigation and evaluation of their own patient care, appraisal and assimilation of scientific evidence, and improvements in patient care
4. **Interpersonal and communication skills** that result in effective information exchange and teaming with patients, their families, and other health professionals
5. Professionalism, as manifested through a commitment to carrying out professional responsibilities, adherence to ethical principles, and sensitivity to a diverse patient population
6. Systems-based practice, as manifested by actions that demonstrate an awareness of and responsiveness to the larger context and system of health care and the ability to effectively call on system resources to provide care that is of optimal value [emphasis added]

SOURCE: ACGME, 2007a.

certification in internal medicine to complete 3 years of postgraduate training and an additional 2-year fellowship for subspecialization in medical oncology (ABIM, 2006b). ABIM incorporated the six ACGME competencies into its resident evaluation forms, and ACGME asked all residency review committees (RRCs) to make reference to them in their program requirements (Goroll et al., 2004). Program requirements for the medical oncology subspecialty further state that fellows "must have formal instruction, clinical experience, and must demonstrate competence in the prevention, evaluation and management of . . . rehabilitation and psychosocial aspects of clinical management of the cancer patient" (ACGME, 2005). However, very few questions on a typical certification examination in internal medicine or medical oncology directly address psychosocial health services. ABIM estimates that on average, five questions per examination may cover psychosocial or mental health content, but emphasizes that "drawing conclusions about examinee performance in these areas" would be impossible because "scores would be unreliable for such a small number of questions."[11]

Family Medicine Residency Training Program   The American Board of Family Medicine (ABFM) also requires candidates for certification in family medicine to complete 3 years of postgraduate training (ABFM, 2006b). Program requirements for family medicine state that residents must become trained in meeting the psychosocial health needs of patients. Specifically, residents must address the "total health care of the individual and family, taking into account social, behavioral, economic, cultural, and biologic dimensions" and become skilled in the "diagnosis and management of psychiatric disorders in children and adults, emotional aspects of non-psychiatric disorders, psychopharmacology . . . and counseling skills" (ACGME, 2006a:16,28).

Pediatric Residency Training Program and Pediatric Hematology-Oncology Fellowship   The American Board of Pediatrics (ABP) similarly requires candidates for certification in pediatrics to complete 3 years of postgraduate training; an additional 3-year fellowship is required for subspecialization in pediatric hematology-oncology (ABP, 2006a). Program requirements in general pediatrics state, in part, that (ACGME, 2006b)

- Residents should "be able to interview patients/families . . . with specific attention to behavioral, psychosocial, environmental, and family unit correlates of disease" (p. 11).

---

[11]Personal communication, P. Poniatowski, ABIM, October 12, 2006.

- The comprehensive experience for all residents should include . . . acute psychiatric, behavioral, and psychosocial problems (p. 19).
- Residents should demonstrate knowledge and skill in management of psychosocial problems that affect children with complex chronic disorders and their families (p. 23).
- Residents should be able to serve as a member of a multidisciplinary team "since no one individual has all the needed expertise to attend to the medical, psychological, and social needs of patients" (p. 42).

Approximately 3 percent of questions on the general pediatrics certifying examination pertain to psychosocial issues and problems, such as family issues, chronic illness, and handicapping conditions (ABP, 2007). ABP emphasizes that there are many other aspects of psychosocial health services that subspecialty trainees need to learn that cannot be tested in a multiple-choice examination, but could be learned through clinical training during residency.[12]

Psychiatry Residency Training Program   Because psychiatric services are by definition psychosocial health services, the written and oral examinations given by the American Board of Psychiatry and Neurology (ABPN) can reasonably be expected to address psychosocial health services.[13] For these clinicians, a greater issue is the extent to which psychiatrists are knowledgeable about and qualified to address the effects of acute or chronic illness on mental health. Accordingly, program requirements in psychiatry state that clinical education should give residents experience in "the diagnosis and management of mental disorders in patients with multiple comorbid medical disorders" and "opportunities to apply psychosocial rehabilitation techniques and to evaluate and treat differing disorders in a chronically ill patient population" in a variety of clinical settings (ACGME, 2007b:15,16). However, such experiences may be inadequate to prepare psychiatrists to care for individuals with serious complex health conditions. As noted in Chapter 6, in 2003 ABMS approved a new subspecialty in psychosomatic medicine to address in particular the care of the "complex medically ill" (Lyketsos et al., 2001:5).

---

[12]Personal communication, James Stockman, MD, ABP, October 9, 2006, and Jean Robillard, MD, ABP Sub-Board of Pediatric Hematology-Oncology, October 12, 2006.

[13]Although this may not ensure that psychiatrists have competency in all aspects of psychosocial health services such as communication skills, assessment of social issues affecting the patient, competency working with an interdisciplinary team, or implementation of the psychosocial plan.

Continuing Education and Ongoing Certification of Competency

U.S. jurisdictions (states, territories, and the District of Columbia) granting licenses to physicians require renewal of those licenses every 1, 2, or 3 years. Virtually all require completion and reporting of a specified number of hours of continuing medical education (CME) (12–50 hours per year) as part of license renewal. Some areas have also imposed content requirements (e.g., in geriatric medicine or palliative care) (AMA, 2006). Traditionally, CME has taken place through a lectures-at-a-conference format; however, this method has consistently been found ineffective as a means of changing clinical practice (Bero et al., 1998; Davis et al., 1999; Parochka and Paprockas, 2001). As a result, CME is being reconceptualized as "a more continuous process with more emphasis on self-assessment and continuous improvement and less on attending traditional lecture courses" (Goroll et al., 2004:908).

In addition, physicians with certification in a specialty are required to be recertified periodically. Similar to the changing conceptualization of CME, the specialty recertification process for physicians has evolved from periodic testing to a more continuous "maintenance of certification" (MOC) process (ABMS, 2006). Developed by ABMS and its Member Boards, the MOC process involves the assessment and improvement of practice performance by physicians in every specialty (Batmangelich and Adamowski, 2004; Miller, 2006). Each Member Board will be required to develop specific mechanisms for assessing evidence of diplomates' competency in specific areas (Pugh, 2003), as shown through ABIM's Practice Improvement Module (PIM), ABFM's Maintenance of Certification Program for Family Physicians (MC-FP) (ABFM, 2006a), ABP's Program for Maintenance of Certification in General Pediatrics (PMCP-G®) and in Pediatric Subspecialties (PMCP-S®) (ABP, 2006a), and ABPN's MOC program (ABPN, 2006a). Within such programs, topics related to psychosocial health services could be incorporated in such mechanisms as self-assessment modules, used to evaluate knowledge, and performance-in-practice modules, used for peer review.

Registered Nurses

There are three major educational paths to becoming a registered nurse (RN): obtaining a 2-year associate's degree in nursing from a community or junior college, a 3-year hospital-based diploma, or a 4-year baccalaureate degree in nursing from a college or university (IOM, 2004b). All state boards of nursing except those of North Dakota and New York accept these three educational paths as appropriate academic preparation for RN licensure (Kovner and Knickman, 2005).

Associate and Baccalaureate Nursing Education

Two different organizations accredit nursing education programs. The National League for Nursing Accrediting Commission (NLNAC) accredits practical nursing, diploma, associate's, baccalaureate, master's, and doctoral programs and schools. The Commission on Collegiate Nursing Education (CCNE), an autonomous arm of the American Association of Colleges of Nursing (AACN), also accredits programs offering baccalaureate and master's degrees in nursing.

NLNAC does not require nursing educational institutions to teach specific knowledge or skills to achieve accreditation. Rather, each institution is to identify the knowledge and skills to be acquired by students through its curriculum at each level of education it provides. NLNAC then verifies that the school is meeting the educational objectives it has set for itself. NLNAC does require, however, that each school's curriculum meet specific standards; for example,

> Curriculum developed by nursing faculty flows from the nursing education unit philosophy/mission through an organizing framework into a logical progression of course outcomes and learning objectives to achieve desired program objectives/outcomes.
>
> Program design provides opportunity for students to achieve program objectives and acquire skills, values, and competencies necessary for nursing practice. (NLNAC, 2006:15)

Although not requiring that specific knowledge and skills be taught, NLNAC does require accredited schools to build their curricula around guidelines for nursing practice selected from among those established by a number of recognized nursing organizations. For example, NLNAC supports the Pew Health Professions Commission's 21 *Competencies for the Twenty-First Century* as the basis for preparing practitioners to meet evolving health care needs,[14] and recommends as guidance a set of core competencies, a number of which address psychosocial health services (see Box 7-4). With respect to all of the core competencies it identifies, NLNAC states: "It is essential that each nursing program interpret these skills and competencies in the content, context, function, and structure of their program" (NLNAC, 2006:84).

AACN identifies nurses as "practice[ing] from a holistic base and incorporate[ing] bio-psycho-social and spiritual aspects of health" (AACN,

---

[14]NLNAC also recognizes other statements, including but not limited to the competencies published in *Health Professions Education: A Bridge to Quality* (IOM, 2003), the National Task Force on Quality Nurse Practitioner Education's *Criteria for Evaluation of Nurse Practitioner Programs* (2002), and the National Association of Clinical Nurse Specialists' 2004 *Statement on Clinical Nurse Specialist Practice and Education*.

BOX 7-4
Selected NLNAC Core Competencies Addressing
Psychosocial Health Services

Nurses should

- care for community's health and have broad understanding of determinants of health (i.e., environment, socioeconomic conditions, behavior, genetics)
- incorporate the psychosocial-behavioral perspective into a full range of clinical practice competencies
- emphasize primary and secondary preventive strategies (i.e., occupational health, wellness centers, self-care programs, and health education and health promotion programs)
- involve patients and families in the decision-making processes
- help individuals, families, and communities maintain and promote healthy behavior
- provide counseling for patients in situations where ethical issues arise

SOURCE: NLNAC, 2006.

1998:5). Accordingly, topics related to psychosocial health services are to be woven in throughout the nursing curriculum.[15] More specifically, baccalaureate curricula are required to incorporates knowledge and skills identified in *The Essentials of Baccalaureate Education for Professional Nursing Practice* (AACN, 1998), which includes core competencies pertaining to psychosocial health services (examples are presented in Box 7-5).

CCNE's accreditation standards require that baccalaureate curricula incorporate knowledge and skills identified in *The Essentials of Baccalaureate Education for Professional Nursing Practice* and (for master's curricula) knowledge and skills identified in *The Essentials of Master's Education for Advanced Practice Nursing* (CCNE, 2003).

Licensure

Graduates who have completed any of the above three educational paths must pass the National Council Licensure Examination for RNs (NCLEX-RN), administered by the National Council of State Boards of Nursing (NCSBN), to become licensed as an RN. Approximately 6–12 percent of questions on the NCLEX-RN are devoted to "psychosocial

---

[15]Personal communication, Joan Stanley, AACN, November 9, 2006.

BOX 7-5
Selected Core Competencies from
The Essentials of Baccalaureate Education

Graduates must have the knowledge and skills to

- adapt communication methods to patients with special needs, e.g., sensory or psychological disabilities
- provide relevant and sensitive health education information and counseling to patients
- perform a holistic assessment of the individual across the lifespan, including a health history that includes spiritual, social, cultural, and psychological assessment, as well as a comprehensive exam
- assess physical, cognitive, and social functional ability of the individual in all developmental stages, with particular attention to changes due to aging
- provide teaching, and emotional and physical support in preparation for therapeutic procedures
- foster strategies for health promotion, risk reduction, and disease prevention across the life span
- assess and manage physical and psychological symptoms related to disease and treatment
- anticipate, plan for, and manage physical, psychological, social, and spiritual needs of the patient and family/caregiver
- demonstrate sensitivity to personal and cultural influences on the individual's reactions to the illness experience and end of life
- coordinate and manage care to meet the special needs of vulnerable populations, including the frail elderly, in order to maximize independence and quality of life
- coordinate the health care of individuals across the lifespan utilizing principles and knowledge of interdisciplinary models of care delivery and case management
- understand how human behavior is affected by culture, race, religion, gender, lifestyle, and age
- provide holistic care that addresses the needs of diverse populations across the lifespan
- understand the effects of health and social policies on persons from diverse backgrounds
- recognize the need for and implement risk-reduction strategies to address social and public health issues, including societal and domestic violence, family abuse, sexual abuse, and substance abuse

SOURCE: AACN, 1998.

integrity" (which includes behavioral interventions, coping mechanisms, family dynamics, mental health concepts, psychopathology, religious and spiritual influences on health, and support systems). Another 13–19 percent relate to "management of care" (content includes continuity of care, referrals, and collaboration with interdisciplinary teams), and 6–12 percent to "health promotion and maintenance" (which includes self-care, lifestyle choices, principles of teaching and learning, health screening, health promotion programs, and disease prevention) (NCSBN, 2006a). However, recent revisions to the exam reduced the content on "psychosocial integrity" (Stuart, 2006), which suggests a decreased focus on psychosocial issues.

The scope of practice of RNs is defined by the state in which the nurse practices. Currently, 20 states participate in a Nurse Licensure Compact Agreement, whereby a nurse with a license in his/her state of residency is allowed to practice in another, subject to each state's practice law and regulation (NCSBN, 2006b).[16] All states require nurses to renewal their license periodically, which sometimes requires continuing education.

Specialty Certification and Continued Competency

Nurses can obtain specialty certification from various organizations to focus their practice in a certain field. For example, the American Nurses Credentialing Center (ANCC), a subsidiary of the American Nurses Association, certifies nursing specialties such as psychiatric nursing and mental health. The Oncology Nursing Certification Corporation (ONCC) also offers examinations in oncology nursing for care of both pediatric and adult patients, including exams for certification as an Oncology Certified Nurse (OCN), Certified Pediatric Oncology Nurse (CPON), Advanced Oncology Certified Nurse Practitioner (AOCNP), and Advanced Oncology Certified Clinical Nurse Specialist (AOCNS) (ONCC, 2006). Thirty-six percent of the content of the test for certification as an OCN addresses knowledge of "quality-of-life" issues, including (but not limited to) pain; fatigue; sleep disorders; coping (risk factors, prevention, and management); spiritual distress; financial concerns; emotional distress; social dysfunction; loss and grief; anxiety; altered body image; cultural issues; loss of personal control; depression; survivorship issues; sexuality (risk factors, prevention, and management); reproductive issues; supportive care; dying and death; local, state, and national resources; and rehabilitation. Eight percent of the content of the CPON certification examination addresses psychosocial issues, and an additional 8, 3, and 6 percent, respectively, addresses growth and development, health promotion, and end-of-life care. Fifteen

---

[16]Colorado, Kentucky, and New Jersey have enacted but not yet implemented the compact agreement (National Council of State Boards of Nursing, 2006).

percent of the AOCNP examination addresses "psychosocial management," including risk factors for psychosocial disturbances (e.g., comorbidities, specific treatments, lack of social support); assessment techniques; sexuality; pharmacological interventions (e.g., anxiolytics, antidepressants); nonpharmacological interventions (e.g., relaxation techniques, hypnosis, biofeedback, art/music therapy); coping methods; family dynamics; and diversity (e.g., cultural, lifestyle, and religious factors). Sixteen percent of the AOCNS examination similarly addresses psychosocial management (ONCC, 2007a,b,c,d).

Evidence of continued competency is not yet uniformly required of licensed nurses. The most recent (2004–2006) data collected by NCSBN show that 13 states have no requirements for demonstration of "continued competence" for licensed nurses. The 31 states that do report using a variety of mechanisms for ensuring continued competency require peer review (4), continuing education (25), periodic refresher courses (5), minimal practice (11), assessment of continued competence (4), and other mechanisms (6). Twelve states require specific subject matter—such as AIDS, child abuse, domestic violence, end of life, law and rules, pain management, and pharmacology—to be addressed through continuing education (NCSBN, undated).

Social Workers

The practice of social work includes "helping people obtain tangible services; counseling and psychotherapy with individuals, families, and groups; helping communities or groups provide or improve social and health services . . . [and] requires knowledge of human development and behavior; of social and economic, and cultural institutions; and of the interaction of all these factors" (NASW, 2007b:1). Although social workers can practice with a bachelor's, master's, or doctoral degree, the master of social work (MSW) is the most common academic requirement for licensure. Obtaining an MSW degree usually requires 2 years of postundergraduate study and field placements/practica (Morris et al., 2004). Educational preparation for the different degrees varies in conceptualization and design, content, program objectives, and expected knowledge and skills (CSWE, 2004).

Baccalaureate and Master's Degrees in Social Work

Baccalaureate programs in social work prepare graduates for generalist professional practice; master's programs in social work prepare graduates for advanced professional practice in an area of concentration. The Council on Social Work Education (CSWE) accredits both degree programs in the United States (CSWE, 2004). Since social work is the primary profession for the delivery of social services, its accreditation standards, like those for the discipline of psychiatry, can be assumed to be psychosocial in their orientation. Less certain is the extent to which these accreditation standards facilitate the preparation of social workers in the knowledge, skills, and abilities required to address psychosocial needs when dealing with individuals with complex medical conditions such as cancer. CSWE's accreditation standards do not evidence substantial attention to psychosocial needs in the presence of illness. For example, a previous IOM report (IOM, 2006) documented that most schools of social work fail to provide students with basic knowledge of alcohol- and drug-use issues, and that a significant factor contributing to this situation is that accreditation standards do not mandate that curricula contain substance-use content (Straussner and Senreich, 2002).

Licensure

The Association of Social Work Boards (ASWB) develops and maintains four categories of social work licensure examinations—at the bachelor's, master's, advanced generalist, and clinical levels. Approximately 14 percent of questions on the bachelor's-level exam are assigned to "human development and behavior in the environment," with one of its six dimensions addressing "impact of crises and changes." Eleven percent of the master's-level examination addresses "assessment, diagnosis, and intervention planning," of which "biopsychosocial history and collateral data" is one of five dimensions (ASWB, 2006a).

Specialization and Continuing Education

Additionally, many social workers specialize in a particular area of practice, and a variety of organizations issue voluntary credentials and specialty certifications for those individuals who have a bachelor of social work (BSW) degree or an MSW. For example, the National Association of Social Workers (NASW) issues many specialty certifications, including the Certified Social Worker in Health Care (C-SWHC). Social workers who hold the C-SWHC have a current NASW membership; an MSW degree from an institution accredited by CSWE; 2 years and 3,000 hours of paid, supervised, post-MSW health care social work experience; an evaluation from an approved supervisor and a reference from an MSW colleague; and an Academy of Certified Social Workers (ACSW) or Diplomate in Clinical Social Work (DCSW) credential and/or a current state MSW-level license or a passing score on an ASWB MSW-level exam. They also must agree to adhere to the NASW Code of Ethics and the NASW Standards for Continuing Professional Education, and are subject to the NASW adjudication process (NASW, 2007a).

The Association of Oncology Social Work (AOSW) provides a definition for oncology social workers' scope of practice, has established voluntary standards for practice, and serves as an educational resource. It defines oncology social work as providing "psychosocial services to patients, families, and significant others facing the impact of a potential or actual diagnosis of cancer," such as "stress and symptom management, care planning, case management, system navigation, education and advocacy" (AOSW, 2001:1). Similarly, the Association of Pediatric Oncology Social Work (APOSW) is a membership organization for individuals engaged in clinical social work in the field of pediatric oncology. It promotes knowledge and skill competency in part though its continuing education programs. The Board of Oncology Social Work Certification additionally offers Oncology Social Work Certification (OSW-C) to individuals who have graduated from a CSWE accredited program; have 3 years of post-master's degree work in oncology social work or a related field, such as palliative or end-of-life care; hold licensure in good standing and membership in AOSW or APOSW; have three professional statements of support; can show evidence of involvement in extramural service, education, or research activities; and have agreed to uphold AOSW Standards of Practice and NASW Code of Ethics. Certification renewal requires evidence of continued relevant work, licensure, and fulfillment of continuing education requirements.[17] The American Cancer Society (ACS) awards students in MSW programs advanced training grants to provide psychosocial services to people with cancer and their families (ACS, 2006). Finally, nearly every jurisdiction requires continuing education courses for renewal of social work licenses, although these requirements vary from one jurisdiction to another, for example, in the number of hours or types of courses required (ASWB, 2006b).

Mental Health Providers

Psychosocial health services also are offered by licensed mental health providers, such as psychologists and counselors, who address psychological health as the primary purpose of their intervention. Because, as with psychiatrists, their services are by definition "psychological," their education and training can reasonably be expected to address psychosocial health care. For these practitioners, as for psychiatrists and social workers, the issue is how well prepared they are to serve those with acute or chronic health problems (especially when these problems can be life-threatening) and how well they are prepared to carry out key psychosocial interventions, such as assessing social issues affecting the patient, coordinating care, and working with an interdisciplinary team.

---

[17]Personal communication, Ginny Vaitones, Board of Oncology Social Work Certification, August 21, 2007.

Psychologists

In 2004, the United States had 85,000 psychologists trained at the doctoral level, the standard educational path for practice as an independent clinical psychologist.[18] To become a licensed clinical psychologist, graduates of doctoral programs also must complete supervised postdoctoral training (Olvey and Hogg, 2002).

Clinically oriented graduate programs are organized and accredited in three categories: clinical psychologist preparation, counseling, and school psychologist preparation. Psychologists can remain generalists or develop an area of expertise within these broad categories. Most relevant to the provision of psychosocial health services to medically ill patients and their families is the specialty of clinical health psychology, discussed in more detail below. Other relevant specialties include neuropsychology, rehabilitation psychology, and pediatric psychology. Just over 5,000 members of the American Psychological Association (APA) list a medically related interest area.[19]

Clinical health psychology has been a major area of growth, and part of the psychology discipline's organized effort to broaden its scope from a *mental health* to a *health* profession. It was formally recognized by APA as a specialty in the professional practice of psychology in 1997. There are 68 doctoral programs across clinical, counseling, and school psychology with an emphasis in health or medically related areas (APA, 2006b). There are 201 predoctoral internships with a major rotation in health psychology and 381 with a minor rotation, plus an additional 51 postdoctoral fellowships that incorporate training on this topic (http://www.appic.org/directory/).

Accreditation   Accreditation of educational programs for psychologists is managed by the APA's Committee on Accreditation. The aim is to ensure that each program has ". . . clearly defined and appropriate objectives and maintains conditions under which their achievement can reasonably be expected. It encourages improvement through continuous self-study and review" (http://www.apa.org/ed/accreditation/). Accreditation is offered for doctoral programs, pre- and postdoctoral internships, and specialty postdoctoral internships. The latter are limited in number and include a focus on clinical child psychology (3), clinical health psychology (5), clinical neuropsychology (11), and rehabilitation psychology (1). (Doctoral accreditation encompasses master's-level training, but accreditation is not

---

[18]Individuals with a master's degree in psychology also can practice under the direction of a doctoral-prepared psychologist, or independently as school psychologists or counselors (APA, 2003; Duffy et al., 2004).
[19]Personal communication, Cynthia Belar, PhD, Executive Director for Education, American Psychological Association, October 18, 2006.

available for terminal master's programs.) The doctoral accreditation standards require that students be "exposed to the current body of knowledge in . . . biological aspects of behavior . . ." (APA, 2005:12). However, there is no additional detail regarding this standard. Pre- and postdoctoral standards contain no reference to this domain of knowledge.

Licensure   The Examination for Professional Practice in Psychology (EPPP) was developed and is updated by the Association of State and Provincial Psychology Boards (ASPPB). This standardized exam is used by every jurisdiction in the United States and Canada except Puerto Rico and portions of Quebec. Many jurisdictions complement the EPPP with written and oral exams that assess clinical competence and knowledge of local mental health law. Licensing is generic for the practice of psychology and does not distinguish among clinical, counseling, and health psychologists. Only one state offers a license to practice in a specialty area of the discipline.

ASPPB conducts a practice analysis every 6–10 years, including a survey of practicing psychologists, in order to update the exam. From the ASPPB's perspective, the objective of the national exam and the licensing process is to ensure a minimum level of competence and public safety. The objective is *not* to change or advance the field.[20]

Each EPPP comprises 225 multiple-choice questions (ASPPB, 2006), 11 percent of which focus on the content area "biological bases of behavior." Issues related to the impact of disability constitute just 1 of 26 areas covered under the content area "social and multicultural bases of behavior" (12 percent of the exam). Numerous other content areas have some potential relevance: "cognitive-affective bases of behavior" (13 percent); "growth and lifespan development" (13 percent); "assessment and diagnosis" (14 percent); and "treatment, intervention, and prevention" (15 percent). While a significant portion of the exam focuses on the biological bases of behavior, experts in health psychology view this content as a necessary but largely insufficient knowledge base on the biopsychosocial interrelationships that must be understood in order to practice in a medically related specialty.

Certification   The American Board of Professional Psychology (ABPP) certifies psychologists in 13 specialty areas, including clinical health psychology, clinical neuropsychology, and rehabilitation psychology. Board certification is not a requirement for practice in any jurisdiction or service organization, and it has not been pursued by the vast majority of psycholo-

---

[20]Personal communication, Stephen DeMers, EdD, Executive Director, Associations of State and Provincial Psychology Boards, October 5, 2006.

gists. Currently, there are only an estimated 3,000 board-certified psychologists in the United States.

Those seeking board certification in the area of clinical health psychology may specialize in any number of areas, including prevention, health promotion, public health, pain management, weight reduction, smoking cessation, and/or the psychological aspects of chronic illness. Board certification requires a degree from an APA-approved graduate program, plus licensure and two years of postdoctoral training or supervised experience in clinical health psychology. The elements of the certification process include review of qualifications, review of a work sample, an oral exam focused on the work sample and ethics, and endorsement by colleagues. Board-certified experts review the candidate and make a determination regarding certification. There are no competency sets or explicit standards used as criteria.

It has been difficult to interest health psychologists in applying for certification. Military psychologists constitute the one group that has promotion/salary incentives tied to certification. There are only an estimated 100 psychologists certified in this specialty.[21]

Graduate training   Training in clinical health psychology during graduate study usually involves a number of additional required courses focused on this specialty, plus an advanced clinical placement working with medically ill individuals. This advanced placement follows basic training in core clinical skills. Graduate training in psychology at the doctoral level involves required and elective courses, complemented by supervised clinical experience. Other than limited didactic content on the biological bases of behavior, general students in these programs are usually not exposed to didactic or substantive experiential training related to chronic medical illnesses and the psychosocial aspects of care for persons with these illnesses.

Pre/postdoctoral internships   A 1-year predoctoral internship is required for graduation from an APA-approved doctoral training program. Postdoctoral internships are optional, but are often the vehicle selected by recent graduates to obtain specialty training and the supervised experience necessary to apply for licensure.

To explore the nature of internship training related to cancer care, a request for information was circulated nationally by the Association of Psychology Postdoctoral and Internship Centers to its member programs. A total of 18 responses were received, most of which briefly summarized one program's training activities. By and large, these internships appear to involve supervised clinical experience working with cancer patients and

---

[21]Personal communication, Douglas Tynan, PhD, Chair, Board of Clinical Health Psychology, American Board of Professional Psychology, October 26, 2006.

their families in hospital settings. Additional elements of the training may involve selected readings, while a few sites offer a related course. Though asked, respondents did not identify competency sets or model curricula related to this training.

A noteworthy exemplar is Children's Hospital of Philadelphia, with its Psychology Training Programs in Pediatric Oncology (http://www.chop.edu/hc_professionals/psych_edu.shtml). Pre- and postdoctoral training is offered, as well as supervised experiences for graduate students. These programs provide opportunities for outpatient-, school-, and community-based work in addition to hospital-based training.

Competencies and curricula Core curricular components in graduate-level clinical health psychology were first specified through a national consensus conference in 1983 (Stone, 1983). These core components centered on the social, biological, and psychological bases of health and disease; health policy, systems, and organizations; health assessment, consultation, and intervention; health research methods; ethical, legal, and professional issues; and interdisciplinary collaboration (Belar, 1990). In 1997, Belar and colleagues developed a model for self-assessment of knowledge and skills by health psychologists that drew from the content areas identified in the original consensus conference (Belar et al., 2001). The Society for Pediatric Psychology also recently published a set of recommendations for training in the subspecialty of clinical child psychology (Spirito et al., 2003), which articulate a dozen suggested "domains of training."

Conclusions The psychology profession has seen rapid growth, expanding the potential pool of mental health professionals who can respond to the psychosocial needs of cancer patients; clear growth has occurred as well in health-related specialties, including health psychology, neuropsychology, and rehabilitation psychology. However, accreditation standards for training in psychology are very general and have limited direct applicability to psychosocial aspects of serious, complex medical illness. While accreditation standards are often referenced in the health care workforce literature as potential levers of change in efforts to influence curricula (IOM, 2003), it is difficult to envision how the current standards in this profession, given their general nature, could be modified to effect substantive change in training programs on the issues addressed in this report. Moreover, board certification does not play a major role in the field of psychology and therefore is an unlikely vehicle for effecting change.

In comparison with accreditation standards, the content domains in the national licensing exam (EPPP) are relatively specific. While the biological bases of behavior are covered, it is possible to envision adding specificity in this area addressing the psychosocial aspects of illness and recovery. Doing so might influence curricula design in graduate programs. However, it could conflict with the generalist nature of the exam and the aim of reflecting current rather than optimal practice.

A training focus on cancer appears to occur principally through supervised experience in cancer care settings. Any call for additional core or basic training should probably focus on the psychosocial aspects of chronic illnesses generally rather than cancer in particular. The knowledge and skill gained through basic training in medical illness and its psychosocial effects could then be applied during additional supervised clinical experience with unique populations of chronically ill individuals, such as persons with cancer. However, training activity in this profession, as in much of medicine, tends to be organized around hospital settings and funded through hospital-based activities. This situation serves as a barrier to the development and delivery of psychosocial services to medically ill patients in nonhospital community settings.

A striking finding is that there appear to be no detailed competency sets or model curricula related to cancer care in use within this profession; there is merely a brief list of "core curricular areas" from a seminal 1983 health psychology conference. The development, dissemination, and adoption of competency sets and model curricula are potential high-yield interventions for advancing training in the psychosocial aspects of illness. In addition to the absence of clear competencies and curricula, other apparent barriers to improved education and training in this area include the absence of funding for training and a lack of qualified faculty.

Counselors

Requirements to become a licensed counselor include completing a master's degree in counseling, passing a state-recognized exam, adhering to ethical codes and standards, and completing continuing education (BLS, 2006a). Professional educational programs in counseling voluntarily undergo review by an accrediting body, such as the Commission on Rehabilitation Education (CORE), which accredits graduate programs in Rehabilitation Counselor Education (RCE) (CORE, 2006), or the Commission on the Accreditation of Counseling and Related Educational Programs (CACREP), which accredits a variety of master's degree programs, including family, community, gerontological, and mental health counseling (CACREP, 2006). Licensed counselors may become certified by the Commission of Rehabilitation Counselor Certification, which grants the credential Certified Rehabilitation Counselor (CRC) (CCRC, 2006), or by the National Board for Certified Counselors (NBCC), which grants the general practice credential National Certified Counselor (NBCC, 2006).

Pastoral Counselors

A diagnosis of cancer or another serious illness can challenge a person's spiritual as well as physical and psychological well-being. During illness and recovery, patients and their families may explore ways to address these difficulties by seeking pastoral counselors—ministers who integrate religious resources with insights from the behavioral sciences—to assist them with coping. The American Association of Pastoral Counselors (AAPC) accredits pastoral counselor training programs and credentials individuals in the discipline. To become a certified pastoral counselor, a candidate must possess a bachelor's, master's, or doctoral degree in divinity; become ordained or recognized by identified faith groups; maintain an active relationship to a local religious community; complete a supervised self-reflective pastoral experience; spend 3 years in ministry; and complete an AAPC-approved Training Program in Pastoral Counseling. Pastoral counselors are then able to work with a state license (AAPC, 2005).

EDUCATIONAL BARRIERS TO PSYCHOSOCIAL HEALTH CARE

The above discussion indicates that there is likely inconsistency in the extent to which the educational curricula studied by predominantly medically focused health care providers address psychosocial health care (and conversely the extent to which the curricula studied by predominantly psychosocial health care providers address the effects of illness on psychosocial functioning). Confounding the ability to understand and redress this inconsistency are the limited information systems available to collect data on how educational standards are translated into hours or methods of instruction, the content of such instruction, or the resulting skills of the workforce. Therefore, it is not possible to know with any certainty the characteristics of the education these health care providers receive on psychosocial issues, or the actual competency in assessing and addressing psychosocial needs they develop as a result of their education.

As discussed in Chapters 1 and 4, however, there is compelling evidence that the psychosocial needs of patients are not being adequately identified (Passik et al., 1998; McDonald et al., 1999; Fallowfield et al., 2001; Keller et al., 2004; President's Cancer Panel, 2004; Maly et al., 2005; Merckaert et al., 2005; USA Today et al., 2006; IOM, 2007). Also as discussed previously, a range of interrelated factors—including how work in clinical practices is designed and how incentives from payers and oversight organizations operate—can impede the health care workforce's identification of psychosocial needs and delivery of psychosocial services. Yet limitations of the content and methods of professional education and training play a role as well. In addition to a possible underemphasis on psychosocial issues in health professions education, education that does not prepare clinicians to practice in today's work environments, a lack of faculty or knowledge by faculty about what needs to be taught, and ineffective approaches to education can adversely affect the development of needed competencies.

Barriers to Education

Gap Between Health Professions Education and the Current Practice Environment

There are broad concerns about health professions education that go far beyond the lack of emphasis on biopsychosocial models of illness and recovery. Experts in education and health care delivery have concluded that clinical education has not kept pace with the shift in patient demographics and desires, changing expectations for the workforce within health systems, evolving practice requirements and staffing arrangements, the continuous flood of new information, the focus on quality improvement, and new technologies. Accordingly, they have called for the restructuring of health professions education to make it more relevant to twenty-first century health care (IOM, 2001, 2003). The IOM has recommended an intensive focus on five core competencies as the cornerstones of health professions education and improved workforce performance (IOM, 2003:4):

- *Patient-centered care*—Identify, respect, and care about patient differences, values, preferences, and expressed needs; relieve pain and suffering; coordinate continuous care; listen to, clearly inform, communicate with, and educate patients; share decision making and management; and continuously advocate disease prevention, wellness, and promotion of healthy lifestyles, including a focus on population health.
- *Work in interdisciplinary teams*—Cooperate, collaborate, communicate, and integrate care in teams to ensure that care is continuous and reliable.
- *Employ evidence-based practice*—Integrate best research with clinical expertise and patient values for optimum care, and participate in learning and research activities to the extent feasible.
- *Apply quality improvement*—Identify errors and hazards in care; understand and implement basic safety design principles, such as standardization and simplification; continually understand and measure quality of care in terms of structure, process, and outcomes in relation to patient and community needs; and design and test interventions to change processes and systems of care, with the objective of improving quality.

- *Utilize informatics*—Communicate, manage knowledge, mitigate error, and support decision making using information technology.

The current weaknesses in health professions education in these five areas impede the delivery of psychosocial services to cancer patients in very concrete ways. Inattention to patient differences, values, preferences, and concerns contributes to psychosocial needs being undetected and unaddressed. Difficulties in communicating hamper collaboration with patients and families and undermine shared decision making about strategies for meeting psychosocial needs. The absence of skills related to interdisciplinary, team-based care creates a barrier to establishing the linkages with other professionals that are essential in connecting patients and families to available psychosocial resources. A tendency to rely on clinical tradition rather than evidence leaves the workforce unaware of emerging evidence on the effectiveness of psychosocial services and unfamiliar with new practice guidelines that are drawn from that evidence. A lack of familiarity with informatics creates an aversion to innovative, computer-assisted methods for the critical tasks of screening and assessment of psychosocial needs.

Inconsistent Use of Competencies to Guide Training

In response to growing concerns about the abilities of health professionals to keep up with the rapid pace of clinical developments and changes in health care systems, many health professions groups are undertaking initiatives to rethink the competencies their clinicians need to practice effectively. ACGME, for example, has launched a major, multiyear initiative to identify, better develop, and assess the competency of physicians in residency training (Swing, 2002). The Council identified six general competencies addressing patient care, medical knowledge, practice-based learning and improvement, interpersonal and communication skills, professionalism, and systems-based practice (http://www.acgme.org/outcome/). ACGME required the committees that establish accreditation criteria for residencies in each specialty to incorporate these general competencies into their requirements. In a graduated fashion, residency programs are being required to define the specific knowledge, skills, and attitudes that make up each general competency; to redesign their programs to teach the competencies; and to formally assess the competency of their residents. There is emerging evidence that these requirements have had an impact on training programs. For example, Weissman and colleagues (2006) found that psychiatric residency programs provide didactic and supervised clinical experience in evidence-based psychotherapies much more frequently than do graduate-level psychology or social work programs. In the latter two fields, accreditation standards are less prescriptive regarding the teaching of evidence-based practices.

This focus on competency identification is occurring broadly in other disciplines as well. Various mental health professions are developing competency models in such disciplines as marriage and family therapy, psychology, advanced practice psychiatric nursing, and psychiatric rehabilitation. Cross-disciplinary competencies are being developed for practice with specific populations, such as children and adults with severe mental illness. Other initiatives have focused on competencies for special treatment approaches, such as recovery-oriented care, peer support, and culturally competent care (Hoge et al., 2005a). The inadequate delivery of psychosocial health care in oncology suggests that there also may be benefits to specifying the competencies necessary for providing psychosocial services to medically ill patients in general, and to cancer patients in particular.

There are existing resources and some positive developments that could be used to advance the use of core competencies for the psychosocial care of cancer patients and their families. C-Change (http://www.c-changetogether.org), a coalition of federal and state government agencies, cancer centers, professional organizations, private businesses, nonprofit groups, and business leaders and individuals in the private sector whose missions relate to cancer research, control, and/or patient advocacy, has undertaken a major initiative to strengthen the core competencies of the cancer care workforce. The goal of this initiative is to develop and disseminate basic cancer care competencies to the *general* health care workforce—that not specializing in oncology. This focus on the nonspecialist workforce is deliberate, based on data showing an expanding need for oncology care that is not accompanied by as expansive a growth in the specialty oncology workforce. C-Change recognizes that the general health care workforce, as well as the specialty oncology workforce, needs to be competent in delivering cancer care (Smith and Lichtveld, 2007).

C-Change has already defined a set of core workforce competencies, many of which address the psychosocial services and interventions recommended in the committee's model and standard for care (see Box 7-6). C-Change plans to work with pilot sites to implement the competencies in 2007. Based on the results of this pilot test and evaluation, in 2008 C-Change plans to pursue national dissemination of the core competencies through academic, health care, and professional organizations, as well as through comprehensive cancer control coalitions. The core competencies and to-be-developed curriculum resources will be able to be integrated into (1) basic health professions education curricula used at academic institutions, (2) continuing education programs and licensing requirements of health professional societies, and (3) worksite training programs offered by employers of health professionals (Smith and Lichtveld, 2007).

The set of five competencies recommended by the IOM (2003) and the set of six general competencies required by ACGME (Swing, 2002) also can contribute to the development of core psychosocial competencies, as does a model for self-assessment of knowledge and skills by health psychologists described by Belar and colleagues (2001). Similarly, Division 54 of the APA recommended 12 areas of training in pediatric psychology, which could easily be translated into competency domains (Spirito et al., 2003). The Memorial-Sloan Kettering Cancer Center has identified specific competencies for its Fellowship in Psycho-Oncology and Psychosomatic Medicine within each of the six ACGME categories and is sharing these competencies with similar programs around the country.[22] For example, a core competency for fellows in the "systems-based practice competency" involves the following: "Demonstrates a knowledge of community resources available to patients for continuing psychiatric care, care for family members, support and information and advocacy services for cancer patients/survivors, and hospice/palliative care resources" (Memorial-Sloan Kettering Cancer Center, 2007:4). As discussed earlier, the subspecialty of psychosomatic medicine also was recently approved as a subspecialty in psychiatry by ACGME, and the program requirements for this subspecialty indirectly identify essential competencies (http://www.acgme.org/acWebsite/RRC_400/400_prIndex.asp). The Academy of Psychosomatic Medicine has organized a committee that is charged with developing more specific competencies for this area of practice, which will serve as yet another resource.[23]

Finally, the model for providing psychosocial services to cancer survivors and their families detailed in Chapter 4 should inform efforts to specify the competencies relevant to providing psychosocial services for all members of the workforce. It provides clear direction regarding the types of core competencies that should be considered essential in future efforts to develop comprehensive competency sets and related curricula. These include knowledge and skills in the following:

- Communication with patients and families
- Screening
- Needs assessment
- Care planning and coordination
- Illness self-management
- Collaboration across disciplines/specialties and work in teams

---

[22]Personal communication, Andrew J. Roth, MD, Attending Psychiatrist, Department of Psychiatry and Behavioral Sciences, Memorial Sloan-Kettering Cancer Center, March 21, 2007.

[23]Personal communication, William S. Breitbart, MD, Chief, Psychiatry Service, Department of Psychiatry and Behavioral Sciences, Memorial Sloan-Kettering Cancer Center, March 21, 2007.

BOX 7-6
Selected C-Change Psychosocial Core Competencies

DOMAIN I: CONTINUUM OF CARE. Within the context of the professional discipline and scope of practice, a health care professional should . . .

Prevention and Behavioral Risks . . .
Incorporate the shared decision-making process into cancer risk-reduction counseling.

Treatment
    a. Access cancer treatment information specific to cancer location and type.
    b. Describe the available cancer treatment modalities. . . .
    d. Describe options to manage disease and treatment-related symptoms.
    e. Manage disease and treatment-related symptoms.
    f. Refer for treatment of disease and treatment-related symptoms.
    g. Provide emotional support to patients.
    h. Refer for mental health services.

Post Treatment
    b. Assess that resources for cancer services and insurance coverage are consistent with current recommendation.
    c. Assist patients and families in navigating the health care system following cancer treatment.
    d. Guide patients with cancer and their families toward support systems and groups.
    e. Provide ongoing health services that meet age and gender recommendations.
    f. Recognize the importance of survivorship in a long-term cancer care plan at the conclusion of active treatment.
    g. Manage continuing and late effects of cancer and cancer treatment.
    j. Refer survivors to rehabilitation services.
    k. Provide support for cancer survivors and their families and caregivers as they cope with daily living, including lifestyle, employment, school, sexual relationships, fertility issues, and personal intimacy.

Pain Management
    a. Explain how cancer pain differs from other types of pain.
    b. Describe the methods used to diagnosis cancer pain throughout the progression of the disease.
    c. Differentiate between acute and chronic pain symptoms.

- Linking of patients to psychosocial services
- Outcome assessment
- Informatics (to support screening, needs assessment, planning, care coordination, service provision, and outcome assessment)

d. Describe the characteristics used to assess cancer pain: frequency, intensity, and site.
e. Perform a cancer pain assessment.
f. Explain the different treatment options for cancer pain.
g. Perform a pain-related history taken during a physical examination.
h. Manage cancer-related pain and analgesic side effects.

DOMAIN III: COLLABORATION AND COMMUNICATION.
A. Participate Within an Interdisciplinary Cancer Care Team
  1. Define interdisciplinary care.
  2. Describe the contribution of each professional perspective in the development of cancer care plan.
  3. Consider the financial implications for recommended cancer care.
  4. Refer patients to an oncology social worker for financial guidance and resource navigation.
  5. Consider the resource challenges of the agency in implementing a treatment plan.

B. Incorporate Psychosocial Communication Strategies in Conveying Cancer Information
  1. Refer patients to mental health, psychosocial, and support services.
  2. Recognize the signs and symptoms of cancer-related depression and anxiety.
  3. Explain the management of depression and anxiety in patients with cancer.
  4. Explain the useful copying [sic] mechanisms following a cancer diagnosis.

C. Incorporate Cross-Cultural Communication Strategies in Conveying Cancer Information
  1. Identify cultural subgroups in a given patient population.
  2. Define culture-specific beliefs and practices.
  3. Communicate cancer care information that is sensitive to religious and spiritual beliefs and practices.

D. Describe Common Ethical and Legal Issues in Cancer Care
  1. Adhere to HIPAA policies, procedures, and regulations.
  2. Access institutional and other ethics resources.
  3. Advocate for the use of advanced directives, including the right to refuse care.
  4. Justify the need for informed consent in cancer research.

SOURCE: Smith and Lichtveld, 2007.

Elaboration is required for each of these content areas, specifying behavioral descriptors for the underlying knowledge, skills, and attitudes required for (1) different sectors of the workforce (e.g., paraprofessional case manager versus medical oncologist), (2) different stages of development (e.g., completion of training versus independent practice), and (3) different

levels of competence (exceptional, acceptable, substandard). Such sophisti-
cation in competency identification and assessment is required to move the
field beyond the common and limited practice of simply listing generic competencies with no specificity or behavioral anchors (Hoge et al., 2005b).

Competency-based approaches offer a flexible foundation for staff development and assessment. Traditional approaches, in which qualifications
or abilities are inferred from degrees, certification, licensure, discipline, or
job description, lack specificity regarding skills and are of little utility when
assessing skills that are shared by multiple segments of the workforce. Case
management, for example, is a skill that can be performed by nondegreed
paraprofessionals, such as navigators, or by highly trained professionals,
such as master's-prepared social workers or medical oncologists. Conceptualizing case management as a function or competency, defined by clear
behavioral descriptors and several levels of expertise, would provide for
greater utility and flexibility in providing training in and assessing workforce capacities.

Faculty Needs

Identified educational competencies are necessary but insufficient for
the development of student/trainee knowledge and skills. Sufficient numbers of faculty who themselves possess the requisite attitudes, knowledge,
and skills are required to teach the competencies. Faculty development
programs are widely used to help train a critical mass of faculty in areas
identified as deficient, such as education about substance use (Haack and
Adger, 2002). Some professions, such as nursing, additionally suffer from
an inadequate supply of faculty generally. Faculty development programs
that attend to both numbers and expertise are needed to ensure the application of the competencies across health professions schools.

Effective Teaching Practices

Competency identification and curriculum development provide a foundation for training and education. However, they must be combined with
effective teaching practices to achieve the desired learning outcomes (Stuart
et al., 2004). A substantial evidence base exists in medicine regarding effective teaching and skill development approaches (Davis et al., 1999). The
principal finding of research in this area is that didactic or noninteractive,
single-session lectures and workshops constitute the most common training approaches in continuing education and much of preservice education,
but have virtually no effect in changing the practice behaviors of trainees (Mazmanian and Davis, 2002; Bloom, 2005). Davis and colleagues
(1999) argue that the evidence on this issue is so strong that continuing

education credit should probably not be offered for most continuing education events.

Oxman and colleagues (1995) conclude there is no single magic bullet for achieving skill development and change in practice behaviors among learners. Combining multiple teaching strategies, each proven to have small effects on practice behavior, represents an evidenced-based approach to teaching. Such strategies include interactive or experiential methods; outreach visits, sometimes referred to as academic detailing; reminders; auditing of practice behaviors with the provision of feedback to the learner; the use of opinion leaders; and patient-mediated interventions (Soumerai, 1998; Borgiel et al., 1999; Davis et al., 1999; O'Brien et al., 2003). Examples of some of these strategies are presented below.

Combined, multiple teaching strategies   The Communication Skills Teaching and Research (Comskil) Lab at Memorial Sloan-Kettering Cancer Center is currently training fellows from nonpsychiatric medical specialties in communication skills. To date, 39 fellows have been trained around six core modules: (1) Breaking Bad News, (2) Shared Decision Making About Treatment Options, (3) Responding to Patient Anger, (4) Discussing Prognosis, (5) Discussing the Transition from Curative to Palliative Care, and (6) Shared Decision Making About "Do Not Recussitate" Orders.

The Comskil training program was developed using best practices that have been established for communication skills training. Before attending a module, participants receive a booklet summarizing the literature and skill recommendations. Each 2½- to 3-hour training module consists of a didactic presentation, exemplary video clips demonstrating skills, and a small-group role play session in which learners have the opportunity to practice with a trained actor playing the role of a patient. Immediate video playback of this role play encourages review, experimentation, and reinforcement of new skills. Each session is cofacilitated by a medical/surgical and a psychosocial facilitator.

Assessment and feedback are essential to the Comskil experience. Before attending their first Comskil training module, participants are video recorded in their outpatient consultations with two patients, with the patient's permission. These recordings are analyzed using a coding system based on the Comskil curriculum to assess participants' baseline. Participants receive feedback letters, based on this coding, that describe their current clinical communication strengths, as well as areas for improvement. Following training, participants are again video recorded in their consultations with two patients. The recordings are analyzed, and feedback letters are sent to participants describing their strengths, improvements, and areas in need of continued improvement.

Interactive, multicomponent education postlicensure   The Individual Cancer Assistance Network (ICAN) initiative of the National Association of Social Workers, CancerCare, the American Psychosocial Oncology Society (APOS), and Bristol-Meyers Squibb Foundation uses interactive strategies to train social workers and other mental health professionals to provide "cancer-sensitive" counseling to individuals with cancer. ICAN's 8-hour face-to-face, interactive, experiential training program comprises discussion and knowledge- and skill-building activities encompassing clinicians' monitoring of their own attitudinal and emotional responses to cancer; psychosocial issues relevant to cancer patients, including stress management, coping, quality-of-life concerns, grief, and hope; and ongoing case consultation support. Skill-building activities address biopsychosocial assessment, counseling methods, relaxation techniques, collaborative care, and resource utilization. Evaluations of the ICAN program found that participants rated the program highly with respect to increasing their knowledge and making them better prepared to serve cancer patients (Blum et al., 2006). As of the end of 2006, more than 20,000 people from at least 68 countries had taken the online courses offered by APOS and NASW; 75 percent of these participants had taken and passed the continuing education credit exams; and more than 400 social workers had participated in the day-long in-person training sessions hosted by NASW state chapters. Most recently, the ICAN program implemented a train-the-trainer format, and 20 participants were trained to deliver the curriculum to at least 20 colleagues in their communities.[24]

Interdisciplinary, experiential, statewide education   In response to a study revealing a high level of unmet psychosocial needs among cancer patients in the state, Pennsylvania's Cancer Control Program commissioned the development of a statewide continuing education program for health professionals working with cancer patients (Barg et al., 1993). Priorities of the program were to (1) enhance provider knowledge about psychosocial services, as well as pain and symptom control; (2) develop and distribute consumer guides to community resources to increase the use of existing support services; and (3) increase effective provider communication with patients and their families. Responsibility for curriculum content, methods, and implementation was shared by the University of Pennsylvania, University of Pittsburgh, Hershey Medical Center, and Lehigh Valley-Allentown Cooperative Cancer Center. The 3-day curriculum for health professionals was delivered at more than 20 sites across the state, and involved transmitting knowledge and using experiential educational strategies such as role

---

[24]Personal communication, Patricia Doykos Duquette, PhD, Bristol-Myers Squibb Foundation, New York, December 14, 2006.

playing, exercises in communication and problem solving, and analysis of ethical dilemmas. An interdisciplinary approach to care was modeled through the use of teams, comprising a nurse and social worker, to deliver the continuing education program. The majority of participants were nurses, complemented by social workers, nutritionists, clergy, and pharmacists. Evaluation revealed measurable changes in psychosocial assessments, interventions, and referrals taking place at attendees' workplaces.

Learning collaborative In conjunction with The Robert Wood Johnson Foundation, the American Association of Medical Colleges launched an Academic Chronic Care Collaborative to improve care of persons with chronic conditions who receive their care in academic health systems and to ensure that clinical education occurs in an exemplary clinical environment. Teams from 22 academic medical centers are participating in the initiative and have reported significantly enhanced clinical processes and outcomes for persons with diabetes, chronic obstructive pulmonary disease, and childhood asthma. In addition, their redesign of resident training produced new evidence-based approaches to trainees' experiences and evaluation, as well as new insights into how to revitalize primary care in these settings (AAMC, 2006a).

CONCLUSIONS AND RECOMMENDATION

The committee concludes that the health care workforce's attention to psychosocial needs may be inadequate for a number of reasons. As discussed in other chapters, practice environments may not be designed or organized to support efforts to identify and meet these needs. Policies of insurers and others also may create disincentives to attend to psychosocial health care. However, health professions education and training shape clinicians before they enter the workforce and are key determinants of clinicians' attitudes, knowledge, and skills. Continuing education and maintenance-of-competency initiatives also help as new knowledge and care methods develop. Thus, professional education and training should not be ignored as a factor influencing the practices of health care providers.

With respect to workforce training and development, the committee identifies the following factors as possible impediments to the provision of psychosocial health services:

- lack of clarity about the competencies the workforce should optimally possess to provide the services;
- the absence of well-developed curricula built around clearly defined competencies;

- inadequate numbers of faculty qualified to train and mentor students in psychosocial skills; and
- insufficient specificity in accreditation and licensing standards regarding competencies in and curricula on psychosocial care.

Moreover, the lack of information systems to track developments in education and training hampers the identification of effective educational approaches. Significant efforts are needed to ensure appropriate education and training of practitioners. Educational accrediting organizations, licensing bodies, and professional societies should examine their standards, licensing, and certification criteria with an eye to developing them as fully as possible in accordance with the standard of care set forth in this report. The committee further makes the following recommendation.

Recommendation: Workforce competencies.

a. Educational accrediting organizations, licensing bodies, and professional societies should examine their standards and licensing and certification criteria with an eye to identifying competencies in delivering psychosocial health care and developing them as fully as possible in accordance with a model that integrates biomedical and psychosocial care.

b. Congress and federal agencies should support and fund the establishment of a Workforce Development Collaborative on Psychosocial Care during Chronic Medical Illness. This cross-specialty, multidisciplinary group should comprise educators, consumer and family advocates, and providers of psychosocial and biomedical health services and be charged with

  – identifying, refining, and broadly disseminating to health care educators information about workforce competencies, models, and preservice curricula relevant to providing psychosocial services to persons with chronic medical illnesses and their families;

  – adapting curricula for continuing education of the existing workforce using efficient workplace-based learning approaches;

  – drafting and implementing a plan for developing the skills of faculty and other trainers in teaching psychosocial health care using evidence-based teaching strategies; and

  – strengthening the emphasis on psychosocial health care in educational accreditation standards and professional licensing and certification exams by recommending revisions to the relevant oversight organizations.

c. Organizations providing research funding should support assessment of the implementation in education, training, and clinical practice of the workforce competencies necessary to provide psychosocial care and their impact on achieving the standard for such care.

The committee proposes a sequence of three steps to foster both immediate and increasing attention to this workforce need.

First, to catalyze the process, the National Institutes of Health (NIH) and other components of the Department of Health and Human Services (DHHS) should jointly convene a meeting of stakeholders in psychosocial health care to identify, summarize, and develop a distribution plan regarding currently available competencies, curricula, and model training approaches. This group should also develop the recommended membership and 2-year work plan for the proposed Workforce Development Collaborative.

As a second step, DHHS should establish a full-time managerial position within its Health Resources and Services Administration (HRSA) with responsibility for improving the provision of psychosocial health services to individuals with chronic medical illnesses and their families. This individual should convene a multiagency federal working group to coordinate federal efforts on this agenda. At a minimum, the group should include representatives from HRSA, the Office of Behavioral and Social Sciences Research (OBSSR) within NIH, the Centers for Medicare and Medicaid Services (CMS), the Agency for Healthcare Research and Quality (AHRQ), and the Substance Abuse and Mental Health Services Administration (SAMHSA).

The third step in this process should involve appropriation or allocation of federal funds to establish and support the operation of the Workforce Development Collaborative. Once convened, the Collaborative would pursue activities to further develop competencies and curricula, improve the skills of faculty, and influence the strengthening of accreditation standards. The Collaborative should give consideration to using small "challenge grants" to stimulate competency and curriculum development, following the model being used by the Picker Institute (http://www.pickerinstitute. org) to stimulate best practices in graduate medical education on patient-centered care.

Congressional action and support for these recommended steps would be optimal, providing robust support for fully realizing the objectives identified. However, action on these recommendations can and should be taken by the federal agencies even in the absence of congressional action.

Moreover, action can be taken independently by educational leaders in the private sector as described in recommendation a above:

a. Educational accrediting organizations, licensing bodies, and professional societies should examine their standards and licensing and certification criteria with an eye to identifying competencies in delivering psychosocial health care and developing them as fully as possible in accordance with a model that integrates biomedical and psychosocial care.

Finally, the committee notes that it is most common to call upon health professionals to incorporate necessary psychological and social content into their curricula, but that a similar need exists in the social service professions to incorporate content on biological stressors, including chronic illnesses, into their curricula.

REFERENCES

AACN (American Association of Colleges of Nursing). 1998. *The essentials of baccalaureate education for professional nursing practice.* http://www.aacn.edu/Education/pdf/BaccEssentials98.pdf (accessed July 11, 2007).

AAFP (American Academy of Family Physicians). 2006. *Facts about AAFP.* http://www.aafp.org/online/en/home/aboutus/theaafp/aafpfacts.html (accessed October 22, 2006).

AAMC (Association of American Medical Colleges). 1998. *Report I. Learning objectives for medical student education.* Washington, DC: AAMC.

AAMC. 2006a. *Academic chronic care collaborative congress.* Seattle, WA. October 26–27, 2006. http://www.aamc.org/patientcare/iicc/congress.htm (accessed January 22, 2007).

AAMC. 2006b. *Medical school graduation questionnaire.* http://www.aamc.org/data/gq/allschoolsreports/2006.pdf (accessed November 14, 2006).

AAP (American Academy of Pediatrics). 2006. *AAP at-a-glance.* http://www.aap.org/75/profile/aapprofile-complete.pdf (accessed September 20, 2006).

AAPC (American Association of Pastoral Counselors). 2005. *Training programs in pastoral counseling.* http://www.aapc.org/index.cfm (accessed July 12, 2007).

AAPC. 2006. *About pastoral counseling.* http://www.aapc.org/about.cfm (accessed December 16, 2006).

ABFM (American Board of Family Medicine). 2006a. *About the Maintenance of Certification Program for Family Physicians (MC-FP).* https://www.theabfm.org/MOC/InstructionManualMC-FP.pdf (accessed December 4, 2006).

ABFM. 2006b. *Certification.* https://www.theabfm.org/cert/cert.aspx (accessed September 20, 2006).

ABFM. 2006c. *Diplomate statistics.* https://www.theabfm.org/about/stats.aspx (accessed September 20, 2006).

ABIM (American Board of Internal Medicine). 2006a. *Number of diplomates.* http://www.abim.org/resources/dnum.shtm (accessed October 1, 2006).

ABIM. 2006b. *Policies and procedures for certification, July 2006.* https://www.abim.org/resources/publications/D04.pdf (accessed November 19, 2006).

ABMS (American Board of Medical Specialties). 2006. *Maintenance of Certification (MOC).* http://www.abms.org/About_Board_Certification/MOC.aspx (accessed July 11, 2007).

ABMS. 2007. *American Board of Medical Specialties board certification editorial background.* http://www.abms.org/News_and_Events/Media_Newsroom/pdf/ABMS_EditorialBackground.pdf (accessed November 19, 2007).

ABP (American Board of Pediatrics). 2006a. *A comprehensive overview of the board certification process for generalist and subspecialist pediatricians.* https://www.abp.org/ABPWebSite/ (accessed October 3, 2006).

ABP. 2006b. *Number of diplomate certificates granted through December 2005.* https://www.abp.org/stats/numdips.htm (accessed November 12, 2006).

ABP. 2007. *General Pediatrics Certifying Examination—General pediatrics content outline* https://www.abp.org/certinfo/genpeds/gpoutline.pdf (accessed on November 19, 2007).

ABPN (American Board of Psychiatry and Neurology, Inc.). 2006a. *ABPN maintenance of certification program.* http://www.abpn.com/moc.htm (accessed December 4, 2006).

ABPN. 2006b. *Certification statistics.* http://www.abpn.com/cert_statistics.htm (accessed October 22, 2006).

ACGME (Accreditation Council for Graduate Medical Education). 2005. *Program requirements for fellowship education in medical oncology.* http://www.acgme.org/acWebsite/downloads/RRC_progReq/147pr705_u806.pdf (accessed November 15, 2006).

ACGME. 2006a. *Program requirements for graduate medical education in family medicine.* http://www.acgme.org/acWebsite/downloads/RRC_progReq/120pr706.pdf (accessed July 10, 2007).

ACGME. 2006b. *Program requirements for residency education in pediatrics.* http://www. acgme.org/acWebsite/downloads/RRC_progReq/320pr01012006.pdf (accessed November 15, 2006).

ACGME. 2007a. *ACGME outcome project.* http://www.acgme.org/outcome/ (accessed October 12, 2006).

ACGME. 2007b. *Program requirements for residency education in psychiatry.* http://www. acgme.org/acWebsite/downloads/RRC_progReq/400pr07012007_TCC.pdf (accessed November 15, 2006).

ACP (American College of Physicians). 2006. *About the American College of Physicians.* http://www.acponline.org/college/aboutacp/aboutacp.htm (accessed October 1, 2006).

ACS (American Cancer Society). 2006. *Master's training grants in clinical oncology social work.* http://www.cancer.org/docroot/res/content/res_5_2x_masters_training_grants_in_clinical_oncology_social_work.asp?sitearea=res (accessed December 15, 2006).

AMA (American Medical Association). 2006. *State medical licensure requirements and statistics, 2006.* https://catalog.ama-assn.org/Catalog/product/product_detail.jsp?productId =prod240140# (accessed July 11, 2007).

AOSW (Association of Oncology Social Work). 2001. *AOSW oncology social work standards of practice.* http://www.aosw.org/html/prof-standards.php (accessed September 11, 2007).

APA (American Psychological Association). 2003. *Psychology: Scientific problem solvers—careers for the 21st century.* http://www.apa.org/students/brocure/brochurenew.pdf (accessed June 28, 2005). Washington, DC: American Psychological Association.

APA. 2006a. *About APA.* http://www.apa.org/about/ (accessed September 5, 2007).

APA. 2006b. *Graduate study in psychology.* Washington, DC: APA Books.

APA, Committee on Accreditation. 2005. *Guidelines and principles for accreditation of programs in professional psychology.* Washington, DC: APA.

ASCO (American Society of Clinical Oncology). 2006. *About ASCO.* http://www.asco.org (accessed October 22, 2006).

ASPHO (American Society of Pediatric Hematology/Oncology). 2006. *A career in pediatric hematology-oncology?* http://www.aspho.org/files/public/PHO_Brochure_PDF.pdf (accessed October 22, 2006).

ASPPB (Association of State and Provincial Psychology Boards). 2006. *Information for candidates: Examination for professional practice in psychology.* Montgomery, AL: ASPPB.

Astin, J., T. Goddard, and K. Forys. 2005. Barriers to the integration of mind-body medicine: Perceptions of physicians, residents, and medical students. *Explore: The Journal of Science and Healing* 1(4):278–283.

Astin, J. A., K. Soeken, V. Sierpina, and B. Clarridge. 2006. Barriers to the integration of psychosocial factors in medicine: Results of a national survey of physicians. *Journal of the American Board of Family Medicine* 19(6):557–565.

ASWB (Association of Social Work Boards). 2006a. *Examination content outlines.* http:// www.aswb.org/exam_info_NEW_content_outlines.shtml (accessed December 4, 2006).

ASWB. 2006b. *Social work continuing education.* http://www.aswb.org/education/ (accessed December 4, 2006).

Barg, F. K., R. McCorkle, C. Jepson, J. Downes, G. G. Ferszt, D. Malone, and K. M. McKeehan. 1993. A statewide plan to address the unmet psychosocial needs of people with cancer. *Journal of Psychosocial Oncology* 10(4):55–77.

Batmangelich, S., and S. Adamowski. 2004. Maintenance of certification in the United States: A progress report. *The Journal of Continuing Education in the Health Professions* 24(3):134–138.

Belar, C. 1990. Issues in training clinical health psychologists. *Psychology and Health* 4(1): 31–37.

Belar, C. D., R. Brown, L. Hersch, L. Hornyak, R. H. Rozensky, E. Sheridan, R. Brown, and G. W. Reed. 2001. Self-assessment in clinical health psychology: A model for ethical expansion of practice. *Professional Psychology: Research and Practice* 32(2):135–141.

Bero, L., R. Grilli, J. Grimshaw, E. Harvey, A. Oxman, and M. Thomson. 1998. Closing the gap between research and practice: An overview of systematic reviews of interventions to promote the implementation of research findings. The Cochrane effective practice and organization of care review group. *British Medical Journal* 317(7156):465–468.

Bloom, B. S. 2005. Effects of continuing medical education on improving physician clinical care and patient health: A review of systematic reviews. *International Journal of Technology Assessment in Health Care* 21(3):380–385.

BLS (Bureau of Labor Statistics). 2006a. *Occupational outlook handbook, 2006–07 edition, counselors.* http://www.bls.gov/oco/ocos067.htm (accessed October 22, 2006).

BLS. 2006b. *Occupational outlook handbook, 2006–07 edition, physicians and surgeons.* http://www.bls.gov/oco/ocos074.htm (accessed October 22, 2006).

BLS. 2006c. *Occupational outlook handbook, 2006–07 edition, psychologists.* http://www. bls.gov/oco/ocos056.htm (accessed October 22, 2006).

BLS. 2006d. *Occupational outlook handbook, 2006–07 edition, social workers.* http://www. bls.gov/oco/ocos060.htm (accessed October 22, 2006).

Blum, D., E. Clark, P. Jacobsen, J. Holland, M. J. Monahan, and P. D. Duquette. 2006. Building community-based short-term psychosocial counseling capacity for cancer patients and their families: The Individual Cancer Assistance Network (ICAN) model. *Social Work in Health Care* 43(4):71–83.

Borgiel, A., J. Williams, D. Davis, E. Dunn, N. Hobbs, B. Hutchison, C. Wilson, J. Jensen, J. O'Neil, and M. Bass. 1999. Evaluating the effectiveness of 2 educational interventions in family practice. *Canadian Medical Association Journal* 161(8):965–970.

CACREP (Commission on the Accreditation of Counseling and Related Educational Programs). 2006. *Commission on the Accreditation of Counseling and Related Educational Programs.* http://www.cacrep.org (accessed December 10, 2006).

CCNE (Commission on Collegiate Nursing Education). 2003. *Standards for accreditation of baccalaureate and graduate nursing programs: Amended October 2003.* http://www. aacn.nche.edu/Accreditation/NewStandards.htm (accessed July 12, 2007).

CORE (Council on Rehabilitation Education). 2007. *CORE—Council on Rehabilitation Education.* http://www.core-rehab.org (accessed on November 19, 2007).

CRCC (Commission of Rehabilitation Counselor Certification). 2006. *Commission of Rehabilitation Counselor Certification.* http://www.crccertification.com/pages/10certification. html (accessed December 15, 2006).

CSWE (Council on Social Work Education). 2004. *Educational policy and accreditation standards.* http://www.cswe.org/NR/rdonlyres/111833A0-C4F5-475C-8FEB-EA740FF4D9F1/ 0/EPAS.pdf (accessed July 12, 2007).

Davis, D., M. T. O'Brien, N. Freemantle, F. Wolf, P. Mazmanian, and A. Taylor-Vaisey. 1999. Impact of formal continuing medical education: Do conferences, workshops, rounds, and other traditional continuing education activities change physician behavior or health care outcomes? *Journal of the American Medical Association* 282(9):867–874.

DHHS (Department of Health and Human Services). 1999. *Mental health: A report of the Surgeon General.* Rockville, MD: DHHS. http://www.surgeongeneral.gov/library/mentalhealth/pdfs/c8.pdf (accessed November 19, 2007).

Duffy, F. F., J. C. West, J. Wilk, W. E. Narrow, D. Hales, J. Thompson, D. A. Regier, J. Kohout, G. M. Pion, M. M. Wicherski, N. Bateman, T. Whitaker, E. I. Merwin, D. Lyon, J. C. Fox, K. R. Delaney, N. Hanrahan, R. Stockton, J. Garbelman, J. Kaladow, T. W. Clawson, S. C. Smith, D. M. Bergman, W. F. Northey, L. Blankertz, A. Thomas, L. D. Sullivan, K. P. Dwyer, M. S. Fleischer, C. R. Woodruff, H. F. Goldsmith, M. J. Henderson, J. J. Atay, and R. W. Manderscheid. 2004. Mental health practitioners and trainees. In *Mental health, United States, 2002.* DHHS Publication No. (SMA) 3938. Edited by R. W. Manderscheid and M. J. Henderson. Rockville, MD: DHHS Substance Abuse and Mental Health Services Administration. Pp. 327–368.

Engel, G. L. 1977. The need for a new medical model: A challenge for biomedicine. *Science* 196(4286):129–136.

Erikson, C., E. Salsberg, G. Forte, S. Bruinooge, and M. Goldstein. 2007. Future supply and demand for oncologists: Challenges to assuring access to oncology services. *Journal of Oncology Practice* 3(2):79–86.

Fallowfield, L., D. Ratcliffe, V. Jenkins, and J. Saul. 2001. Psychiatric morbidity and its recognition by doctors in patients with cancer. *British Journal of Cancer* 84(8):1011–1015.

FSMB and NBME (Federation of State Medical Boards of the United States, Inc., and National Board of Medical Examiners). undated-a. *United States medical licensing exam: Step 1 content outline, general principles, 1996–2005.* http://www.usmle.org/step1/s1princ.htm (accessed July 10, 2007).

FSMB and NBME. undated-b. *United States medical licensing exam: Step 3. Purpose and content.* http://www.usmle.org/step3/clincon.htm (accessed July 10, 2007).

Goroll, A. H., C. Sirio, F. D. Duffy, R. F. LeBlond, P. Alguire, T. A. Blackwell, W. E. Rodak, and T. Nasca. 2004. A new model for accreditation of residency programs in internal medicine. *Annals of Internal Medicine* 140(11):902–909.

Grumbach, K. 2002. Fighting hand to hand over physician workforce policy. *Health Affairs* 21(5):13–27.

Haack, M., and H. Adger. 2002. *Strategic plan for interdisciplinary faculty development: Arming the nation's health professional workforce for a new approach to substance use disorders.* Dordrecht, The Netherlands: Kluwer Academic/Plenum Publishers.

Hoge, M. A., J. A. Morris, and M. E. Paris. 2005a. Special issue: Competency development in behavioral health. *Administration and Policy in Mental Health* 32(5/6):485–488.

Hoge, M. A., J. A. Morris, A. S. Daniels, L. Y. Huey, G. W. Stuart, N. Adams, M. Paris, E. Goplerud, C. M. Horgan, L. Kaplan, S. A. Storti, and J. M. Dodge. 2005b. Report of recommendations: The Annapolis coalition conference on behavioral health workforce competencies. *Administration and Policy in Mental Health* 32(5/6):651–663.

Hoge, M. A., J. A. Morris, A. S. Daniels, G. W. Stuart, L. Y. Huey, and N. Adams. 2007. *An action plan on behavioral health workforce development.* Cincinnati, OH: The Annapolis Coalition on the Behavioral Health Workforce.

Horowitz, S., S. Miller, and P. Miles. 2004. Board certification and physician quality. *Medical Education* 38(1):10–11.

HRSA (Health Resources and Service Administration). 2004. *What is behind HRSA's projected supply, demand, and shortage of registered nurses?* ftp://ftp.hrsa.gov/bhpr/workforce/behindshortage.pdf (accessed September 4, 2007).

HRSA. 2006. *The registered nurse population. Findings from the March 2004 National Sample Survey of Registered Nurses.* ftp://ftp.hrsa.gov/bhpr/workforce/0306rnss.pdf (accessed September 5, 2007).

IOM (Institute of Medicine). 2001. *Crossing the quality chasm: A new health system for the 21st century.* Washington, DC: National Academy Press.

IOM. 2003. *Health professions education: A bridge to quality.* A. Greiner and E. Knebel, eds. Washington, DC: The National Academies Press.

IOM. 2004a. *Improving medical education: Enhancing the behavioral and social science content of medical school curricula.* P. Cuff and N. Vanselow, eds. Washington, DC: The National Academies Press.

IOM. 2004b. *Keeping patients safe: Transforming the work environment of nurses.* A. E. K. Page, ed. Washington, DC: The National Academies Press.

IOM. 2006. *Improving the quality of health care for mental and substance-use conditions.* Washington, DC: The National Academies Press.

IOM. 2007. *Implementing cancer survivorship care planning.* Washington, DC: The National Academies Press.

IOM and NRC. 2006. *From cancer patient to cancer survivor: Lost in transition.* M. Hewitt, S. Greenfield, and E. Stovall, eds. Washington, DC: The National Academies Press.

Keller, M., S. Sommerfeldt, C. Fischer, L. Knight, M. Riesbeck, B. Löwe, C. Herfarth, and T. Lehnert. 2004. Recognition of distress and psychiatric morbidity in cancer patients: A multi-method approach. *Annals of Oncology* 15(8):1243–1249.

Kovner, A., and J. Knickman. 2005. *Health care delivery in the United States.* 8th ed. New York: Springer Publishing Company.

LCME (Liaison Committee on Medical Education). 2006a. *Functions and structure of a medical school: Standards for accreditation of medical education programs leading to the M.D. Degree.* http://www.lcme.org/standard.htm (accessed September 21, 2006).

LCME. 2006b. *Overview: Accreditation and the LCME.* http://www.lcme.org/overview.htm (accessed November 13, 2006).

Leach, D. 2001. Changing education to improve patient care. *Quality in Health Care* 10(Supplement II):ii54–ii58.

Lyketsos, C., J. Levenson, and Academy of Psychosomatic Medicine Task Force for Subspecialization. 2001. Proposal for recognition of "psychosomatic medicine" as a psychiatric subspecialty. *Academy of Psychosomatic Medicine.* http://www.apm.org/subspecialty/ABPNsubspecialtyproposal.pdf (accessed April 6, 2007).

Maly, R. C., Y. Umezawa, B. Leake, and R. A. Silliman. 2005. Mental health outcomes in older women with breast cancer: Impact of perceived family support and adjustment. *Psycho-Oncology* 14(7):535–545.

Mazmanian, P., and D. Davis. 2002. Continuing medical education and the physician as a learner: Guide to the evidence. *Journal of the American Medical Association* 288(9):1057–1060.

McDonald, M. V., S. D. Passik, W. Dugan, B. Rosenfeld, D. E. Theobald, and S. Edgerton. 1999. Nurses' recognition of depression in their patients with cancer. *Oncology Nursing Forum* 26(3):593–599.

Memorial-Sloan Kettering Cancer Center. 2007 (unpublished). *Core competency evaluation for fellows in psycho-oncology/psychosomatic medicine.*

Merckaert, I., Y. Libert, N. Delvaux, S. Marchal, J. Boniver, A.-M. Etienne, J. Klastersky, C. Reynaert, P. Scalliet, J.-L. Slachmuylder, and D. Razavi. 2005. Factors that influence physicians' detection of distress in patients with cancer. Can a communication skills training program improve physicians' detection? *Cancer* 104(2):411–421.

Miller, S. 2006. ABMS' maintenance of certification: The challenge of continuing competence. *Clinical Orthopaedics and Related Research* 449:155–158.

Morris, J., E. Goplerud, and M. Hoge. 2004 (unpublished). *Workforce issues in behavioral health*. Institute of Medicine.

NASW (National Association of Social Workers). 2006. *About NASW*. http://www. socialworkers.org/nasw (accessed September 20, 2006).

NASW. 2007a. *Certified social worker in health care (C-SWHC)*. http://www.socialworkers. org/credentials/specialty/C-SWHC.asp (accessed July 12, 2007).

NASW. 2007b. *Practice*. http://www.socialworkers.org/practice/default.asp (accessed July 12, 2007).

National Council of State Boards of Nursing. 2006. *Nurse licensure compact (NLC)*. https:// www.ncsbn.org/158.htm (accessed December 10, 2006).

NBCC (National Board for Certified Counselors). 2006. *General information of the national certified counselors credential*. http://www.nbcc.org/ncc_credential (accessed December 15, 2006).

NCSBN (National Council of State Boards of Nursing). undated. *Member board profiles: Continued competency*. https://www.ncsbn.org/Continued_Competency(1).pdf (accessed July 12, 2007).

NCSBN. 2006a. *NCLEX-RN test plan, effective April 2007*. https://www.ncsbn.org/RN_Test_ Plan_2007_Web.pdf (accessed December 9, 2006).

NCSBN. 2006b. *Nurse Licensure Compact (NLC)*. https://www.ncsbn.org/158.htm (accessed December 10, 2006).

New Freedom Commission on Mental Health. 2003. *Achieving the promise: Transforming mental health care in America. Final Report*. DHHS Publication Number SMA-03-3832. Rockville, MD: DHHS.

NLNAC (National League for Nursing Accrediting Commission, Inc.). 2006. *NLNAC accreditation manual with interpretive guidelines by program type for post secondary and higher degree programs in nursing*. http://www.nlnac.org/manuals/NLNACManual2006. pdf (accessed July 11, 2007).

O'Brien, M. T., N. Freemantle, A. Oxman, F. Wolf, D. Davis, and J. Herrin. 2003. Continuing education meetings and workshops: Effects on professional practice and health care outcomes. *Cochrane Database of Systematic Reviews* (1).

Olvey, C., and A. Hogg. 2002. Licensure requirements: Have we raised the bar too far? *Professional Psychology: Research & Practice* 33(3):323–329.

ONCC (Oncology Nursing Certification Corporation). 2006. *About ONCC*. http://www.oncc. org/about/ (accessed September 24, 2006).

ONCC. 2007a. *Get certified: 2007 AOCNP® test blueprint*. http://www.oncc.org/getcertified/ TestInformation/aocnp/06blueprint.shtml (accessed July 12, 2007).

ONCC. 2007b. *Get certified: 2007 AOCNS® test blueprint*. http://www.oncc.org/getcertified/ testinformation/AOCNS/06blueprint.shtml (accessed July 12, 2007).

ONCC. 2007c. *Get certified: 2007 CPON® test blueprint*. http://www.oncc.org/getcertified/ TestInformation/cpon/06blueprint.shtml (accessed July 12, 2007).

ONCC. 2007d. *Get certified: 2007 OCN® test blueprint*. http://www.oncc.org/getcertified/Tes- tInformation/ocn/06Blueprint.shtml (accessed July 12, 2007).

ONS (Oncology Nursing Society). 2006. *ONS homepage*. http://www.ons.org (accessed September 28, 2006).

Oxman, A., M. T. O'Brien, D. Davis, and R. Haynes. 1995. No magic bullets: A systematic review of 102 trials of interventions to improve professional practice. *Canadian Medical Association Journal* 153(10):1423–1431.

Parochka, J., and K. Paprockas K. 2001. A continuing medical education lecture and workshop, physician behavior, and barriers to change. *Journal of Continuing Education in the Health Professions* 21(2):110–116.

Passik, S., W. Dugan, M. McDonald, and B. Rosenfeld. 1998. Oncologists' recognition of depression in their patients with cancer. *Journal of Clinical Oncology* 16(4):1594–1600.

President's Cancer Panel. 2004. *Living beyond cancer: Finding a new balance. President's Cancer Panel 2003–2004 annual report.* Bethesda, MD: National Cancer Institute, National Institutes of Health, U.S. Department of Health and Human Services.

Pugh, M. 2003. Refining the paradigm: The transition from recertification to maintenance of certification. *Annals of Family Medicine* 1(1):56–58.

Reinhardt, E. 2002. Dreaming the American dream: Once more around on physician workforce policy. *Health Affairs* 21(3):28–32.

Smith, A. P., and M. Y. Lichtveld. 2007. A competency-based approach to expanding the cancer care workforce. *Nursing Economics* 25(2):110–118.

Snyderman, R., G. F. Sheldon, and T. A. Bischoff. 2002. Gauging supply and demand: The challenging quest to predict the future physician workforce. *Health Affairs* 21(1):167–168.

Soumerai, S. B. 1998. Principles and uses of academic detailing to improve the management of psychiatric disorders. *Internal Journal of Psychiatry in Medicine* 28(1):81–96.

Spirito, A., R. Brown, E. D'Angelo, A. Delamater, J. Rodrigue, and L. Siegel. 2003. Society of pediatric psychology task force report: Recommendations for the training of pediatric psychologists. *Journal of Pediatric Psychology* 28(2):85–98.

Stone, G. 1983. National working conference on education and training in health psychology. *Health Psychology* 2(Supplement 5):1–153.

Straussner, S. L., and E. Senreich. 2002. Educating social workers to work with individuals affected by substance use disorders. In *Strategic plan for interdisciplinary faculty development: Arming the nation's health professional workforce for a new approach to substance use disorders.* Edited by M. Haack and H. Adger. Dordrecht, The Netherlands: Kluwer Academic/Plenum Publishers. Pp. 319–340.

Stuart, G. 2006. Guest editorial: What is the NCLEX really testing? *Nursing Outlook* 54(1):1–2.

Stuart, G., J. Tondora, and M. Hoge. 2004. Evidence-based teaching practice: Implications for behavioral health. *Administration and Policy in Mental Health* 32(2):107–130.

Swing, S. R. 2002. Assessing the ACGME general competencies: General considerations and assessment methods. *Academic Emergency Medicine* 9(11):1278–1288.

USA Today, Kaiser Family Foundation, and Harvard School of Public Health. 2006. *National Survey of Households Affected by Cancer: Summary and chartpack.* Menlo Park, CA, and Washington, DC: USA Today, Kaiser Family Foundation, and Harvard School of Public Health.

USMLE (U.S. Medical Licensing Examination). 2006. *2007 USMLE bulletin of information.* http://www.usmle.org/bulletin/2007/2007bulletin.pdf (accessed October 23, 2006).

Waldstein, S. R., S. A. Neumann, D. A. Drossman, and D. H. Novack. 2001. Teaching psychosomatic (biopsychosocial) medicine in United States medical schools: Survey findings. *Psychosomatic Medicine* 63(3):335–343.

Weissman, M., H. Verdeli, M. Gameroff, S. Bledsoe, K. Betts, L. Mufson, H. Fitterline, and P. Wickramaratne. 2006. National survey of psychotherapy training in psychiatry, psychology, and social work. *Archives of General Psychiatry* 63:925–934.

Yuen, J., R. Breckman, R. Adelman, C. Capello, V. LoFaso, and R. Carrington. 2006. Reflections of medical students on visiting chronically ill older patients in the home. *Journal of the American Geriatrics Society* 54(11):1778–1783.

8

A Research Agenda

CHAPTER SUMMARY

In addition to taking the actions described in the previous chapters, improving the delivery of psychosocial health services will require targeted research. This research should aim to clarify the efficacy and effectiveness of new and existing services, including identifying subpopulations who benefit from specific services and the circumstances in which given services are most effective. Health services research also is needed to identify more effective and efficient ways of delivering these services to various populations in different geographic locations and with varying levels of resources. As discussed in Chapter 3, the economical production, interpretation, and application of research findings would be improved by a taxonomy and nomenclature for psychosocial health services that would be shared across disciplines.

A TAXONOMY AND NOMENCLATURE FOR PSYCHOSOCIAL HEALTH SERVICES

The committee reiterates the importance of the recommendation made in Chapter 3 for the development of a standardized, transdisciplinary taxonomy and nomenclature for psychosocial health services:

Recommendation: Standardized nomenclature. To facilitate research on and quality measurement of psychosocial interventions, the National Institutes of Health (NIH) and the Agency for Healthcare Research and Quality (AHRQ) should create and lead an initiative to develop a standardized, transdisciplinary taxonomy and nomenclature for psychosocial health services. This initiative should aim to incorporate this taxonomy and nomenclature into such databases as the National Library of Medicine's Medical Subject Headings (MeSH), PsycINFO, CINAHL (Cumulative Index to Nursing and Allied Health Literature), and EMBASE.

As discussed in Chapter 3, the absence of a commonly understood vocabulary to describe psychosocial health services and interventions hinders the identification, interpretation, analysis, and application of evidence of effective delivery of those services. Developing a language that can be used across professions and disciplines is critical to the production of better evidence to support the delivery of effective psychosocial health services, which are themselves multidisciplinary and multiprofessional.

EFFECTIVENESS AND HEALTH SERVICES RESEARCH

Although evidence described in Chapters 3, 4, and 5 supports the health care benefits of providing psychosocial health services and points to ways of doing so effectively, there are still many unanswered questions. Key questions remain about how to address certain psychosocial health problems most effectively, as well as how to deliver services most efficiently to the various individuals who need them.

Effectiveness Research

As is the case in biomedical care, providing effective psychosocial services to all who need them is hindered in part by limitations of the knowledge base. For the past three decades, the National Cancer Institute (NCI) and other private organizations that fund cancer research have supported a wide range of psychosocial research studies involving cancer patients and their families. However, the challenge with cancer is that it is not a single disease (prostate cancer, for example, is different from lung cancer in its impact), and even for a particular cancer site, individuals' specific psychosocial health care needs may vary (e.g., in early-stage versus advanced disease). Given that there are more than 100 specific cancer types, it is therefore difficult to generalize about the benefits of particular psychosocial interventions, as their efficacy may vary based on the cancer site or phase of disease. Increasingly, research studies have focused on homogeneous samples of patients, making interpretation of outcomes more salient. For these reasons, psychosocial research with cancer patients is more challenging than that focused on more homogeneous diseases, such as asthma, diabetes, or heart disease.

For some psychosocial problems, research has not yet identified effective services to resolve them. In other cases, evidence that a remedy works effectively for some populations does not necessarily mean that the same remedy is effective for (is generalizable to) all people in all situations. Moreover, evidence is frequently not as clear as one would like it to be. Findings can be mixed, with evidence of the effectiveness of a service being found in one study but not being replicated in others. Additionally, evidence that a given service is effective does not exclude the possibility that another service is more effective for the same problem or equally effective at lower cost. In such cases, research continues to be needed even for services and interventions whose efficacy is supported by research findings. All of these situations are found in the array of evidence pertaining to psychosocial health services.

Identification of Effective Interventions

For some psychosocial health problems faced by cancer patients, research has not yet identified efficacious remedies. For example, as discussed in Chapter 3, research does not well inform clinicians about how to address effectively continued tobacco use among cancer patients, cognitive impairment among adults treated for cancer, and difficulties with school reentry for children treated for cancer. Further, although cancer is recognized as having a large impact on family members, they are rarely the subject of or included in research on psychosocial health care (Helgeson, 2005). More commonly, research points to the effectiveness of specific psychosocial services, but offers limited evidence about whether a broad spectrum of patients (and family members) benefit equally from those services in all situations.

Determination of Effectiveness in Different Populations and Scenarios

Questions about the effectiveness of many psychosocial services have evolved from addressing whether given services are effective to addressing for whom and under what circumstances specific services are needed and effective (Helgeson et al., 2000; Zebrack and Zeltzer, 2003; Cohen, 2004; Helgeson, 2005; Stanton, 2005). Effectiveness research on psychosocial health services has most often focused on women with breast cancer at the middle to upper middle socioeconomic levels without regard to the amount of psychosocial stress they are experiencing. Services need to be tested with men, in patients with sites of cancer other than breast, across different stages of cancer, with patients experiencing different types and levels of psychosocial needs and stress, and with those from different cultural and socioeconomic backgrounds.

Variables that moderate treatment effects need to be better understood as well (Helgeson, 2005). For example, many individuals diagnosed with cancer report manageable psychological distress that resolves over time without the need for formal services. Other research has found that patients with the highest levels of distress often show the greatest reduction in symptoms when provided psychosocial services (Andrykowski and Manne, 2006; Antoni et al., 2006). Research conducted with individuals with varying availability of social supports has found that the effectiveness of different types of psychosocial services can depend on the nature and extent of those supports (Cohen, 2004). Because of such findings, experts point to the need for a new generation of research on the effectiveness of psychosocial health services (Helgeson, 2005) involving "increasingly careful a priori consideration of the nature of the samples, interventions, and outcomes involved, as well as theory-guided examinations of mechanisms for the obtained effects" (Stanton, 2005:4819). Particular attention should be paid to socially disadvantaged populations, examining the effects of socioeconomic status and race/ethnicity on the risk for psychosocial problems and on the impact of interventions on these problems. Such work should also take into account developmental issues, particularly for children with cancer, and the effectiveness of interventions at different life stages (Zebrack and Zeltzer, 2003).

Use of More Robust Research Methods

The strength and generalizability of the evidence generated by research are increased by attention to several research design issues. First, the effectiveness of a service is often measured using dimensions of quality of life. Because measures of quality of life are numerous and variable, what one study finds effective may not be interpreted as such by others. The development of standard outcome measures by which the effectiveness of psychosocial services can be measured would increase the understanding and application of research results.

Research using more rigorous research designs is also needed, including use of longer follow-up periods (Helgeson, 2005). For example, with respect to the effects of psychotropic medications used to treat depression and other mental health conditions of patients with cancer, conclusions about effectiveness are limited (see Chapter 3) because of the few randomized controlled trials that have been done. More such trials are needed, using a larger patient cohort that is studied over a longer period of time to properly assess drug efficacy. These trials will likely require multicenter sites. The trials should be limited to patients with significant levels of depressive or anxious symptoms at baseline (e.g., severe adjustment disorder with depressive or anxious symptoms or anxiety, post-traumatic stress disorder, or mood disorder) to ensure an adequate effect size. Studies also are needed that compare one drug with another and with the drug plus a psychosocial intervention.

More multisite research on services targeting children is needed as well. Because cancer in children is rare, most research involves small samples, limiting the conclusions that can be drawn (Patenaude and Kupst, 2005).

Research testing the effects of the receipt of psychosocial health services on physiological and clinical outcomes also could help build the conceptual framework underpinning those services, and point to new interventions and ways to target services and interventions to those who are most vulnerable (Patenaude and Kupst, 2005; Thacker et al., 2007). Such research should address, for example, the links between certain types of stress and immune system functioning and the effects of psychosocial supports on health, such as through changes in endocrine and immunological functioning and mediating physiological pathways.

Health Services Research

Health services research could help identify better ways of implementing some of the interventions necessary for the delivery of psychosocial health services. This research could be accomplished through the large-scale demonstration program recommended in Chapter 5 that would test various approaches to the effective provision of psychosocial health care in accordance with the standard of care set forth in this report. Health services research could also address how to implement components of the model described in Chapter 4 more efficiently and effectively, focusing in particular on methods for improving the patient–provider partnership, the development of better screening and needs assessment tools, comprehensive illness and wellness management interventions, approaches for effectively linking patients with services and coordinating care, and reimbursement arrangements that would support these interventions.

Methods for Improving the Patient–Provider Partnership

As discussed in Chapters 3 and 4, tools and approaches are needed to improve communication between patients and providers and to support patient decision making in the face of a large volume of complex information. Research is needed to develop such tools and approaches for populations at greatest risk (e.g., older adults; those of lower socioeconomic status; and those with comorbid conditions, including psychosocial distress and decreased cognition).

Development of Better Tools for Screening

The screening tools described in Chapter 4 all have somewhat different purposes. For example, the Distress Thermometer and its accompanying Problem List screen for generalized distress and identify emotional, spiritual, physical, family, and practical issues, such as problems with transportation, as sources of distress. PCM 2.0 focuses on role functioning and overall quality of life. Other types of psychosocial health needs not addressed by these instruments include, for example, social isolation/social support, difficulties in navigating the health system, and poor literacy. Health services research should focus on the development of psychosocial screening tools addressing a more comprehensive range of psychological and social stressors that can interfere with the ability of patients and families to manage cancer and its consequences.

Also needed are psychosocial screening tools and approaches for their use that consider the comorbidities frequently experienced by cancer survivors. Data from the 1998–2000 National Health Interview Survey, for example, show that 49 percent of cancer survivors are age 65 or older. Among cancer survivors aged 65 or older, 39 percent report having a diagnosis of heart disease, angina, heart attack, heart condition, or stroke; 13 percent report currently being treated for diabetes (Hewitt et al., 2003). These findings are significant because efforts are under way to understand psychosocial barriers to patients' self-management of these conditions and to apply psychosocial screening instruments developed for individuals with these conditions (Glasgow et al., 2001; Whittemore et al., 2005). The Problem Areas in Diabetes (PAID) instrument, for example, is a 20-item self-administered measure of diabetes-specific emotional distress that has performed well in psychometric testing. It has been found to correlate strongly with "a wide range of theoretically related constructs such as general emotional distress, depression, diabetes self-care behaviors, diabetes coping, and health beliefs" and to be a statistically significant predictor of glycemic control (Polonsky et al., 2006). The Diabetes Self-Management Assessment Tool is another example.

The issue of comorbidity raises a number of questions. Hypothetically, should cancer patients be administered a separate psychosocial screening tool for each of their comorbid conditions? In addition to the burden that multiple screening instruments would likely impose on the patient, screening for psychosocial distress in cancer survivors might not be clinically feasible outside of oncology practices if medical providers had to implement multiple screens to address each patient's unique multiple illnesses. Other questions arise as well. If a clinician cares for an individual with more than one chronic condition, which screening tool or tools should be used? Is there a minimum set of domains that should be included in all screening tools for psychosocial health needs? Is there an ideal set? Could a tool be developed that would address all these domains? Should existing tools be improved to achieve greater utility?

Some of these questions would be addressed if there were a valid psychosocial screening instrument that could be used across multiple chronic conditions. One possibility would be to develop such an instrument along the lines of the NIH Patient-Reported Outcomes Measurement Information System (PROMIS) (http://www.nihpromis.org/default.asp). The goal of this initiative is to develop ways to measure patient-reported symptoms, such as pain and fatigue, and aspects of health-related quality of life across a wide variety of chronic diseases and conditions. The PROMIS initiative establishes a collaborative relationship between NIH and individual research teams in order to

- Develop and test a large repository of items and questionnaires measuring patient-reported outcomes.
- Build a Web-based resource for administering computerized adaptive tests, collecting self-report data, and reporting instant health assessments.
- Evaluate the utility of PROMIS and promote widespread use of the instruments for clinical research and clinical care.
- Sustain the repository and continued development of the PROMIS tools and system for clinical research and practice (NIH, undated).

The network will collaborate on the collection of self-reported data from diverse populations of individuals with a variety of chronic diseases using agreed-upon methods, modes, and questionnaires.

If a less sweeping initiative were desired with respect to screening instruments, research could address, for example, more testing of existing screening instruments, testing of the effectiveness of cancer-focused screening instruments for other chronic conditions and vice versa, and ways to incorporate quality-of-life measures into screening instruments. Use of screening instruments in conjunction with comprehensive needs assessment also should be addressed.

Development of Better Needs Assessment Instruments

Chapter 4 presents the results of a systematic appraisal (Wen and Gustafson, 2004) of needs assessment instruments for cancer that identifies 17 patient and 7 family instruments for which information is available on their reliability, validity, burden, and psychometric properties. Across these instruments, many problems are noted, including wide variation in the needs addressed,[1] inconsistency in domains within the instrument and in items included in similarly named domains, a lack of evidence of sensitivity to change over time, failure to examine reading levels, and failure to address the period after initial treatment for cancer. The authors express their doubt as to whether any one instrument could be developed to address all areas of interest, but recommend that a common set of domain terms be adopted to form the core of needs assessment and that agreement be reached on some items to be placed in the domains. Research also is recommended to address obstacles to the practice of needs assessment, to identify characteristics of effective performance of needs assessment, and to establish the relative importance and significance of identified needs. As with the questions posed above with respect to screening, questions about how best to conduct needs assessment in the presence of comorbidities also require attention.

Comprehensive Illness and Wellness Management Interventions

As described in Chapters 3 and 4, comprehensive illness self-management programs have been found to be effective in improving patient knowledge, skills, and confidence in managing a number of chronic illnesses, such as diabetes, asthma, heart disease, lung disease, stroke, and arthritis. Some of these programs also have been found to be effective in improving health outcomes (Lorig et al., 2001; Bodenheimer et al., 2002; Lorig and Holman, 2003; Chodosh et al., 2005). Yet while particular interventions have been developed and found to be effective in helping cancer patients manage individual symptoms, such as pain and fatigue, comprehensive illness and health management programs similar to those that exist for individuals with other chronic illnesses have not been developed and tested in individuals living with the diagnosis and sequelae of cancer. Research to this end is needed.

Approaches for Effectively Linking Patients with Services and Coordinating Care

Also as discussed in Chapter 4, the various mechanisms used to link patients with services delivered by different health and human service providers (e.g., structured referral arrangements and formal agreements with external providers, case management, collocation and clinical integration of services, patient navigators, use of shared electronic health records) have

---

[1]For example: physical, psychological, medical interactions, sexual, coping information, activities of daily living, interpersonal communication, availability and continuity of care, physician competence, support networks, spiritual, child care, family needs, pain/symptom control, home services, having purpose.

varying levels of empirical support. This support does not come from studies of the use of these mechanisms by oncology providers in ambulatory care settings. Because most oncology patients receive their cancer care in outpatient settings, research comparing the effectiveness and cost of using different mechanisms to link patients to psychosocial services and coordinate their care could help inform and redesign oncology practices. Such research also could evaluate the use of different types of personnel (e.g., nurses and social workers with varying levels of education and training and unlicensed, trained workers such as patient care navigators) to perform linkage and coordination activities.

Reimbursement Arrangements That Promote Psychosocial Care

As illustrated in Chapter 6, little information exists outside of Medicare about how group purchasers and health plans provide for psychosocial health care in their contracts with each other and with health care providers. Although there are anecdotal reports of best practices by some health plans and providers, qualitative and quantitative research could better illuminate the reimbursement and other mechanisms used by leading health care providers to address psychosocial health services and their effects on clinicians, work design, and patients and on the delivery of effective psychosocial health care. Such research could also address to what extent mechanisms have been developed for reimbursing for higher-than-average care coordination needs.

Recommendation

Consistent with the above discussion, the committee recommends the following research agenda.

Recommendation: Research priorities. **Organizations sponsoring research in oncology care should include the following areas among their funding priorities:**

- **Further development of reliable, valid, and efficient tools and strategies for use by clinical practices to ensure that all patients with cancer receive care that meets the standard of psychosocial care. These tools and strategies should include**
  - **approaches for improving patient–provider communication and providing decision support to cancer patients;**
  - **screening instruments that can be used to identify individuals with any of a comprehensive array of psychosocial health problems;**

- needs assessment instruments to assist in planning psychosocial services;
- illness and wellness management interventions; and
- approaches for effectively linking patients with services and coordinating care.
- Identification of more effective psychosocial services to treat mental health problems and to assist patients in adopting and maintaining healthy behaviors, such as smoking cessation, exercise, and dietary change. This effort should include
  - identifying populations for whom specific psychosocial services are most effective, and psychosocial services most effective for specific populations; and
  - development of standard outcome measures for assessing the effectiveness of these services.
- Creation and testing of reimbursement arrangements that will promote psychosocial care and reward its best performance.

Research on the use of these tools, strategies, and services should also focus on how best to ensure delivery of appropriate psychosocial services to vulnerable populations, such as those with low literacy, older adults, the socially isolated, and members of cultural minorities.

REPORT EVALUATION

As part of this study, NIH requested that the Institute of Medicine make recommendations for how the impact of this report could be evaluated. The committee believes that evaluation activities could be useful in promoting action on all the recommendations made in this report and in designing future studies. Accordingly, the committee makes the following recommendation.

Recommendation. Promoting uptake and monitoring progress. The National Cancer Institute/NIH should monitor progress toward improved delivery of psychosocial services in cancer care and report its findings on at least a biannual basis to oncology providers, consumer organizations, group purchasers and health plans, quality oversight organizations, and other stakeholders. These findings could be used to inform an evaluation of the impact of this report and each of its recommendations. Monitoring activities should make maximal use of existing data collection tools and activities.

This recommendation could be implemented using a variety of approaches. For example, to determine the extent to which patients with cancer receive psychosocial health care consistent with the standard of care and its implementation as set forth in Chapters 4 and 5, respectively, the Department of Health and Human Services (DHHS) could

- Conduct an annual, patient-level, process-of-care evaluation using a national sample and validated, reliable instruments, such as the Consumer Assessment of Healthcare Providers and Systems (CAHPS) instruments.
- Add measures of the quality of psychosocial health care for patients (and families as feasible) to existing surveys, such as the Centers for Disease Control and Prevention's Behavioral Risk Factor Surveillance System (BRFSS).
- Conduct annual practice surveys to determine compliance with the standard of care.
- Monitor and document the emergence of performance reward initiatives (e.g., content on psychosocial care in requests for proposals [RFPs] and pay-for-performance initiatives that specifically include incentives for psychosocial care).

For the committee's recommendation on patient and family education (see Chapter 5), NCI could

- Routinely query patient education and advocacy organizations about their efforts to educate patients with cancer and their family caregivers that they should expect, and request when necessary, cancer care that meets the standard of care recommended in this report.
- Assess whether patients and caregivers show greater knowledge of how oncology providers should address their psychosocial needs (the standard of care) and whether they report more receipt of psychosocial health services as part of their cancer care. Surveys could be used to gather this information and would indicate the extent to which cancer care is meeting the standard of care.
- Use an annual patient-level, process-of-care evaluation (such as CAHPS) to identify patient education experiences.

For the committee's recommendation on dissemination and uptake of the standard of care (see Chapter 5), DHHS could determine whether NCI, the Centers for Medicare & Medicaid Services (CMS), and AHRQ had conducted demonstration projects and how they had disseminated the findings from those demonstrations.

For the committee's recommendation on support from payers (see Chapter 6), NCI and/or advocacy, provider, or other interest groups could

- Survey national organizations (e.g., America's Health Insurance Plans, the National Business Group on Health) about their awareness of and/or advocacy activities related to the recommendations in this report and the initiation of appropriate reimbursement strategies/activities.
- Monitor and document the emergence of performance reward initiatives (e.g., RFP content on psychosocial care, pay-for-performance that specifically includes incentives for psychosocial care).
- Evaluate health plan contracts and state insurance policies for coverage, copayments, and carve-outs for psychosocial services.
- Assess coverage for psychosocial services for Medicare beneficiaries.

For the committee's recommendation on quality oversight (see Chapter 6), DHHS could

- Examine the funding portfolios of NIH, CMS, AHRQ, and other public and private sponsors of quality-of-care research to evaluate the funding of quality measurement for psychosocial health care as part of cancer care.
- Query organizations that set standards for cancer care (e.g., National Comprehensive Cancer Network, American Society of Clinical Oncology, American College of Surgeons' Commission on Cancer, Oncology Nursing Society, American Psychosocial Oncology Society) and other standards-setting organizations (e.g., National Quality Forum, National Committee for Quality Assurance, URAC, the Joint Commission) to determine the extent to which they have
  - created oversight mechanisms used to measure and report on the quality of ambulatory cancer care (including psychosocial health care);
  - incorporated requirements for identifying and responding to psychosocial health care needs into their protocols, policies, and standards in accordance with the standard of care put forth in this report; and
  - used performance measures of psychosocial health care in their quality oversight activities.

For the committee's recommendation on workforce competencies (see Chapter 7), DHHS could

- Monitor and report on actions taken by Congress and federal agencies to support and fund the establishment of a Workforce

Development Collaborative on Psychosocial Care during Chronic Medical Illness.

- Review board exams for oncologists and primary care providers to identify questions relevant to psychosocial care.
- Review accreditation standards for educational programs used to train health care personnel to identify content requirements relevant to psychosocial care.
- Review certification requirements for clinicians to identify those requirements relevant to psychosocial care.
- Examine the funding portfolios of NIH, CMS, AHRQ, and other public and private sponsors of quality-of-care research to quantify the funding of initiatives aimed at assessing the incorporation of workforce competencies into education, training, and clinical practice and their impact on achieving the standard for psychosocial care.

For the committee's recommendation on standardized nomenclature and research priorities (see Chapter 3 and this chapter, respectively), DHHS could

- Report on NIH/AHRQ actions to develop a taxonomy and nomenclature for psychosocial health services.
- Examine the funding portfolios of public and private research sponsors to assess whether funding priorities included the recommended areas.

REFERENCES

Andrykowski, M. A., and S. L. Manne. 2006. Are psychological interventions effective and accepted by cancer patients? I. Standards and levels of evidence. *Annals of Behavioral Medicine* 32(2):93–97.

Antoni, M. H., S. K. Lutgendorf, S. W. Cole, F. S. Dhabhar, S. E. Sephton, P. G. McDonald, M. Stefanek, and A. K. Sood. 2006. The influence of bio-behavioral factors on tumor biology: Pathways and mechanisms. *Nature Reviews. Cancer* 6(3):240–248.

Bodenheimer, T., K. Lorig, H. Holman, and K. Grumbach. 2002. Patient self-management of chronic disease in primary care. *Journal of the American Medical Association* 288(19): 2469–2475.

Chodosh, J., S. C. Morton, W. Mojica, M. Maglione, M. J. Suttorp, L. Hilton, S. Rhodes, and P. Shekelle. 2005. Meta-analysis: Chronic disease self-management programs for older adults. *Annals of Internal Medicine* 143(6):427–438.

Cohen, S. 2004. Social relationships and health. *American Psychologist* 59(8):676–684.

Glasgow, R. E., D. J. Toobert, and C. D. Gillette. 2001. Psychosocial barriers to diabetes self-management and quality of life. *Diabetes Spectrum* 14(1):33–41.

Helgeson, V. S. 2005. Recent advances in psychosocial oncology. *Journal of Consulting and Clinical Psychology* 73(2):268–271.

Helgeson, V. S., S. Cohen, R. Schultz, and J. Yasko. 2000. Group support interventions for women with breast cancer: Who benefits from what? *Health Psychology* 19(2): 107–114.

Hewitt, M., J. H. Rowland, and R. Yancik. 2003. Cancer survivors in the United States: Age, health, and disability. *Journal of Gerontology* 58(1):82–91.

Lorig, K. R., and H. Holman. 2003. Self-management education: History, definition, outcomes, and mechanisms. *Annals of Behavioral Medicine* 26(1):1–7.

Lorig, K. R., P. Ritter, A. L. Stewart, D. S. Sobel, B. W. Brown, A. Bandura, V. M. Gonzalez, D. D. Laurent, and H. R. Holman. 2001. Chronic disease self-management program: 2-year health status and health care utilization outcomes. *Medical Care* 39(11): 1217–1223.

NIH (National Institutes of Health). undated. *Primary goals of PROMIS*. http://www. nihpromis.org/Web%20Pages/Goals.aspx?PageView=Shared (accessed September 12, 2007).

Patenaude, A. F., and M. J. Kupst. 2005. Psychosocial functioning in pediatric cancer. *Journal of Pediatric Psychology* 30(1):9–27.

Polonsky, W. H., B. J. Anderson, P. A. Lohrer, G. Welch, A. M. Jacobson, J. E. Aponte, and C. E. Schwartz. 2006. *RCMAR measurement tools: Problem areas in diabetes (PAID)*. Resource Centers for Minority Aging Research (RCMAR). http://www.musc.edu/dfm/ RCMAR/PAID.html (accessed January 9, 2007).

Stanton, A. L. 2005. How and for whom? Asking questions about the utility of psychosocial interventions for individuals diagnosed with cancer. *Journal of Clinical Oncology* 23(22):4818–4820.

Thacker, P. H., S. K. Lutgendorf, and A. K. Sood. 2007. The neuroendocrine impact of chronic stress on cancer. *Cell Cycle* 6(4):430–433.

Wen, K.-Y., and D. H. Gustafson. 2004. Needs assessment for cancer patients and their families. *Health and Quality of Life Outcomes* 2:11.

Whittemore, R., G. D. E. Melkus, and M. Grey. 2005. Metabolic control, self-management and psychosocial adjustment in women with type 2 diabetes. *Journal of Clinical Nursing* 14(2):195–203.

Zebrack, B., and L. Zeltzer. 2003. Quality of life issues and cancer survivorship. *Current Problems in Cancer* 27(4):198–211.

Appendix A

Committee Member Biographies

Nancy E. Adler, PhD, is professor of psychology, Departments of Psychiatry and Pediatrics, University of California, San Francisco (UCSF), where she is also vice-chair of the Department of Psychiatry, and director of the Center for Health and Community. She received a BA from Wellesley College and a PhD in psychology from Harvard University. After serving as assistant and associate professor at the University of California, Santa Cruz, she went to UCSF to initiate a graduate program in health psychology. She has served as director of that program, a National Institute of Mental Health (NIMH)-sponsored postdoctoral program in Psychology and Medicine: An Integrative Research Approach, and a new postdoctoral Health and Society Scholars Program funded by The Robert Wood Johnson Foundation. Dr. Adler is a fellow of the American Psychological Society and the American Psychological Association (APA). She has served as president of the APA's Division of Population and Environmental Psychology and received its Superior Service Award. She is a member of the Society for Experimental Social Psychology, the Academy of Behavioral Medicine Research, and the Society for Behavioral Medicine. She has been awarded the UCSF Chancellor's Award for Advancement of Women; the George Sarlo Prize for Excellence in Teaching; and the Outstanding Contribution to Health Psychology Award from the APA's Division of Health Psychology. She is a member of the Institute of Medicine (IOM) and was named a national associate of the National Academies. She also serves on the Advisory Committee to the Director of the National Institutes of Health (NIH). Dr. Adler's earlier research examined the utility of decision models for understanding health behaviors, with a particular focus on reproductive

health. Her current work examines the pathways from socioeconomic status to health. As director of the MacArthur Foundation Research Network
on Socioeconomic Status and Health, she coordinates research spanning
social, psychological, and biological mechanisms by which socioeconomic
status influences health. Within the network she has focused on the role of
subjective social status in health.

Rhonda J. Robinson-Beale, MD, is chief medical officer, Clinical Program
Effectiveness and Quality, for United Behavioral Health (UBH). In this position, she manages a staff of clinicians and professionals solely dedicated
to quality, clinical program design and implementation, learning and consultation, and behavioral health informatics. She is an experienced behavioral health practitioner with more than 20 years of experience in diverse
treatment and research settings who recognizes the value of integrating
behavioral, medical, pharmacy, and disability programs to treat the needs
of the whole patient. Dr. Robinson-Beale joined the legacy UBH company
PacifiCare Behavioral Health in October 2005 as chief medical officer. She
assumed her new duties as chief medical officer of UBH during the compa-
nies' brief integration period. Her extensive background includes lead clinical positions at national behavioral and health organizations such as Cigna
Behavioral Health, Blue Cross Blue Shield of Michigan, and Health Alliance
Plan. During her tenure at Cigna, she was responsible for the organization's
clinical direction, particularly in the area of clinical integration across
pharmacy, behavioral, and medical programs. During the past 10 years,
Dr. Robinson-Beale has authored more than 17 papers that have informed
audiences about behavioral health integration, selected quality initiatives,
diagnosis and management of behavioral health conditions in the primary
care setting, disease management models, substance abuse and pregnancy,
dual diagnosis, and management of psychiatric care for HIV patients. She
is a graduate of Wayne State University School of Medicine in Detroit and
the University of Michigan, Ann Arbor.

Diane S. Blum, MSW, is executive director of CancerCare, Inc., a national
nonprofit organization that provides free professional support services,
including counseling, education, financial assistance, and practical help,
to people with cancer and their loved ones. Prior to joining CancerCare as
director of social service, Ms. Blum served as a social work supervisor at the
Memorial Sloan-Kettering Cancer Center and the Dana Farber Cancer Institute. Co-founder of the National Alliance of Breast Cancer Organizations,
she is a founder of National Breast Cancer Awareness Month and serves as
editor-in-chief of *People Living with Cancer*, the American Society of Clinical Oncology's (ASCO) website for patients and the public. Additionally,
she serves on committees of the IOM, ASCO, and the National Association
of Social Work and is a member of the editorial boards of five oncology-

related publications. Ms. Blum's awards include the Lifetime Achievement Award from the Board of Sponsors of National Breast Cancer Awareness Month, the Special Recognition Award from the National Coalition for Cancer Survivorship, the Republic Bank Breast Cancer Research Foundation Award, and the Special Recognition Award of the American Society of Clinical Oncology. Ms. Blum has written and lectured extensively on the psychosocial needs of cancer patients and their families. Her research has been published in a variety of medical journals, including the *American Journal of Hospice and Palliative Care*, the *Journal of Psychosocial Oncology*, the *Journal of Pain and Symptom Management*, and the *Annals of Internal Medicine*. She received a bachelor's degree from the University of Rochester and a master's degree from the School of Social Welfare at the State University of New York, Buffalo.

Patricia A. Ganz, MD, a medical oncologist, received her BA magna cum laude from Radcliffe College (Harvard University) in 1969 and her MD from the University of California, Los Angeles (UCLA) in 1973. She subsequently completed her training in internal medicine and hematology-oncology at UCLA Medical Center, where she also served as chief resident in medicine. She has been a member of the faculty of the UCLA School of Medicine since 1978 and the UCLA School of Public Health since 1992. Since 1993 she has been director of the Division of Cancer Prevention and Control Research at the Jonsson Comprehensive Cancer Center. In 1999 she was awarded an American Cancer Society Clinical Research Professorship for "enhancing patient outcomes across the cancer control continuum." In 2006 she was awarded funding to lead UCLA's Cancer Survivorship Center of Excellence as part of the LIVESTRONG™ Survivorship Center of Excellence Network. Dr. Ganz is a pioneer in the assessment of quality of life in cancer patients and is active in clinical trials research with the National Surgical Adjuvant Breast and Bowel Project. She has focused many of her clinical and research efforts in the areas of breast cancer and its prevention, and was a member of the National Cancer Institute's (NCI) Progress Review Group on Breast Cancer. At the Jonsson Cancer Center, she directs the UCLA Family Cancer Registry and Genetic Evaluation Program. Her other major areas of research include cancer survivorship and late effects of cancer treatment, cancer in the elderly, and quality of care for cancer patients. She is an associate editor for the *Journal of Clinical Oncology*, the *Journal of the National Cancer Institute*, and *CA-A Journal for Clinicians*. She currently serves on the NCI Board of Scientific Advisors and recently completed a term on the Board of Directors of ASCO.

Sherry Glied, PhD, is professor and chair of the Department of Health Policy and Management of Columbia University's Mailman School of Public Health. She holds a BA in economics from Yale University, an MA in economics from the University of Toronto, and a PhD in economics from Harvard University. In 1992–1993, she served as a senior economist for health care and labor market policy to the President's Council of Economic Advisers under Presidents Bush and Clinton. She was a participant in President Clinton's Health Care Task Force and headed working groups on global budgets and on the economic impacts of the health plan. Her research on health policy has focused on the financing of health care services in the United States. She is the author of recently published articles and reports on women's health insurance, expansions of children's health insurance, Medicaid managed care, and the role of insurance in hospital care. Dr. Glied is past recipient of a Robert Wood Johnson Investigator Award, through which she has been studying the U.S. employer-based health insurance system. Her work in mental health policy has focused on the problems of women and children. She is a member of the MacArthur Foundation's Network on Mental Health Policy, the IOM, the board of AcademyHealth, and the National Academy of Social Insurance and a research associate of the National Bureau of Economic Research. In 2004 Professor Glied served as chair of the AcademyHealth Annual Research Meeting. She was the 2004 winner of Research!America's Eugene Garfield Economic Impact of Health Research Award. She is a senior associate editor of *Health Services Research*; an associate editor of the *Journal of Health Politics, Policy, and Law*; a member of the editorial board of the *Milbank Quarterly*; and a member of the editorial committee of the *Annual Review of Public Health*.

Jessie Gruman, PhD, is founder and president of the Center for the Advancement of Health, an independent, nonpartisan Washington-based policy institute funded by the John D. and Catherine T. MacArthur Foundation; the Annenberg Foundation; and others, including the W. K. Kellogg Foundation and the Atlantic Philanthropies. Since it was established in 1992, the Center has worked to ensure that people are able to meet the demands placed on them by health information that is increasingly complex, health professionals who are increasingly specialized and pressed for time, and health care that is increasingly brilliant but chaotic. Dr. Gruman has worked on this same set of concerns in the private sector (AT&T), the public sector (National Institutes of Health), and the voluntary health sector (American Cancer Society). She received her undergraduate degree from Vassar College and her PhD in social psychology from Columbia University. She is a professorial lecturer in the School of Public Health at The George Washington University and serves on the boards of trustees of the Advisory Panel on Medicare Education of the U.S. Department of Health and Human Services, the Public Health Institute, the Sallan Foundation, and the Center for Information Therapy, among others. Dr. Gruman is a fellow of the Society of Behavioral Medicine and has received the Society's awards for distinguished service and Leadership in Translation of Research to Practice. She was recognized for outstanding service by the APA and was honored by Research!America for her leadership in advocacy for health research. She is the recipient of an honorary doctorate in public policy from Carnegie Mellon University and the Presidential Medal of The George Washington University. She served as executive in residence at Vassar College, serves on the editorial board of *The Annals of Family Medicine*, and is a member of the APA, the Association for Psychological Science, and the Council on Foreign Relations. Dr. Gruman is the author of numerous articles and essays published in scholarly journals and public media. Her book for the general public, *After Shock: What to Do When the Doctor Gives You—or Someone You Love—a Devastating Diagnosis* (Walker Publishing, 2007), is about how people use scientific information to make decisions about their health care.

Michael Hoge, PhD, is professor of psychology in the Psychiatry Department of the Yale University School of Medicine and director of Yale Behavioral Health. He is past chair of the Behavioral Health Professional and Technical Advisory Committee of the Joint Commission on Accreditation of Healthcare Organizations and recipient of the 2001 Moffic Award for Ethical Practice in Public Sector Managed Behavioral Healthcare. Dr. Hoge is an expert in workforce development in behavioral health. He is a founding member of The Annapolis Coalition on the Behavioral Health Workforce, which initiated a national, interprofessional effort to improve the recruitment, retention, and training of individuals who provide prevention and treatment services for persons with mental illnesses and substance use disorders. He is also senior editor of the recently released National Action Plan on Behavioral Health Workforce Development, which was commissioned by the federal Substance Abuse and Mental Health Services Administration. Dr. Hoge has consulted on behavioral health workforce issues for the President's New Freedom Commission on Mental Health, the IOM's Committee on Crossing the Quality Chasm: Adaptation to Mental Health and Addictive Disorders, and multiple states and organizations. He is senior editor of three special journal issues on workforce development in behavioral health and author of numerous peer-reviewed articles on this topic.

Jimmie C. Holland, MD, is attending psychiatrist and holder of the Wayne E. Chapman Chair in Psychiatric Oncology at the Memorial Sloan-Kettering Cancer Center, and professor of psychiatry at Weill Medical College of Cornell University. She is recognized internationally as the founder of the subspecialty of psycho-oncology. Starting in the mid-1970s, she conducted some of the first epidemiological studies related to the prevalence and nature of psychological problems in patients with cancer. In 1977, she established the first Psycho-Oncology Committee as part of the NCI clinical trials group Cancer and Leukemia Group B, serving as chair through 2001. She was founding president of the International Psycho-Oncology Society (1984) and of the American Psychosocial Oncology Society (1986). Dr. Holland was senior editor of the first textbook in psycho-oncology, *The Handbook of Psychooncology* (1989), and of a second text, *Psycho-Oncology* (1998), both published by Oxford University Press. Similarly, she started the first international journal in the field, *Psycho-Oncology*, in 1992, and continues as its co-editor. Dr. Holland and Sheldon Lewis co-authored a book aimed at helping patients and their families cope with cancer—*The Human Side of Cancer*, published in 2000 by HarperCollins. As chair of the National Comprehensive Cancer Network's Panel on Management of Distress, Dr. Holland has worked since the Panel's inception in 1997 to promulgate the first clinical practice guidelines for psychosocial care in cancer. The IOM elected her as a member in 1995, and she served on its National Cancer Policy Board. In 2000, she received the American Psychiatric Association's Presidential Commendation. The American Cancer Society (ACS) awarded her its Medal of Honor for Clinical Research in 1994, as well as the ASCO/ACS Lecture and Award in 2003. The 13th Claude Jacquillat Award for Clinical Cancer Research was presented to her in Paris in 2005. In April 2005, the Joseph Burchenal Award for Clinical Research was granted to Dr. Holland by the American Association for Cancer Research.

Melissa M. Hudson, MD, is a full member of the Department of Oncology at St. Jude Children's Research Hospital. She earned her MD from the University of Texas Medical School in Houston in 1983. She completed a pediatric residency at the University of Texas and then pursued pediatric hematology-oncology fellowship training at the M. D. Anderson Cancer Center. Dr. Hudson joined the St. Jude faculty in 1989. She is currently a member of the Leukemia/Lymphoma Division in the Department of Hematology Oncology. She has been principal investigator of St. Jude pediatric Hodgkin's trials for the past 15 years. These trials have evaluated risk-adapted, response-based combined modality therapy regimens designed to reduce organ dysfunction and subsequent malignancies in long-term survivors. In 1993 Dr. Hudson became director of the After Completion of Therapy Clinic, which supervises the care of more than 5,000 long-term childhood cancer survivors treated in St. Jude trials. She has published widely on her research initiatives in pediatric Hodgkin's disease, late treatment sequelae after childhood cancer, and health education of childhood cancer survivors. She is vice-chair of the Children's Oncology Group Late Effects Steering Committee and co-chair of the Children's Oncology Group Long-Term Follow-Up Guidelines for Survivors of Childhood, Adolescent and Young Adult Cancer. She also serves as pediatric section editor of the journal *Cancer* and on the editorial board of *Pediatric Blood and Cancer* and *ASCO News & Forum*.

Sherrie Kaplan, PhD, is associate dean for the School of Medicine, professor of medicine and executive director, Center for Health Policy Research, University of California, Irvine (UCI). She came to UCI from Tufts University School of Medicine and the Harvard School of Public Health, where she received the outstanding professor award for multiple consecutive years. Dr. Kaplan received her undergraduate, MPH, MSPH, and PhD from the University of California, Los Angeles, the latter in a joint program between public health and measurement psychology. One of the eminent social scientists in medicine, she is currently professor of medicine at the UCI School of Medicine. In her distinguished academic career, Dr. Kaplan has pioneered a number of areas of research. She has done ground-breaking research demonstrating that patients can be taught to participate effectively in medical decisions, with positive effects on their health outcomes. Her work on the application of psychometric techniques to assessment of the performance of varying levels of the health care system, from health care organizations to individual physicians, has made her a national expert on this current and controversial topic. Well known for her work in the development of measures of the quality of technical and interpersonal care, health status, and quality of life, particularly for vulnerable populations, she is now working on an innovative project among minority populations using community-based minority "coaches" to train patients to participate effectively in chronic disease care, and is developing and modifying measures for assessing the project's impact on quality of care and quality of life.

Alicia K. Matthews, PhD, is a clinical psychologist and associate professor in the Department of Public Health, Mental Health, and Administrative Nursing at the University of Illinois at Chicago. Her primary research interests are in cancer prevention and control, psychosocial adjustment to illness, and identification of the sociocultural predictors of mental and physical health outcomes in African American and other underserved populations. She has conducted funded research studies examining information seeking and treatment decision making among newly diagnosed African American cancer patients, factors associated with quality of life in lesbian women with breast cancer, prevalence and predictors of anxiety among survivors of breast cancer, evaluation of a education program on breast and cervical cancer education targeting African American lesbian and bisexual women, and mental illness stigma in members of the African American community.

Ruth McCorkle, PhD, has over 28 years of experience in cancer control and psychosocial oncology research. She is a national and international leader in cancer nursing and education and cancer control research. She was the first research chair of the Oncology Nursing Society, and is a charter member of the Oncology Nursing Society, the International Society of Nurses in Cancer Care, and the American Psychosocial Oncology Society. She has served on the board of directors of all three organizations and is currently president of the latter. Dr. McCorkle has served as a member of the study sections of the National Cancer Institute and the National Institute of Nursing Research. She was on the Board of Scientific Advisors for NCI and is currently on the External Scientific Advisory Board of the Children's Oncology Group. In the early 1980s, she obtained the first nonmedical NCI Institutional Research Training Grant and opened the door for other nonmedical fields to become competitive in securing funding. She was elected to the American Academy of Nursing in 1970 and the IOM in 1990 and recently served on the committee to review NIH centers. Dr. McCorkle is Florence S. Wald Professor of Nursing and has twice been designated an American Cancer Society Professor (1986–1991, 1992–1996). She is director of Yale's Center for Excellence in Chronic Illness Care and was chair of the School of Nursing's doctoral program from 1998 to 2004. Dr. McCorkle has won numerous awards recognizing her outstanding contributions to nursing science and oncology nursing. She has done landmark research on the psychosocial ramifications of cancer, testing the effects of a specialized nursing intervention program on helping patients and caregivers manage the consequences of cancer and its treatment, enhancing their quality of life, and improving their survival. In 1988, she received the Outstanding Research Award from the Pennsylvania Nurses Association. She was recognized again in 1993 as Nurse Scientist of the Year by the American Nurses Association and in 1994 received the Distinguished Research Award from the Oncology Nursing Society. In 2004, she was elected to the Connecticut Academy of Science and Engineering. Most recently, she was awarded the Distinguished Scholar in Nursing by the College of Nursing, New York University.

Harold Alan Pincus, MD, is vice chair of the Department of Psychiatry and associate director of the Irving Institute for Clinical and Translational Research at Columbia University and director of Quality and Outcomes Research at New York-Presbyterian Hospital. He also serves as senior scientist at the RAND Corporation. Previously, he was director of RAND-University of Pittsburgh Health Institute and executive vice chairman of the Department of Psychiatry at the University of Pittsburgh, where he still maintains an adjunct professorship. He is director of The Robert Wood Johnson Foundation's National Program on Depression in Primary Care: Linking Clinical and Systems Strategies and the Hartford Foundation's National Program on Building Interdisciplinary Geriatric Research Centers.

Dr. Pincus has also served as deputy medical director of the American Psychiatric Association and founding director of its Office of Research, and as executive director of the American Psychiatric Institute for Research and Education. Prior to joining the American Psychiatric Association, he was special assistant to the director of the National Institute of Mental Health. Dr. Pincus has had a particular research interest in the practice of evidence-based medicine; quality improvement; and the relationships among general medicine, mental health, and substance abuse, developing and empirically testing models of those relationships. He currently maintains a small private practice specializing in major affective disorders and has spent one evening a week for 22 years at a public mental health clinic, caring for patients with severe mental illness. Dr. Pincus graduated from the University of Pennsylvania and received his medical degree from Albert Einstein College of Medicine in New York.

Lee S. Schwartzberg, MD, FACP, is a senior partner and medical director at the West Clinic, a 29-physician oncology, hematology, and radiology practice in Memphis, Tennessee. He received fellowship training in medical oncology and hematology at the Memorial Sloan-Kettering Cancer Center, where he also served as chief medical resident and was a founding member of the institutional ethics committee. Dr. Schwartzberg is a clinical professor of medicine at the University of Tennessee College of Medicine. He is founder and medical director for the Baptist Centers for Cancer Care Cancer Genetics Program and the Stem Cell Transplant Program. He also serves as chair of the Baptist Comprehensive Breast Center multidisciplinary program. His major research interests are new therapeutic approaches to breast cancer, targeted therapy, and supportive care. Dr. Schwartzberg was principal investigator for the Baptist Cancer Institute Community Clinical Oncology Program from 1995 to 2000. Since then he has focused his research interests as president of the Accelerated Community Oncology Research Network (ACORN). Dr. Schwartzberg was awarded the 2004 Jefferson Award for community service. He is founding editor-in-chief of the journal *Community Oncology* and serves on the editorial board of the *Journal of Supportive Oncology*. He has authored more than 60 research papers and maintains a private practice in medical oncology.

Edward H. Wagner, MD, MPH, FACP, is a general internist/epidemiologist and director of the MacColl Institute for Healthcare Innovation at the Center for Health Studies (CHS) Group Health Cooperative. His research and quality improvement work focus on improving the care of seniors and others with chronic illness. Since 1998, he has directed Improving Chronic Illness Care, a national program of The Robert Wood Johnson Foundation. He and his MacColl Institute colleagues developed the Chronic Care

Model, which has now been used in quality improvement programs worldwide. He also is principal investigator of the Cancer Research Network, an NCI-funded cancer research consortium of 13 HMO-based research programs. He has written two books and more than 250 publications. He serves on the editorial boards of *Health Services Research*, the *British Medical Journal*, the *Journal of Cancer Survivorship*, and the *Journal of Clinical Epidemiology*.

Terrie Wetle, PhD, is associate dean of medicine for public health and public policy at Brown Medical School and is professor of community health. She was most recently deputy director, National Institute on Aging at NIH. Formerly, she was director for the Braceland Center for Mental Health and Aging at the Institute of Living and associate professor of community medicine and health care, University of Connecticut Health Center School of Medicine. She is former associate director of the Division on Aging and assistant professor of medicine at Harvard Medical School. At Yale, she was director of the Program in Long Term Care Administration and assistant professor of epidemiology and public health. She previously worked in federal government as a social policy analyst for the Administration on Aging, Department of Health and Human Services, and in local government as director of an area agency on aging in Portland, Oregon. She is past president of the Gerontological Society of America and is currently president of the American Federation for Aging Research. Her research interests include social gerontology, the organization and financing of health care, ethical issues in geriatric care and public health, and end-of-life care. She has more than 200 scientific publications and serves on the editorial boards of several journals. Her most recent edited books are *Financing Long Term Care: The Integration of Public and Private Roles* and *Improving Aging and Public Health Research: Qualitative and Mixed Methods*.

Appendix B

Study Methods

A variety of different strategies were used to carry out this study. Although not explicitly stated in the committee's multifocal scope of work (found at the end of this appendix), the initial, linchpin activity was to define "psychosocial services." The committee's next logical activity was to operationalize this definition by identifying and defining the specific services it encompasses. The importance of this effort was heightened by direction from the National Institutes of Health (NIH) that the identification of models for the delivery of psychosocial services (Task 4 in the scope of work) was of paramount interest. To identify models of service delivery, the committee needed to delineate clearly just what services were to be delivered. Third, underlying the identification of psychosocial services and service delivery models was the committee's commitment to identifying *effective* services and delivery models—those that had empirical evidence to support their ability to bring about positive change in individuals' health care and health. The methods the committee used to undertake these three activities, as well as the tasks specified in the study's scope of work, are discussed below.

DEFINING PSYCHOSOCIAL SERVICES

The committee searched for and located a limited number of definitions of psychosocial services. These definitions and their varying conceptual underpinnings are presented below.

Review of Existing Definitions

"Psychosocial support" is identified by multiple parties as an essential component of quality cancer care (American Psychosocial Oncology Society, undated; National Breast Cancer Centre and National Cancer Control Initiative, 2003; IOM and NRC, 2004; President's Cancer Panel, 2004; Association of Community Cancer Centers, 2006). However, there does not appear to be a commonly shared definition or listing of the various types of psychosocial services or a conceptual framework underpinning various definitions.

Psychosocial services literally could be interpreted as referring to all psychological (mental health, emotional issues) services, as well as all services needed to address adverse social conditions. However, several expert bodies explicitly identify several other dimensions of psychosocial needs/services. The Association of Community Cancer Centers (2006:25), for example, defines psychosocial oncology care (which it also refers to as "psychosocial distress management services") as services "to address the psychological, emotional, *spiritual*, social, *and practical* aspects that patients and their families have as a consequence of cancer and its treatment [emphasis added]." The Institute of Medicine (IOM) report *Improving Palliative Care for Cancer* (IOM and NRC, 2001) also identifies spiritual, religious, and existential distress separately from psychosocial distress. Are spiritual, religious, and existential concerns mutually exclusive and conceptually different? Are "psychological" and "emotional" concerns? Should they and "practical concerns" be included separately as components of a definition of psychosocial services?

The IOM report *Meeting Psychosocial Needs of Women with Breast Cancer* (IOM and NRC, 2004:70–71) presents "brief descriptions of the *full range* of psychosocial services [emphasis added]." However, it then discusses only "basic social and emotional support," which "focuses on adjustment to diagnosis, apprehension regarding treatment, and existential concerns," and psychoeducational approaches; cognitive and behavioral interventions, such as guided imagery, biofeedback, progressive muscle relaxation, and meditation; psychotherapeutic interventions, such as group therapy and counseling; pharmacological interventions; and complementary therapies, such as yoga and massage. It contains no discussion of social services addressing such practical concerns as transportation, child care, financial problems, work, or educational problems.

Australia's Clinical Practice Guidelines for the Psychosocial Care of Adults with Cancer define a psychosocial intervention as "treatment that is intended to address psychological, social, and *some* spiritual needs [emphasis added]" but does not clarify which spiritual issues are and are not to be addressed (National Breast Cancer Centre and National Cancer Control Initiative, 2003:212). The recent IOM publication *From Cancer Patient to Cancer Survivor: Lost in Transition* includes "behavioral" issues in its definition of psychosocial services, that is

> services relating to the psychological, social, behavioral, and spiritual aspects of cancer, including education, prevention and treatment of problems in these areas. (IOM and NRC, 2006:482)

The report addresses the need for behavioral interventions in such areas as smoking cessation, physical activity, nutrition and diet, and weight management. It also reviews the use of complementary and alternative medicine.

The inclusion of behavioral issues is consistent with the scope of issues addressed by the American Psychosocial Oncology Society (APOS) in its mission statement: to "advance the science and practice of psychosocial care for people with cancer . . . in the areas of psychological, social, behavioral, and spiritual aspects of cancer" (American Psychosocial Oncology Society, undated). The inclusion of these issues is also consistent with the American Psychological Association's definition of psychology:

> Psychology is the study of the mind and behavior. The discipline embraces all aspects of the human experience . . . "the understanding of behavior" is the enterprise of psychologists. (American Psychological Association, 2006)

However, this definition is not wholly consistent with a definition of behavioral medicine that conversely subsumes psychosocial issues:

> Behavioral Medicine is the interdisciplinary field concerned with the development and integration of behavioral, psychosocial, and biomedical science knowledge and techniques relevant to the understanding of health and illness, and the application of this knowledge and these techniques to prevention, diagnosis, treatment and rehabilitation. (SBM, 2006:1)

NIH notes that "there has been a lack of definitional clarity to several concepts and terms such as palliative care, end of life care, and hospice care" (NIH, 2004:3). In its review of definitions of psychosocial services, the committee also found a similar need for better definitional and conceptual clarity regarding "psychosocial services."

Conceptual Framework

The committee sought to use a definition that had a conceptual and empirical basis. Conceptual frameworks considered included (1) the list of "psychosocial and environmental problems" contained in the American Psychiatric Association's *Diagnostic and Statistical Manual of Mental*

Disorders (DSM-IV-TR), (2) the National Comprehensive Cancer Network's (NCCN) *Clinical Practice Guidelines for Distress Management*, (3) illness self-management approaches, (4) conceptual models of health-related quality of life, and (5) other frameworks.

Frameworks

DSM-IV-TR list of psychosocial and environmental problems　*DSM-IV-TR*, used by clinicians to diagnose and plan treatment for both mental *disorders* and less serious mental health *problems*, includes assessment of psychosocial and environmental problems that may affect diagnosis, treatment, and prognosis as one of five dimensions (axes)[1] to be evaluated when planning treatment. It categorizes Psychosocial and Environmental Problems in Axis IV as

- **Problems with primary support group**—e.g., death of a family member; health problems or discord in family; separation, divorce, estrangement; abuse or neglect.
- **Problems related to the social environment**—e.g., death or loss of a friend, inadequate social support, living alone, discrimination.
- **Educational problems**—e.g., literacy, school achievement, disruptions to education.
- **Occupational problems**—e.g., unemployment, potential job loss, difficult work conditions.
- **Housing problems**—e.g., homeless, unsafe or inadequate housing.
- **Economic problems**—e.g., inadequate income for routine life needs, difficulty paying for health care.
- **Problems with access to health care**—e.g., inadequate health insurance, transportation problems, geographic hardship accessing care.
- **Problems related to interactions with the legal system**—e.g., arrest or fear of arrest, use of illegal substances, incarceration.
- **Other psychosocial and environmental problems**—e.g., no telephone, exposure to natural disaster or violence, unavailability of social service agencies.

The American Psychiatric Association describes this categorization and *DSM-IV-TR*'s multiaxial assessment approach as a "format for organizing and communicating clinical information, for capturing the complexity

---

[1]The other four axes are Axis I, Clinical Disorders and Other Conditions that may be a focus of clinical psychiatric care; Axis II, Personality Disorders and Mental Retardation; Axis III, General Medical Conditions; and AXIS V, Global Functioning.

of clinical situations, and for describing the heterogeneity of individuals presenting with the same diagnosis. In addition, the multiaxial system promotes the application of the biopsychosocial model in clinical, educational, and research settings" (APA, 2000:27).

National Comprehensive Cancer Network (NCCN) *Clinical Practice Guidelines for Distress Management* The IOM report *Meeting Psychosocial Needs of Women with Breast Cancer* (IOM and NRC, 2004) indicates that psychosocial services are those services intended to alleviate "psychosocial distress." It defines psychosocial distress in cancer as "an unpleasant *emotional* experience that may be psychological, social, or spiritual in nature [emphasis added]" (p. 2) or "an unpleasant experience of an emotional, psychological, social or spiritual nature that interferes with the ability to cope with cancer treatment" (p. 12). It notes that such distress exists along a continuum ranging from the normal and often expected feelings of fear, worry, sadness, and vulnerability related to cancer and its treatment to more severe and disabling symptoms, such as severe anxiety or major depression.

The definition of distress in *Meeting Psychosocial Needs of Women with Breast Cancer* is based on that contained in the NCCN *Clinical Practice Guidelines for Distress Management* (NCCN, 2006). These consensus-based guidelines, developed by 20 of the nation's comprehensive cancer centers, use the word "distress" "to characterize the psychosocial aspects of patient care" (p. MS-2) because "it is more acceptable and less stigmatizing than 'psychiatric,' 'psychosocial,' or 'emotional'; sounds 'normal' and less embarrassing; [and] can be defined and measured by self report" (p. DIS-1). These guidelines define such distress as "a multifactorial, unpleasant *emotional* experience of a psychological (cognitive, behavioral, emotional), social, and/or spiritual nature that may interfere with the ability to cope effectively with cancer, its physical symptoms, and its treatment" [emphasis added] (p. DIS-2). Thus, the NCCN definition distinguishes among at least three sources of psychosocial distress: (1) psychological problems (cognitive, behavioral, and emotional), (2) social problems, and (3) spiritual problems. However, NCCN's screening tool to detect significant levels of patient distress additionally addresses other sources of distress, including practical problems, such as transportation and child care, and physical problems, such as pain, difficulty breathing, fever, changes in urination, and dry/itchy skin.

Illness self-management programs A variety of programs and interventions have been developed to assist individuals in managing a wide range of chronic illnesses. These programs are often referred to as "illness self-management" programs. Self-management is defined as an individual's "ability to manage the symptoms, treatment, physical and psychosocial consequences and lifestyle changes inherent in living with a chronic condition" (Barlow et al., 2002:178). This term is associated most often with conditions such as diabetes mellitus whose severity and progression can be significantly affected by lifestyle changes. There is now considerable evidence for many (noncancer) chronic diseases that interventions directed at improving patients' knowledge, skills, and confidence in managing their illness improves outcomes (Chodosh et al., 2005).

One particular illness self-management approach that has an explicitly stated conceptual model and has been empirically validated for a variety of chronic illnesses (e.g., heart disease, lung disease, stroke, and arthritis) is that of Stanford University (Stanford University School of Medicine, 2006). The Stanford model addresses the day-to-day tasks and skills necessary to live successfully with a chronic illness, including behavioral health practices, social and interpersonal role functioning, and emotional management (Lorig and Holman, 2003). These tasks and skills pertain, for example, to monitoring illness symptoms; using medications appropriately; practicing behaviors conducive to good health in such areas as nutrition, sleep, and exercise; employing stress reduction practices and managing negative emotions; using community resources appropriately; communicating effectively with health care providers; and practicing health-related problem solving and decision making. This model has been shown to reduce pain and disability, lessen fatigue, decrease needed visits to physicians and emergency rooms, and increase self-reported energy and health (Bodenheimer et al., 2000; Lorig et al., 2001; Lorig and Holman, 2003). Illness self-management also is one of the essential components of the Chronic Care Model, which can help inform the development of a conceptual framework.

Health-related quality of life Conceptual models developed to describe the variety of effects cancer has on psychological health, functional abilities, family relationships and other social roles, and important aspects of life also underpin numerous instruments designed to measure health-related quality of life (HRQOL). Examples of these instruments include "generic" instruments used to assess problems for any type of illness, such as the Short Form Health Survey (SF) instruments of the Medical Outcomes Study, and instruments used specifically to assess problems occurring in patients with cancer. These latter instruments (developed for research purposes) include, for example, the Cancer Rehabilitation Evaluation System, the European Organization for Research and Treatment of Cancer Quality of Life Questionnaire, Functional Assessment of Cancer Therapy (FACT) instruments, and the Quality of Life Breast Cancer Instrument (IOM and NRC, 2004). However, the committee that authored the IOM report *From Cancer Patient to Cancer Survivor: Lost In Transition* found no agreed-upon conceptual model for HRQOL, although these instruments frequently address physical, psychological, social, and spiritual domains.

Need for Face Validity

The committee sought a definition that, in addition to being conceptually sound, would have face validity to cancer patients and oncology practitioners. In numerous reports on cancer care reviewed by the committee, cancer patients, their families and informal caretakers, health care providers, and researchers identify many nonbiological adverse consequences of cancer and its treatment, and describe cancer survivors' need for various types of nonmedical assistance in addressing these consequences. These problems and needs were used to inform the committee's development of a definition of psychosocial services for the present study. These problems and needs, discussed in Chapter 1 of this report, include emotional and mental health problems, developmental problems, cognitive problems, problems in performing activities of daily living, problems in fulfilling family and social roles and relationships, problems in employment, financial and health insurance issues, spiritual and existential needs, problems in adopting and maintaining good health behaviors, and other needs.

Definition

The committee considered and deliberated on the above varying definitions and conceptual frameworks at and subsequent to its first meeting. The committee acknowledged that there is a vast array of adverse psychological and social events in people's lives, but that not all of these events may have implications for health or health care. For example, engagement in illegal activity is a serious social problem but may not have implications for patients' health care (unless, for example, they are incarcerated or suffer emotional distress as a result of their activity). Many people also receive psychosocial services for reasons unrelated (or less directly related) to health care. For example, children in the juvenile justice and child welfare systems receive psychosocial services partly in an effort to help them avoid prosecution and the repetition of illegal behaviors and to strengthen their family.

The committee determined that, to be understandable across multiple health and human services sectors, its definition should refer to the subset of psychosocial services that can help improve health and health care. Accordingly, the committee adopted the following as its definition:

> Psychosocial health services are psychological and social services and interventions that enable patients, their families, and health care providers to

optimize biomedical health care and to manage the psychological/behavioral and social aspects of illness and its consequences so as to promote better health.

For the reasons given above, this definition uses the wording "psychosocial *health* services" to make clear that it refers to services that "enable patients, their families, and health care providers to optimize biomedical health care and to manage the psychological, social, and behavioral aspects of *illness*" as opposed to those psychosocial services that might enable individuals to meet other goals, such as strengthening family functioning or avoiding incarceration. The committee also decided to adopt the wording "psychological/behavioral" because of the lack of consistent usage of "psychological" and "behavioral" in the scientific community; for example, the American Psychological Association subsumes behavior under psychology, while others use "behavioral" as the umbrella term. The committee's definition also includes but distinguishes between psychosocial *services* (i.e., activities or tangible goods directly received by and benefiting the patient or family) and psychosocial *interventions* (activities that enable the provision of those services, such as needs assessment, referral, or care coordination).

IDENTIFYING EFFECTIVE PSYCHOSOCIAL HEALTH SERVICES AND MODELS OF SERVICE DELIVERY

Effective Psychosocial Health Services

The committee identified effective psychosocial health services by first identifying the psychosocial health needs experienced by cancer patients. Psychosocial needs were identified by examining peer-reviewed periodical literature and prior authoritative reports addressing this topic, including the following:

DHHS (Department of Health and Human Services). 2003. *Achieving the promise: Transforming mental health care in America.* New Freedom Commission on Mental Health Final Report. DHHS Publication No. SMA-03-3832. Rockville, MD: DHHS.
Holland, J. C., B. Andersen, M. Booth-Jones, W. Breitbart, M. Dabrowski, M. Dudley, S. Fleishman, P. Fobair, G. Foley, C. Fulcher, D. Greenberg, C. Greiner, G. Handzo, J. Herman, P. Jacobsen, S. Knight, M. Levy, R. McAllister-Black. M. Riba, J. Schuster, N. Slatkin, A. Valentive, J. Weinberg, and M. Zevon. 2003. NCCN distress management clinical practice guidelines in oncology. *Journal of the National Comprehensive Cancer Network* 1:344–374.

IOM (Institute of Medicine). 1999. *Ensuring quality cancer care.* Edited by M. Hewitt and J. V. Simone. Washington, DC: National Academy Press.

IOM. 2000. *Bridging disciplines in the brain, behavioral, and clinical sciences.* Edited by T. C. Pellmar and L. Eisenberg. Washington, DC: National Academy Press.

IOM. 2006. *Improving the quality of health care for mental and substance-use conditions.* Washington, DC: The National Academies Press.

IOM and NRC (National Research Council). 2000. *Enhancing data systems to improve the quality of cancer care.* Washington, DC: National Academy Press.

IOM and NRC. 2001. *Interpreting the volume-outcome relationship in the context of cancer care.* Washington, DC: National Academy Press.

IOM and NRC. 2001. *Improving palliative care for cancer.* Edited by K. M. Foley and H. Gelband. Washington, DC: National Academy Press.

IOM and NRC. 2001. *Crossing the quality chasm: A new health system for the 21st century.* Washington, DC: National Academy Press.

IOM and NRC. 2003. *Childhood cancer survivorship: Improving care and quality of life.* Edited by M. Hewitt, S. L. Weiner, and J. V. Simone. Washington, DC: The National Academies Press.

IOM and NRC. 2004. *Meeting psychosocial needs of women with breast cancer.* Edited by M. Hewitt, R. Herdman, and J. C. Holland. Washington, DC: The National Academies Press.

IOM and NRC. 2005. *Assessing the quality of cancer care: An approach to measurement in Georgia.* Edited by J. Eden and J. V. Simone. Washington, DC: The National Academies Press.

IOM and NRC. 2006. *From cancer patient to cancer survivor: Lost in transition.* Edited by M. Hewitt, S. Greenfield, and E. Stovall. Washington, DC: The National Academies Press.

National Breast Cancer Centre and National Cancer Control Initiative. 2003. *Clinical practice guidelines for the psychosocial care of adults with cancer.* http://www.nhmrc.gov.au/publications/synopses/_files/cp90.pdf.

NIH (National Institutes of Health). 2004. Symptom management in cancer: Pain, depression and fatigue. The National Institutes of Health State-of-the-Science Conference. *Monographs Journal of the National Cancer Institute* 32.

NIH (National Institutes of Health). 2004. *Statement on improving end-of-life care.* Paper read at National Institutes of Health State-of-the-Science Conference, December 6–8, 2004, Bethesda, MD.

President's Cancer Panel. 2004. *Living beyond cancer: Finding a new balance.* President's Cancer Panel 2003–2004 annual report. Bethesda, MD: National Cancer Institute, National Institutes of Health, U.S. Department of Health and Human Services.

From this literature, the committee was able to distinguish among the psychosocial health problems encountered by cancer patients and their families. These include problems in (1) coping with emotions accompanying disease and treatment; (2) comprehensively managing their illness; (3) changing specific behaviors to minimize the impact of disease; (4) obtaining material and logistical resources, such as transportation, needed to manage the illness; (5) managing disruptions in work, school, and family life; and (6) managing financial burdens. The committee initially identified 38 services that could potentially be effective in addressing these problems. The committee then undertook systematic searches for evidence of the effectiveness of these services and reviews of this evidence.

The large number of psychosocial services in question and the committee's desire to be thorough in its search for evidence led to very large sets of evidence to review. To make the evidence review manageable, the committee used a serial search strategy (illustrated in Table B-1) that gave priority to both (1) reviewing interventions that have been specifically tested in populations of cancer survivors, and (2) making use of existing systematic reviews, where available.

Each search first aimed to identify meta-analyses and systematic reviews pertaining to the effectiveness of the intervention when provided to cancer survivors (Strategy A). If this effort generated sufficient information for reviewers' assessment of evidence, the search for evidence ended, and reviewers assessed the evidence obtained. If Strategy A provided no or insufficient evidence, the search was expanded to Strategy B, which additionally sought evidence from individual controlled and observational studies with cancer survivors, and meta-analyses and systematic reviews of the effectiveness of the service in populations with conditions other than cancer. Single studies of the service in populations with conditions other than cancer were given lowest priority. The search parameters included English-language ar-

TABLE B-1 Serial Search Strategies

Type of Study	Intervention Tested in Cancer Survivors	Intervention Tested in Populations with Other Conditions
Meta-analyses and Systematic Reviews	Strategy A	Strategy B
Single Controlled or Observational Studies	Strategy B	Strategy C

ticles published from 1980 to 2007 in Medline, PsychInfo, CINAHL, and EMBASE databases. When known, evidence from books, book chapters, and other governmental or nongovernmental evidence reports not indexed in Medline, PsychInfo, CINAHL, and EMBASE was included. Each evidence review involved two reviewers who examined individual studies and the evidence in the aggregate with the aid of standard evidence reporting and scoring forms. Each review team made a determination of the extent to which the evidence showed the intervention to be effective in addressing the identified need. Search terms for each of the 38 candidate services are available from IOM study staff.

When undertaking this review, the committee again encountered a lack of clarity in the terminology used to refer to psychosocial services (discussed above for psychosocial services in the aggregate and in Chapter 3 with respect to individual services). The absence of some definitions, other overlapping definitions and constructs, and the absence of evidence for some services led the committee to "collapse" its list of psychosocial services to the final list of 15 listed in Table B-2.

The findings of the committee's evidence reviews are included in Chapter 3. The committee hopes that the development of a taxonomy and nomenclature for psychosocial health services and the use of stronger research methods will in the future enable more efficient and effective identification, retrieval, and analyses of evidence. The committee is concerned that the absence of a controlled vocabulary for psychosocial health services may have led to inadvertent omission of some relevant evidence in its analyses of the effectiveness of individual psychosocial health services.

Effective Models of Service Delivery

The committee defined the term "models"—as used in the sponsor's task statement—to mean *interventions* that have been found effective in delivering psychosocial health services to patients with cancer or other serious chronic illnesses *in a community setting*. Interventions should (1) have been used to deliver psychosocial health services consistent with the committee's definition, and (2) have been evaluated and found effective in improving patient outcomes. Identified outcomes of interest included (but were not necessarily limited to) the following:

- Increased survival
- Functional status—improving function or preventing or slowing decline
- Decreased comorbidity (e.g., depression)

TABLE B-2 Psychosocial Needs and Formal[a] Services to Address Them

Psychosocial Need	Health Services
Information about illness, treatments, health, and services	• Provision of information, e.g., on illness, treatments, effects on health, and psychosocial services, and the provision of help to patients/families in understanding and using the information
Help in coping with emotions accompanying illness and treatment	• Peer support programs • Counseling/psychotherapy to individuals or groups • Pharmacological management of mental symptoms
Help in managing illness	• Comprehensive illness self-management/self-care programs
Assistance in changing behaviors to minimize impact of disease	• Behavioral/health promotion interventions, such as: – Provider assessment/monitoring of health behaviors (e.g., smoking, exercise) – Brief physician counseling – Patient education, e.g., in cancer-related health risks and risk-reduction measures
Material and logistical resources, such as transportation	• Provision of resources
Help in managing disruptions in work, school, and family life	• Family and caregiver education • Assistance with activities of daily living (ADLs), instrumental ADLs, chores • Legal protections and services, e.g., under Americans with Disabilities Act and Family and Medical Leave Act • Cognitive testing and educational assistance
Financial advice and/ or assistance	• Financial planning/counseling, including management of day-to-day activities such as bill paying • Insurance (e.g., health, disability) counseling • Eligibility assessment/counseling for other benefits (e.g., Supplemental Security Income, Social Security Disability Income) • Supplement financial grants

[a]The committee notes that, as discussed in Chapters 1 and 2, family members and friends and other informal sources of support are key providers of psychosocial health services. This table includes only formal sources of psychosocial support—those that must be secured through the assistance of an organization or agency that in some way enables the provision of needed services (sometimes at no cost or through volunteers).

- Symptom reduction, either physical (e.g., pain, fatigue) or psychological (e.g., anxiety, depressive symptoms) (recognizing that pain and fatigue can be symptoms of psychological conditions as well)
- Increased adherence to a treatment regimen
- Reduction in avoidable inpatient or emergency department care
- Improvement in an evidence-based aspect of quality health care,

such as improved shared decision making by patients and their health care providers; improved coordination of care across multiple care providers; patients' timely receipt of information on their health status, treatment options, or plan of care; and patients' increased ability to manage their illness
- Improved employment and work performance
- Improved educational performance
- Improved family functioning

The committee used four approaches to identify such interventions:

- Review of previous IOM studies and other expert reports (listed above)
- Gathering of the knowledge of effective interventions among committee members
- Solicitation of recommended effective interventions from other expert organizations and individuals
- A search of the peer-reviewed literature

The committee placed greatest value on identifying models that (1) are clearly defined with respect to their conceptual basis, purpose, and component activities; (2) have been successful in achieving their stated purpose as demonstrated by reliable and valid evidence; and (3) have characteristics that promote their uptake.

The strategy used by the committee to search the peer-reviewed literature is available from the IOM study director. Expert organizations contacted to help identify effective models/interventions included the following:

Academic Chronic Care Collaborative
Academy of Psychosomatic Medicine
Administration on Aging, Department of Health and Human Services (DHHS)
American Cancer Society
American College of Surgeons' Commission on Cancer
American Psychiatric Association
American Psychological Association
American Psychosocial Oncology Society
American Society of Clinical Oncology
American Society of Pediatric Hematology/Oncology
Association of Cancer Online Resources
Association of Community Cancer Centers
Association of Oncology Social Workers
Association of Pediatric Oncology Social Workers

Children's Oncology Group
Health Resources and Services Administration, DHHS
Lance Armstrong Foundation
Leukemia and Lymphoma Society
National Coalition for Cancer Survivorship
National Comprehensive Cancer Network
National Conference of State Legislatures
National Council on Aging
National Initiative for Children's Healthcare Quality
National Quality Forum
Oncology Nursing Society
Robert Wood Johnson Community Partnerships for Older Adults
Substance Abuse and Mental Health Services Administration, DHHS
     Centers for Disease Control and Prevention
Veterans Administration

The committee's search yielded 10 interventions that met its criteria and could serve as models for the delivery of psychosocial health services. These are identified and discussed in Chapter 4.

OTHER TASKS IN STUDY SCOPE OF WORK

The committee's scope of work specified nine tasks (one of which was the identification of models of psychosocial care as described above). The remaining eight called for the following:

- Review of the recommendations of previous IOM and other reports on psychosocial services
- Determination of why the recommendations contained in prior reports were not implemented and of possible ways to address barriers to care
- Documentation of
  - types of services needed/provided
  - availability and use of services
  - who is using services and how they are accessed
  - what patients are told/given as their condition evolves (flow of care)
  - provider capacity
  - how services are paid for in various community settings
- Analysis of reimbursement issues and development of recommendations for change
- Analysis of workforce issues, including current and overall capacity required in the community to meet psychosocial health care needs

and the expertise of various disciplines in the delivery of required services (e.g., psychiatry, psychology, social work, nursing, pastoral care, oncology)

- Identification of best-practice training programs
- Development of an applied clinical research agenda
- Development of a dissemination and implementation plan for demonstration models

Evidence to guide the committee's work in these areas was obtained from three main sources: (1) searches of peer-reviewed publications and grey literature (including the review of previous IOM and other reports identified in Task 1); (2) collection of information from psychosocial service providers from their websites and ad hoc follow-up interviews with organizational personnel; and (3) interviews of experts in specific areas, such as the preparation of the workforce in salient professions, Medicare reimbursement, and quality measurement. The relevant published evidence, individuals interviewed, and organizations contacted are listed in each chapter to which they pertain.

The committee encountered a few instances in which it was not possible to provide the specific outcome requested in certain tasks. For example, Task 6, pertaining to the workforce, requested "estimates of overall capacity required in the community in order to meet need, via modeling or other methods, using existing health workforce data and prevalence data of psychosocial problems." In Chapter 7, the committee describes the absence of reliable data on the knowledge and expertise of various disciplines in the delivery of psychosocial health care. The additional wide variety of licensed and unlicensed providers (as well as informal sources of support), the varying combinations in which they can be deployed across a similarly wide array of psychosocial health services, and the numerous variables that would be required to estimate the current capacity and needs of the workforce brought the committee to the same conclusion as others who have addressed the production of workforce estimates: that efforts to plan the size, composition, and distribution of the nation's workforce are characterized by frequent failures and large forecasting errors. This determination that the production of "estimates of overall capacity required in the community in order to meet need" was not feasible (and perhaps not useful) is discussed in Chapter 7.

The scope of work also requested that the committee, "through interviews and testimony . . . determine why the recommendations contained in prior reports were not implemented." The committee's listing of the many recommendations of previous reports that pertain to psychosocial health services is provided in Appendix C. The committee was not convinced that limited interviews and testimony would best illuminate why these numerous recommendations were not implemented. The committee notes that problems with the successful dissemination and adoption of many types of innovations and guidelines for care are widespread in health care, as well as in other industries. A recent systematic review of the literature revealed multiple factors associated with successful implementation (see Box B-1), whose absence likely hinders the uptake of recommendations. The commit-

---

BOX B-1
Key Factors Associated with Successful
Dissemination and Adoption of Innovations

Characteristics of the Innovation

Innovation more likely to be adopted if it

- Offers unambiguous advantages in effectiveness or cost-effectiveness.
- Is compatible with adopters' values, norms, needs.
- Is simple to implement.
- Can be experimented with on a trial basis.
- Has benefits that are easily observed.
- Can be adapted, refined, modified for adopter's needs.
- Is low risk.
- Is relevant to adopter's current work.
- Is accompanied by easily available or provided knowledge required for its use.

Sources of Communication and Influence

Uptake of innovation influenced by

- Structure and quality of social and communication networks.
- Similarity of sources of information to targeted adopters, e.g., in terms of socio-economic, educational, professional, and cultural backgrounds.
- Use of opinion leaders, champions, and change agents.

External Influences

Uptake of innovation influenced by

- Nature of an organization's relationships with other organizations.
- Nature of an organization's participation in formal dissemination and uptake initiatives.
- Policy mandates.

Linkages Among the Components

Innovation more likely to be adopted if there are

- Formal linkages between developers and users early in development.
- Effective relationships between any designated "change agents" and targeted adopters.

tee took to heart the statement in its scope of work that "the committee will place greater priority on the depth of the analyses and recommendations as opposed to a broader array of less detailed analyses and recommendations" and determined that analysis of the multiple reasons why each recommendation failed to be implemented was not likely to be a fruitful undertaking. The committee therefore did not make determinations about why recom-

Characteristics of Individual Adopters

Uptake of innovation influenced by individual's

- General cognitive and psychological traits conducive to trying innovations (e.g., tolerance of ambiguity, intellectual ability, learning style).
- Context-specific psychological characteristics; e.g., motivation and ability to use the intervention in the given context.
- Finding the intervention personally relevant.

Structural and Cultural Characteristics of Potential Organizational Adopters

Innovation more likely to be adopted if organization

- Is large, mature, functionally differentiated, and specialized; has slack in resources; and has decentralized decision making.
- Can identify, capture, interpret, share, and integrate new knowledge.
- Is receptive to change through strong leadership, clear strategic vision, good management and key staff, and climate conducive to experimentation and risk taking.
- Has effective data systems.
- Is "ready" for change because of difficulties in current situation, fit between organization and innovation, anticipated benefits, internal support and advocacy, available time and resources for change, and capacity to evaluate innovation's implementation.

The Uptake Process

Innovation more likely to be adopted with

- Flexible organizational structure that supports decentralized decision making.
- Leadership and management support.
- Personnel motivation, capacity, and competence.
- Funding.
- Internal communication and networks.
- Feedback.
- Adaptation and reinvention.

SOURCE: Greenhalgh et al., 2004, as presented in IOM, 2006.

mendations made in previous reports were not implemented, but calls attention to the findings contained in Box B-1. The committee used these evidence-based factors in successful uptake to shape its recommendations with respect to psychosocial health care and to guide its dissemination plan and early dissemination activities, and urges others to take these factors into account in planning other dissemination and uptake activities.

The committee was convened by the IOM in May 2006. It gathered evidence and conducted its analyses between May 2006 and May 2007. At the five meetings it held during this period, the committee collected and reviewed evidence from the sources described above. The committee also relied on the efforts of several experts who prepared commissioned papers providing the committee with in-depth reviews of two key issues: "Effects of Distressed Psychological States on Adherence and Health Behavior Change: Cognitive, Motivational, and Social Factors" by M. Robin DiMatteo, Kelly B. Haskard, and Summer L. Williams, all of the University of California, Riverside; and "Stress and Disease" by Sheldon Cohen and Denise Janicki-Deverts, both of Carnegie Mellon University.

The committee's draft report containing its recommendations was completed and sent for external review in July 2007. The report was finalized in September 2007.

PSYCHOSOCIAL SERVICES TO CANCER PATIENTS/FAMILIES IN A COMMUNITY SETTING: SCOPE OF WORK

Scope

The Institute of Medicine will conduct a study of the delivery of the diverse (i.e., not limited to mental health) psychosocial services needed by cancer patients and their families in community settings. The study will produce a report that includes

1. a description of how this broad array of services is provided;
2. existing barriers to access of such care;
3. an analysis of the capacity of the current mental health and oncology provider system to deliver such care, and the resources needed to deliver such care nationwide;
4. available training programs for professionals providing psychosocial and mental health services;
5. recommendations to address these issues; and
6. an "action plan" that focuses, in as much detail as possible, on how to overcome the already well known barriers to cancer survivors' receiving needed psychosocial service.

Methods

The methods (including data collection and analysis) used to undertake the scope of work will be developed through the committee convened by the IOM.

- The committee will place greater priority on the depth of the analyses and recommendations as opposed to a broader array of less detailed analyses and recommendations.
- End-of-life care, is of lesser priority for this study, as it has received other attention in recent IOM reports, and includes additional issues that are beyond the resources of this study.
- A workplan will be developed by the committee at its first meeting.

Study Process

Task 1 Review previous IOM and other report recommendations on this issue, including

- AHRQ evidence-based practice reports.
- DHHS (Department of Health and Human Services). 2003. *Achieving the promise: Transforming mental health care in America*. New Freedom Commission on Mental Health Final Report. DHHS Publication No. SMA-03-3832. Rockville, MD: DHHS.
- Holland, J. C., B. Andersen, M. Booth-Jones, et al. NCCN distress management clinical practice guidelines in oncology. *Journal of the National Comprehensive Cancer Network* 1:344–374.
- IOM (Institute of Medicine). 2000. *Bridging disciplines in the brain, behavioral, and clinical sciences*. Edited by T. C. Pellmar and L. Eisenberg. Washington, DC: National Academy Press.
- IOM. 2001. *Crossing the quality chasm: A new health system for the 21st century*. Washington, DC: National Academy Press.
- IOM and NRC (National Research Council). 2001. *Improving palliative care for cancer*. Edited by K. M. Foley and H. Gelband. Washington, DC: National Academy Press.
- IOM and NRC. 2003. *Childhood cancer survivorship: Improving care and quality of life*. Edited by M. Hewitt, S. L. Weiner, and J. V. Simone. Washington, DC: The National Academies Press.
- IOM and NRC. 2004. *Meeting psychosocial needs of women with breast cancer*. Edited by M. Hewitt, R. Herdman, and J. Holland. Washington, DC: The National Academies Press.
- National Breast Cancer Centre and National Cancer Control Initiative. 2003. *Australian clinical practice guidelines for the*

psychosocial care of adults with cancer. http://www.nhmrc.gov.
au/publications/cphome.htm.
- The National Institutes of Health (NIH) State-of-the-Science Con-
  ference on Symptom Management in Cancer: Pain, Depression and
  Fatigue. *Monographs Journal of the National Cancer Institute, No.
  32,* 2004 (especially the Panel's summary findings, pp. 9–13).
- NIH *State-of-the-science conference on improving end-of-life
  care,* December 6–8, 2004. http://consensus.nih.gov/ta/024/
  024EndOfLifepostconfINTRO.htm.
- Other mental health reports, e.g.,
  - *Interpreting the volume-outcome relationship in the context of
    cancer care* (IOM, 2001).
  - *Enhancing data systems to improve the quality of cancer care*
    (IOM, 2000).
  - *Assessing the quality of cancer care: An approach to measure-
    ment in Georgia* (IOM, 2005).

Task 2 Through interviews and testimony to the committee, determine why
the recommendations contained in prior reports were not implemented,
and possible ways to address barriers to care. Interviews and testimony
will be sought, for example, from cancer survivors; mental health patients
with chronic disease; family members; managed care organizations, Centers for Medicare & Medicaid Services; spiritual leaders/clergy; employers;
specialty provider groups such as the American College of Surgeons; health
care payers/insurers; advocates (cancer and mental health); peer outreach
agencies; community delivery agencies; state health commissioners; and
oncology providers.

Interviews and testimony to the Committee about why recommendations contained in the prior reports were not implemented will be secured
both prior to the first meeting and during the time period encompassed by
the first three committee meetings.

Task 3 Using case histories, key informant studies of providers and patients, or other means, document the

- types of services needed/provided
- availability and use
- who is using services and how they access them
- what they are told/given as condition evolves (flow of care)
- provider capacity
- how services are paid for in various community settings

A strategy for implementing this task will be developed by the Committee at its first meeting. Some of this information will be available from published health services research. However, the committee will need to discuss the best methods to use to attain reliable and generalizable information to answer others of these questions. For example, a large, nationally representative survey would be prohibitively expensive; however, focus groups typically do not provide generalizable information. The committee will address study methods and data sources at its first meeting.

Task 4 Identify and characterize diverse models of psychosocial care for patients and families and the extent of evidence for their success (including models from other chronic diseases, noting parallels to cancer in report), including models from other than major, highly resourced centers. These models will be used to analyze how different barriers to care are addressed, or fail to be addressed. Models will be selected with attention to

- stage/course of disease
- economic disparities
- population
- community
- developmental age of survivor

The committee will identify models of psychosocial care to be analyzed in its first two meetings. The committee will review the evidence about these models at the later half of its five meetings.

Sources looked to for models will include, for example: Sloan Kettering; Mayo Clinic, Kaiser Permanente; HRSA; VA System, Indian Health Service; CCOPS; Moffitt Cancer Center, primary care; and SAMHSA's National Registry of Effective Programs and Practices (NREPP). The committee also will include in its review community service entities, such as CancerCare, Inc., in New York City and larger philanthropic agencies (e.g., the Wellness Community, Gilda's Club) that provide an array of psychosocial support services and also use diverse outreach models (e.g., one-on-one, group, educational, crisis management) and modalities (e.g., telephone, teleconference, and online/virtual access) to deliver these services. It will also look to generic models of care delivery that have been shown to be effective across multiple diagnoses, such as the Chronic Care Model, Illness–Self Management Programs, and disease management programs.

Models for delivering care will address how to address the broad array of factors that influence access to such services such as place of residence (rural versus urban), ethnic and cultural differences, and literacy and language barriers. However, given the complexity of this undertaking, it may not be possible to thoroughly explore diversity/health disparity issues. Especially in looking at successful models, the sponsor is seeking more general models to promote, with the understanding that some of these may need be modified to reach underserved communities.

Task 5 Analyze reimbursement issues and develop recommendations for change, in part, by

- a literature review on reimbursement for mental health services delivery and interview of payers (Medicare, Medicaid, and private insurers) to determine current policy and practices regarding reimbursement; and
- a determination of who is currently underwriting the array of psychosocial services required by cancer patients and families; e.g., service agencies, philanthropy, volunteerism, peer counseling, small service charges, etc.

Task 6 Analyze workforce issues, including

- review literature on current capacity of psychosocial service delivery in community setting.
- develop estimates of overall capacity required in the community in order to meet need, via modeling or other methods, using existing health workforce data and prevalence data of psychosocial problems.
- assess expertise in various disciplines to deliver required services (e.g., psychiatry, psychology, social work, nursing, pastoral care, oncology).

Task 7 Develop training recommendations, including

- Examine literature to identify best practice training programs aimed at improving access in the community.
- Contact professional associations for data on training of oncologists about mental health, on training of mental health specialists about chronic disease.
- Training recommendations should address
  - stigma for both patients and providers;
  - accreditation; questions on licensure board exams (medical, nurse, Social work) in addition to training programs;
  - community care providers, i.e., psychosocial service providers (psychiatrists, psychologists, nurses, rehabilitation specialists, noncancer physicians, social workers, pastoral counselors) not affiliated with cancer treatment centers. The goal is to understand what training may be needed for people who neither work

in cancer clinics or centers nor routinely provide psychosocial services to survivors or their family members, but who might care for cancer patients/survivors/family members in the course of their work; and
– emerging opportunities (e.g., telemedicine training).

Task 8 Review literature to identify gaps in knowledge, and develop an applied clinical research agenda about

- who needs services?
- what type of assessment should be provided?
- what type of services should be provided at various stages of disease course?
- who should deliver services?
- are these interventions effective?
- what kind of follow-up is needed?
- are they cost effective in terms of disease course, other health outcomes, employment, etc.?
- how are services paid for, including for family members?
- what are the emerging opportunities (e.g. technological; length of survival)?

Include specific recommendations where appropriate (e.g., for multi-center trials of health service delivery).

Task 9 Develop a dissemination and implementation plan for successful, replicable, demonstration models.

Product

The committee will produce a report that addresses the above topics and includes

- an action plan with policy objectives and recommendations for various stakeholders including federal agencies;
- successful, replicable, demonstration models of effective, accessible psychosocial service delivery in communities; and
- a plan for the evaluation of impact of the report by a third party— as a part of developing its recommendations, the committee will make recommendations to the sponsor about how the impact of the report could be evaluated.

Timeline

This study will take place over 18 months.

REFERENCES

American Psychological Association. 2006. *About APA.* http://www.apa.org/about/ (accessed June 23, 2006).

American Psychosocial Oncology Society. undated. *APOS mission.* http://www.apos-society. org/about/org/mission.aspx (accessed June 15, 2006).

APA (American Psychiatric Association). 2000. *Diagnostic and statistical manual of mental disorders, Text revision (DSM-IV-TR).* 4th ed. Washington, DC: APA.

Association of Community Cancer Centers. 2006. *Cancer program guidelines.* http://www. accc-cancer.org/PUBS/pubs_cpguidelines2006.pdf (accessed June 1, 2006).

Barlow, J., C. Wright, J. Sheasby, A. Turner, and J. Hainsworth. 2002. Self-management approaches for people with chronic conditions: A review. *Patient Education and Counseling* 48(2):177–187.

Bodenheimer, T., K. Lorig, H. Holman, and K. Grumbach. 2000. Patient self-management of chronic disease in primary care. *Journal of the American Medical Association* 288(19): 2469–2475.

Chodosh, J., S. C. Morton, W. Mojica, M. Maglione, M. J. Suttorp, L. Hilton, S. Rhodes, and P. Shekelle. 2005. Meta-analysis: Chronic disease self-management programs for older adults. *Annals of Internal Medicine* 143(6):427–438.

Greenhalgh, T., G. Robert, F. MacFarlane, P. Bate, and O. Kyriakidou. 2004. Diffusion of innovations in service organizations: Systematic review and recommendations. *The Milbank Quarterly* 82(4):581–629.

IOM (Institute of Medicine). 2006. *Improving the quality of health care for mental and substance-use conditions.* Washington, DC: The National Academies Press.

IOM and NRC (National Research Council). 2001. *Improving palliative care for cancer.* Edited by K. M. Foley and H. Gelband. Washington, DC: National Academy Press.

IOM and NRC. 2004. *Meeting psychosocial needs of women with breast cancer.* Edited by M. Hewitt, R. Herdman, and J. Holland. Washington, DC: The National Academies Press.

IOM and NRC. 2006. *From cancer patient to cancer survivor: Lost in transition.* M. Hewitt, S. Greenfield, and E. Stovall, eds. Washington, DC: The National Academies Press.

Lorig, K., and H. Holman. 2003. Self-management education: History, definition, outcomes, and mechanisms. *Annals of Behavioral Medicine* 26(1):1–7.

Lorig, K. R., P. Ritter, A. A. Stewart, D. Sobel, B. W. Brown, A. Bandura, V. M. Gonzalez, D. D. Laurent, and H. R. Holman. 2001. Chronic disease self-management program: 2-year health status and health care utilization outcomes. *Medical Care* 39(11): 1217–1223.

National Breast Cancer Centre and National Cancer Control Initiative. 2003. *Clinical practice guidelines for the psychosocial care of adults with cancer.* Camperdown, NSW, Australia: National Breast Cancer Centre. http://www.nbcc.org.au/bestpractice/resources/PCA131_clinicalpracticeguid.pdf (accessed on September 14, 2007).

NCCN (National Comprehensive Cancer Network). 2006. *Distress management—version 1.2007.* http://www.nccn.org/professionals/physician_gls/PDF/distress.pdf (accessed September 14, 2007).

NIH (National Institutes of Health). 2004. *Statement on improving end-of-life care.* Paper read at National Institutes of Health State-of-the-Science Conference, December 6–8, 2004, Bethesda, MD. http://consensus.nih.gov/2004/2004EndOfLifeCareSOS024html. htm (accessed September 14, 2007).

President's Cancer Panel. 2004. *Living beyond cancer: Finding a new balance.* President's Cancer Panel 2003–2004 Annual Report. Bethesda, MD: National Cancer Institute, National Institutes of Health, U.S. Department of Health and Human Services.

SBM (Society of Behavioral Medicine). 2006. *Definition.* http://www.sbm.org/about/definition. asp (accessed September 14, 2007).

Stanford University School of Medicine. 2006. *Stanford self-management programs.* http:// patienteducation.stanford.edu/programs/ (accessed June 25, 2006).

Appendix C

Recommendations from Prior Selected Reports

TABLE C-1 Recommendations Addressing Psychosocial Services

Report	Recommendations
	Assure Provision of Psychosocial Services
Improving the Quality of Health Care for Mental and Substance-Use Conditions (IOM, 2006)	**Overarching Recommendation 1** Health care for general, mental, and substance-use problems and illnesses must be delivered with an understanding of the inherent interactions between the mind/brain and the rest of the body.
Ensuring Quality Cancer Care (IOM, 1999)	**Recommendation 4** Ensure the following elements of quality care for each individual with cancer: . . . • an agreed upon care plan that outlines goals of care; • access to the full complement of resources necessary to implement the care plan; . . . • a mechanism to coordinate services; and • **psychosocial support services** and compassionate care.
NCCN Distress Management Clinical Practice Guidelines, (NCCN, 2006)	• Distress should be recognized, monitored, documented, and treated promptly at all stages of disease. • Patients, families, and treatment teams should be informed that management of distress is an integral part of total medical care and provided appropriate information about psychosocial services in the treatment center and the community.

continued

TABLE C-1 Continued

Report	Recommendations
Clinical Practice Guidelines for the Psychosocial Care of Adults with Cancer (National Breast Cancer Centre and National Cancer Control Initiative, 2003)	**Emotional and Social Support** **Guideline:** The extent to which a person with cancer has support and feels supported has been identified as a major factor in their adjustment to the disease. It is essential to check the extent of support available to the patient, to recommend additional support as required and to provide information about where this is available. **Gender and psychosocial support** **Guideline:** Clinicians and the treatment team need to consider that the psychosocial needs of men and women may vary both in extent and how they are expressed. Successful strategies for meeting psychosocial support needs may therefore differ for men and women. Where the delivery method is inappropriate or insensitive, men may simply not participate or not gain a benefit.
Achieving the Promise: Transforming Mental Health Care in America (New Freedom Commission on Mental Health, 2003)	**Recommendation 1.1** Advance and implement a national campaign to reduce the stigma of seeking care and a national strategy for suicide prevention. **Recommendation 1.2** Address mental health with the same urgency as physical health. **Recommendation 2.3** Align relevant federal programs to improve access and accountability for mental health services. **Recommendation 2.4** Create a Comprehensive State Mental Health Plan. **Recommendation 3.1** Improve access to quality care that is culturally competent. **Recommendation 3.2** Improve access to quality care in rural and geographically remote areas. **Recommendation 4.1** Promote the mental health of young children.
Meeting Psychosocial Needs of Women with Breast Cancer (IOM and NRC, 2004)	Breast cancer care clinicians, such as oncologists and other medical professionals, responsible for the care of women with breast cancer should incorporate planning for psychosocial management as an integral part of treatment. They should routinely assess and address psychosocial distress as a part of total medical care.
From Cancer Patient to Cancer Survivor: Lost in Transition (IOM and NRC, 2006)	**Recommendation 6** Congress should support the Centers for Disease Control and Prevention (CDC), other collaborating institutions, and the states in developing comprehensive cancer control plans that include consideration of survivorship care, and promoting the implementation, evaluation, and refinement of existing state cancer control plans.
	Screening
NCCN Distress Management Clinical Practice Guidelines, (NCCN, 2006)	• All patients should be screened for distress at their initial visit, at appropriate intervals, and as clinically indicated especially with changes in disease status (i.e., remission, recurrence, progression). • Screening should identify the level and nature of the distress. • Conduct multi-center trials that explore brief screening instruments. . . .

TABLE C-1 Continued

Report	Recommendations
Clinical Practice Guidelines for the Psychosocial Care of Adults with Cancer (National Breast Cancer Centre and National Cancer Control Initiative, 2003)	Clinic-based protocols should be developed to ensure that all patients are screened for clinically significant anxiety and depression.
Achieving the Promise: Transforming Mental Health Care in America (New Freedom Commission on Mental Health, 2003)	**Recommendation 4.3** Screen for co-occurring mental and substance-use disorders and link with integrated treatment strategies.
Improving the Quality of Health Care for Mental and Substance-Use Conditions (IOM, 2006)	**Recommendation 5-1** To make collaboration and coordination of patients' mental and substance-use health care services the norm, providers of the services should establish clinically effective linkages within their own organizations and between providers of mental health and substance-use treatment. The necessary communications and interactions should take place with the patient's knowledge and consent and be fostered by: • Routine sharing of information on patients' problems and pharmacologic and nonpharmacologic treatments among providers of M/SU treatment. • Valid, age-appropriate screening of patients for comorbid mental, substance-use, and general medical problems in these clinical settings and reliable monitoring of their progress.

Patient-Centered Care

Achieving the Promise: Transforming Mental Health Care in America (New Freedom Commission on Mental Health, 2003)	**Recommendation 2.1** Develop an individualized plan of care for every adult with a serious mental illness and child with a serious emotional disturbance.

continued

TABLE C-1 Continued

Report	Recommendations

Quality Improvement

Improving Palliative Care for Cancer (IOM and NRC, 2001)	Recommendation 6: Best available practice guidelines should dictate the standards of care for both physical and psychosocial symptoms. Care systems, payers, and standard-setting and accreditation bodies should strongly encourage their expedited development, validation, and use. Professional societies, particularly the American Society of Clinical Oncology, the Oncology Nursing Society, and the Society for Social Work Oncology, should encourage their members to facilitate the development and testing of guidelines and their eventual implementation, and should provide leadership and training for nonspecialists, who provide most of the care for cancer patients.
NCCN Distress Management Clinical Practice Guidelines (NCCN, 2006)	• Distress should be assessed and managed according to clinical practice guidelines. • Multidisciplinary institutional committees should be formed to implement standards for distress management. • Clinical health outcomes measurement should include assessment of the psychosocial domain (e.g., quality of life and patient and family satisfaction). • Quality of distress management should be included in institutional continuous quality improvement projects.
Meeting Psychosocial Needs of Women with Breast Cancer (IOM and NRC, 2004)	Providers of cancer care should meet the standards of psychosocial care developed by the American College of Surgeon's Commission on Cancer and follow the National Comprehensive Cancer Center Network's (NCCN) Clinical Practice Guidelines for the Management of Distress.
From Cancer Patient to Cancer Survivor: Lost in Transition (IOM and NRC, 2006)	Recommendation 4 Quality of survivorship care measures should be developed through public/private partnerships and quality assurance programs implemented by health systems to monitor and improve the care that all survivors receive.

Continuity of Care

Living Beyond Cancer: Finding a New Balance (President's Cancer Panel, 2004)	Recommendation 1a Upon discharge from cancer treatment, including treatment of recurrences, every patient should be given a record of all care received and important disease characteristics, this should include, at a minimum: . . . • Psychosocial . . . services provided. • Full contact information on treating institutions and key individual providers. Recommendation 1b Upon discharge from cancer treatment, every patient should receive a follow-up care plan incorporating available evidence–based standards of care. This should include, at a minimum: • Information on possible future need for psychosocial support. • Referrals to specific follow-up care providers, support groups. . . . • A listing of cancer-related resources and information (Internet-based sources and telephone listings for major cancer support organizations).

TABLE C-1 Continued

Report	Recommendations
Clinical Practice Guidelines for the Psychosocial Care of Adults with Cancer (National Breast Cancer Centre [NBCC] and National Cancer Control Initiative [NCCI], 2003)	Clinic-based protocols should be developed to ensure that: • All patients are able to identify a key health professional responsible for continuity of care. • Referral pathways for liaison psychiatry, psychologists, support groups, and relevant allied health professionals are established and known to the team.
From Cancer Patient to Cancer Survivor: Lost in Transition (IOM and NRC, 2006)	**Recommendation 2** Patients completing primary treatment should be provided with a comprehensive care summary and follow-up plan that is clearly and effectively explained. This "Survivorship Care Plan" should be written by the principal providers(s) who coordinated oncology treatment. This service should be reimbursed by third party payors of health care. Such a care plan would summarize critical information needed for the survivor's long term care, including . . . information on the availability of psychosocial services in the community and on legal protections regarding employment and access to health insurance.

continued

TABLE C-1 Continued

Report	Recommendations
Improving the Quality of Health Care for Mental and Substance-Use Conditions (IOM, 2006)	**Recommendation 5-2** To facilitate the delivery of coordinated care by primary care, mental health, and substance-use treatment providers, government agencies, purchasers, health plans, and accreditation organizations should implement policies and incentives to continually increase collaboration among these providers to achieve evidence-based screening and care of their patients with general, mental, and/or substance-use health conditions. The following specific measures should be undertaken to carry out this recommendation:

* Primary care and specialty M/SU health care providers should transition along a continuum of evidence-based coordination models from (1) formal agreements among mental, substance-use, and primary health care providers; to (2) case management of mental, substance-use, and primary health care; to (3) collocation of mental, substance-use, and primary health care services; and then to (4) delivery of mental, substance-use, and primary health care through clinically integrated practices of primary and M/SU care providers. Organizations should adopt models to which they can most easily transition from their current structure, that best meet the needs of their patient populations, and that ensure accountability.
* DHHS should fund demonstration programs to offer incentives for the transition of multiple primary care and M/SU practices along this continuum of coordination models.
* Purchasers should modify policies and practices that preclude paying for evidence-based screening, treatment, and coordination of M/SU care and require (with patients' knowledge and consent) all health care organizations with which they contract to ensure appropriate sharing of clinical information essential for coordination of care with other providers treating their patients.
* Organizations that accredit mental, substance-use, or primary health care organizations should use accrediting practices that assess, for all providers, the use of evidence-based approaches to coordinating mental, substance-use, and primary health care.
* Federal and state governments should revise laws, regulations, and administrative practices that create inappropriate barriers to the communication of information between providers of health care for mental and substance-use conditions and between those providers and providers of general care.

Recommendation 5-3 To ensure the health of persons for whom they are responsible, M/SU providers should:

* Coordinate their services with those of other human-services and education agencies, such as schools, housing and vocational rehabilitation agencies, and providers of services for older adults.
* Establish referral arrangements for needed services.

TABLE C-1 Continued

Report	Recommendations

Patient Education and Illness Self-Management

Living Beyond Cancer: Finding a New Balance (President's Cancer Panel, 2004)

Recommendation 2 Procedures should be established within diverse patient care settings to better inform patients/survivors and their caregivers about available legal and regulatory protections and resources [e.g., pertaining to employment and insurance.].

Recommendation 5a All survivors should be counseled about common psychosocial effects of cancer and cancer treatment and provided specific referrals to available support groups and services.

Clinical Practice Guidelines for the Psychosocial Care of Adults with Cancer (National Breast Cancer Centre and National Cancer Control Initiative, 2003)

Clinic-based protocols should be developed to ensure the following goals:
- Copies of evidence-based information about treatment options are provided to all patients.
- Listings of other information resources which may be of value are provided to all patients.

Achieving the Promise: Transforming Mental Health Care in America (New Freedom Commission on Mental Health, 2003)

Recommendation 2.5 Protect and enhance the rights of people with mental illness.

Meeting Psychosocial Needs of Women with Breast Cancer (IOM and NRC, 2004)

The National Cancer Institute (NCI), the American Cancer Society (ACS), and professional organizations (e.g., American Society of Clinical Oncology, American College of Surgeons, American Association of Colleges of Nursing, American Psychosocial Oncology Society, American Society of Social Work, American Society for Therapeutic Radiology and Oncology, Oncology Nursing Society) need to partner with advocacy groups (e.g., National Breast Cancer Coalition, National Alliance of Breast Cancer Organizations, Wellness Community, National Coalition Cancer Survivorship [NCCS]) to focus attention on psychosocial needs of patients and resources that provide psychosocial services in local communities and nationally.

continued

TABLE C-1 Continued

Report	Recommendations

Public Education

Living Beyond Cancer: Finding a New Balance (President's Cancer Panel, 2004)	**Recommendation 4a** National public education efforts sponsored by coalitions of public and private cancer information and professional organizations and the media (e.g., film, television, print, and broadcast news) should be undertaken to: • Raise awareness of survivor experiences and capabilities, and of the continuing growth of the cancer survivor population. These efforts should seek to enhance understanding of the post-treatment experiences of cancer survivors of various ages and their loved ones and the need for life-long follow-up care. **Recommendation 5c** Providers should include psychosocial services routinely as part of comprehensive cancer care treatment and follow-up care and should be knowledgeable about local resources for such care for patients/survivors, caregivers, and family members. In particular: • The transition from active treatment to social reintegration is crucial and should receive specific attention in survivor's care. • Primary and other health care providers should monitor caregivers, children, and siblings of survivors for signs of psychological distress both during the survivor's treatment and in the post-treatment period.

Care Coordination

NCCN Distress Management Clinical Practice Guidelines (NCCN, 2006)	Licensed mental health professionals and certified pastoral caregivers experienced in psychosocial aspects of cancer should be readily available as staff members or by referral.

Reimbursement

Living Beyond Cancer: Finding a New Balance (President's Cancer Panel, 2004)	**Recommendation 7b** Adequate reimbursement for prosthetics must be provided and it must be recognized that: • Many prostheses must be replaced periodically. • Access to prostheses is an integral part of psychosocial care for cancer. **Recommendation 7c** [Health Insurance] Coverage should be routinely provided for psychosocial services for which there is evidence of benefit both during treatment and post-treatment as needed.
NCCN Distress Management Clinical Practice Guidelines (NCCN, 2006)	Medical care contracts should include reimbursement for services provided by mental health professionals.

TABLE C-1 Continued

Report	Recommendations
From Cancer Patient to Cancer Survivor: Lost in Transition (IOM and NRC, 2006)	**Recommendation 2** Patients completing primary treatment should be provided with a comprehensive care summary and follow-up plan that is clearly and effectively explained. This "Survivorship Care Plan" should be written by the principal providers(s) who coordinated oncology treatment. **This service should be reimbursed by third party payors of health care.** **Recommendation 9** Federal and state policy makers should act to ensure that all cancer survivors have access to adequate and affordable health insurance. Insurers and payors of health care should recognize survivorship care as an essential part of cancer care and design benefits, payment policies, and reimbursement mechanisms to facilitate coverage for evidence-based aspects of care.

Support of Informal Caregivers

Living Beyond Cancer: Finding a New Balance (President's Cancer Panel, 2004)	**Recommendation 5b** A caregiver plan should be developed and reviewed with a survivor's caregiver(s) at the outset of cancer treatment. It should include, at a minimum: • An assessment of the survivors' social and support systems. • A description of elements of patient care for which the caregiver will be responsible. Caregivers should be provided adequate and, as needed, ongoing hands-on training to perform these tasks. • Telephone contacts and written information related to caregiver tasks. • Referral to caregiver support groups or organizations either in the caregiver's local area or to national and online support services. **Recommendation 8a** Qualified providers in the treatment setting should train and assist parents to assume their crucial roles in helping the child with cancer return to school and becoming an educator and advocate with individual teachers and the school system. **Recommendation 8b** Pediatric cancer centers should offer and promote teacher training as a part of their community outreach efforts to help ensure that the needs of pediatric cancer survivors returning to the classroom are met. Internet-based training modules also should be considered to extend the geographic reach of these training efforts. If possible, continuing education units (CEUs) should be provided to participating teachers. **Recommendation 8c** NCI and the Dept. of Education should explore collaborative opportunities to improve the classroom re-entry and re-integration of young people with cancer or other chronic or catastrophic illnesses (e.g., remote learning, teacher training). **Recommendation 9b** As part of the process of transitioning survivors of childhood cancers into the adult care setting, information about young adult support groups, Internet sites, and other sources of information and support specific to this age group should be provided to survivors and their families. **Recommendation 10** Cancer care providers should inform families of cancer patients about supportive services, including special camps for families and siblings.

continued

TABLE C-1 Continued

Report	Recommendations
	Recommendation 12a Family members, primary care providers, cancer specialists, and others who are close to or provide medical care to adolescent and young adult survivors should be made aware that depression, anxiety, or other psychosocial issues may affect the survivor long after treatment ends and should be instructed on how to intervene should the survivor experience such difficulties.
	Recommendation 12b Adolescent and young adult survivors should be taught self-advocacy skills that may be needed to secure accommodations for learning differences resulting from cancer or its treatment. Physicians and other providers should act as advocates for survivors when necessary.
	Recommendation 16 Health care providers must ascertain the strength of an older survivor's social and caregiver support system. This should be assessed at diagnosis, during treatment, and at intervals after treatment is completed. Oncology nurses, nurse practitioners, other advanced practice nurses, physician assistants, social workers, patient navigators, or other non-physician personnel may be best able to make these assessments and arrange assistance and services for survivors who lack adequate support.
	Recommendation 17 Health care providers should not assume that older cancer survivors and their partners are uninterested in sexuality and intimacy. Survivors should be asked directly if they have concerns or are experiencing problems in this area and should receive appropriate referrals to address such issues.

Employment

From Cancer Patient to Cancer Survivor: Lost in Transition (IOM and NRC, 2006)	**Recommendation 8** Employers, legal advocates, health care providers, sponsors of support services, and government agencies should act to eliminate discrimination and minimize adverse effects of cancer on employment, while supporting cancer survivors with short-term and long term limitations in ability to work. The following text follows the recommendation: • Cancer professionals, advocacy organizations, and the NCI and other government agencies should continue to educate employers and the public about the successes achieved in cancer treatment, the improved prospects for survival, and the continued productivity of most patients who are treated for cancer. • Public and private sponsors of services to support cancer survivors and their families should finance programs offering education, counseling, support, legal advice, vocational rehabilitation, and referral for survivors who want to work.

TABLE C-1 Continued

Report	Recommendations
	• Providers who care for cancer survivors should become familiar with the employment rights that apply to survivors who want to work and make available information about employment rights and programs that provide counseling, legal services, and referral.
	• Providers should routinely ask patients who are cancer survivors if they have physical or mental health problems that are affecting their work, with the goal of improving symptoms and referring patients for rehabilitative and other services.
	• Employers should implement programs to assist cancer survivors. Examples include short- and long-term disability insurance, return to work programs, wellness programs, accommodation of special needs, and employee assistance programs.
	• Cancer survivors should tell their physicians when health problems are affecting them at work. Survivors should educate themselves about their employment rights and contact support organizations for assistance and referrals when needed.

Workforce Education

Report	Recommendations
NCCN Distress Management Clinical Practice Guidelines (NCCN, 2006)	Educational and training programs should be developed to ensure that health care professionals and pastoral caregivers have knowledge and skills in the assessment and management of distress.
Clinical Practice Guidelines for the Psychosocial Care of Adults with Cancer (National Breast Cancer Centre and National Cancer Control Initiative, 2003)	Clinic-based protocols should be developed to ensure that all staff working with patients with cancer have participated in relevant communication skills training.
Meeting Psychosocial Needs of Women with Breast Cancer (IOM and NRC, 2004)	• Sponsors of professional education and training programs (e.g., NCI, ACS, American Society of Clinical Oncology [ASCO], Oncology Nursing Society, Association of Oncology Social Work, American Cancer Society-Commission on Cancer, American Psychosocial Society) should support continuing education programs by designing, recommending, or funding them at a level that recognizes their importance in psycho-oncology for oncologists, those in training programs, and nurses and for further development of programs similar to the ASCO program to improve clinician's communication skills; and

continued

TABLE C-1 Continued

Report	Recommendations
	• Graduate education programs for oncology clinicians, primary care practitioners, nurses, social workers, and psychologists should evaluate their capacity to incorporate a core curriculum in psycho-oncology in their overall curriculum taught by an adequately trained faculty in psycho-oncology and to include relevant questions in examination requirements.
From Cancer Patient to Cancer Survivor: Lost in Transition (IOM and NRC, 2006)	**Recommendation 7** The National Cancer Institute (NCI), professional associations, and voluntary organizations should expand and coordinate their efforts to provide educational opportunities to health care providers to equip them to address the health care and quality of life issues facing cancer survivors. (The text below follows the recommendation): Immediate steps to facilitate the development of programs include: • Establish a clearinghouse of available sources of survivorship education and training (and guidelines), with opportunity for feedback. • Appoint an interdisciplinary consortium to review available resources, identify promising approaches, develop new programs, and promote cost-effective approaches. • Increase support of model formal training programs (undergraduate and graduate levels, continuing medical education) that could be adopted by others. By specialty: **Physicians** 1. Add more survivorship-related CME: • The American Board of Medical Specialties' new program, "Maintenance of Certification," will require continuous assurance of professional skills for board-certified physicians. The development of a model on cancer survivorship as part of this program could facilitate the assurance of competence for these and other specialty providers. 2. Improve online survivorship information aimed at health care providers: • Expand physician data query to include more information on survivorship care. • Centralize survivorship guidelines online. • Encourage the development and adoption of evidence-based guidelines. • Ease finding survivorship-related guidelines included in the AHRQ-sponsored guideline clearinghouse (e.g., add the term survivorship to the search engine to pick up surveillance guidelines for cancer). 3. Expand training opportunities to promote interdisciplinary shared care.

TABLE C-1 Continued

Report	Recommendations
	Nurses 1. Increase survivorship content in undergraduate and graduate nursing programs. 2. Expand continuing education opportunities on survivorship for practicing nurses. 3. Increase the number of nursing schools that provide graduate training in oncology. 4. Increase the number of nurses who seek certification in oncology (incentives are needed). 5. Endorse activities of those working to ease the nursing shortage. **Social workers and other providers of psychosocial services** 1. Support efforts of APOS to standardize and promote continuing education. 2. Endorse activities of those working to maintain social services in cancer programs.

Research and Demonstrations

NCCN Distress Management Clinical Practice Guidelines (NCCN, 2006)	Conduct multicenter trials that . . . pilot treatment guidelines.
Meeting Psychosocial Needs of Women with Breast Cancer (IOM and NRC, 2004)	1. Research sponsors (e.g., NCI, ACS) and professional organizations (e.g., American Society of Clinical Oncology, American College of Surgeons, American Association of Colleges of Nursing, American Psychosocial Oncology Society, American Society of Social Work, American Society for Therapeutic Radiology and Oncology, Oncology Nursing Society) need to support efforts in collaboration with advocacy groups (e.g., National Breast Cancer Coalition, National Alliance of Breast Cancer Organizations) to enhance practice environments to promote coordinated, comprehensive, and compassionate care. 2. Research sponsors (e.g., NCI, ACS) should continue to support basic and applied psycho-oncology research. This might include: • Further development of simple, rapid screening tools for identifying the patient with distress in outpatient offices and training of primary oncology teams in diagnosis of distress that exceeds the "expected" and when referral to supportive services should be made; • Studies that assess the relative effectiveness of various psychosocial interventions, using population-based patient samples of adequate size, the timing and duration of intervention, and innovative and inexpensive modes of administration (e.g., Internet-based approaches); • A consensus conference to develop a battery of standard instruments for outcome measures to permit comparison of data from studies carried out by different research groups;

continued

TABLE C-1 Continued

Report	Recommendations
	• Organization of a psychosocial clinical trials group in which a network of researchers could address key questions in multi-center studies that would allow access to large, population-based samples; • Clinical trials of psychosocial interventions that are conducted within routine breast cancer care in which cost and quality of life are outcome measures; and • A registry of ongoing psychosocial research/trials to assist researchers in identifying and tracking new areas of study. 3. The NCI should support a special study to ascertain the use of, and unmet need for, cancer-related supportive care services (including psychosocial services) in the United States. The results of such a study could provide benchmarks against which care can be measured and performance monitored. Such a study would document existing disparities in service use by age, race/ethnicity, geography, and insurance coverage.
Evidence Report on the Occurrence, Assessment, and Treatment of Depression in Cancer Patients (Pirl, 2004)	More research is needed on factors that may cause varying rates of depression and that predict which patients are most at risk. Longitudinal studies are needed to estimate the incidence of depression starting at the time of or, ideally, before diagnosis of cancer. Many instruments with a wide range of complexity are currently being used to measure depressive symptoms. . . . Multiple methods of assessment make it difficult to compare studies. A consensus choice of instruments may help to standardize research on depression that is comorbid with cancer.
From Cancer Patient to Cancer Survivor: Lost in Transition (IOM and NRC, 2006)	**Recommendation 5** The Centers for Medicare and Medicaid Services (CMS), National Cancer Institute (NCI), Agency for Healthcare Research and Quality (AHRQ), the Department of Veterans Affairs (VA), and other qualified organizations should support demonstration programs to test models of coordinated, interdisciplinary survivorship care in diverse communities and across systems of care. **Recommendation 10** The NCI, CDC, AHRQ, CMS, VA, private voluntary organizations such as the American Cancer Society, and private health insurers and plans should increase their support of survivorship research and expand mechanisms for its conduct. New research initiatives focused on cancer patient follow-up are urgently needed to guide effective survivorship care. Research is especially needed to improve understanding of . . . • The cost-effectiveness of alternative models of survivorship care and community-based psychosocial services including: – Survivors' and caregivers' attitudes and preferences regarding outcomes and survivorship care; – Needs of racial, ethnic groups, residents of rural areas, and other potentially underserved groups; and – Supportive and rehabilitation programs.

TABLE C-1 Continued

Report	Recommendations
	• Interventions to improve the quality of life, including: – Family and caregiver needs and access to supportive services. – Mechanisms to reduce financial burdens of survivorship care (e.g., the new Medicare prescription drug benefit should be carefully monitored to evaluate its impact, especially how private plan formularies cover cancer drugs). – Employer programs to meet return-to-work needs. – Approaches to improve health insurance coverage. – Legal protections afforded cancer survivors through the Americans with Disabilities Act (ADA), Family and Medical Leave Act, Health Insurance Portability and Accountability Act (HIPAA), and other laws. • Survivorship research methods including barriers to participation, impact of HIPAA, and methods to overcome challenges of survivorship research (e.g., methods to adjust for bias introduced by nonparticipation; methods to minimize loss-to follow-up).

TABLE C-2 Other Recommendations of Potential Relevance

Report	Recommendations
	Access
Ensuring Quality Cancer Care (IOM, 1999)	**Recommendation 9** Services for the un- and underinsured should be enhanced to ensure entry to, and equitable treatment within, the cancer care system.
	Recommendation 10 Studies are needed to find out why specific segments of the population (e.g., members of certain racial or ethnic groups, older patients) do not receive appropriate cancer care. These studies should measure provider and individual knowledge, attitudes, and beliefs, as well as other potential barriers to access to care.
	Data Systems
Ensuring Quality Cancer Care (IOM, 1999)	**Recommendation 7** A cancer data system is needed that can provide quality benchmarks for use by systems of care (such as hospitals, provider groups, and managed care systems).
Enhancing Data Systems to Improve the Quality of Cancer Care (IOM and NRC, 2000)	**Recommendation 2** Congress should increase support to CDC for the National Program of Cancer Registries (NPCR) to improve the capacity of states to achieve complete coverage and timely reporting of incident cancer cases. NPCR's primary purpose is cancer surveillance, but NPCR, together with SEER, has great potential to facilitate national, population-based assessments of the quality of cancer care through linkage studies and by serving as a sample frame for special studies.
	Recommendation 3 Private cancer-related organizations should join the American Cancer society and the American College of Surgeons to provide financial support for the National Cancer Data Base. Expanded support would facilitate efforts underway to report quality benchmarks and performance data to institutions providing cancer care.
	Recommendation 4 Federal research agencies (e.g., NCI, CDC, AHRQ, Health Care Financing Administration) should support research and demonstration projects to identify new mechanisms to organize and finance the collection of data from cancer care quality studies. Current data systems tend to be hospital based, while cancer care is shifting to outpatient settings. New models are needed to capture entire episodes of care, irrespective of the setting of care.
	Recommendation 5 Federal research agencies (e.g., National Institutes of Health, Food and Drug Administration, CDC, VA) should support public private partnerships to develop technologies, including computer-based patient record systems and intranet-based communication systems, that will improve the availability, quality, and timeliness of clinical data relevant to assessing quality of cancer care.

TABLE C-2 Continued

Report	Recommendations
	Recommendation 7 Federal research agencies (e.g., NCI, AHRQ, VA) should expand support for health services research, especially studies based on the linkage of cancer registry to administrative data and special studies of cases sampled from cancer registries. Resources should also be made available through NPCR and SEER to provide technical assistance to states to help them expand the capability of using cancer registry data for quality improvement initiatives. NPCR should also be supported in its efforts to consolidate state data and link them to national data files.
Achieving the Promise: Transforming Mental Health Care in America (New Freedom Commission on Mental Health, 2003)	**Recommendation 6.1** Use health technology and telehealth to improve access and coordination of mental health care, especially for Americans in remote areas or in underserved populations. **Recommendation 6.2** Develop and implement integrated electronic health record and personal health information systems.

Quality Improvement

Report	Recommendations
Childhood Cancer Survivorship: Improving Care and Quality of Life (IOM and NRC, 2003)	**Recommendation 1** Develop evidence-based clinical practice guidelines for the care of survivors of childhood cancer. The NCI should convene an expert group of consumers, providers, and researchers to review available clinical practice guidelines and agree upon an evidence-based standard for current practice. For areas where bodies of evidence have not been rigorously evaluated, AHRQ Evidence Based Practice Centers should be charged to review the evidence. When evidence upon which to make recommendations is not available, the expert group should identify areas in need of research. **Recommendation 2** Define a minimum set of standards for systems of comprehensive, multidisciplinary follow-up care that link specialty and primary care providers, ensure the presence of such a system within institutions treating children with cancer, and evaluate alternative models of delivery of survivorship care. • The NCI should convene an expert group of consumers, providers, and health services researchers to define essential components of a follow-up system and propose alternative ways to deliver care. Consideration could be given to long-term follow-up clinics, collaborative practices between oncology and primary care physicians, and other models that might be dictated by local practices and resources, patient and family preferences, geography, and other considerations. Any system that is developed should assure linkages between specialty and primary care providers.

continued

TABLE C-2 Continued

Report	Recommendations
	• A set of minimal standards for designation as a late effects clinic should be endorsed and adopted by relevant bodies such as Children's Oncology Group (COG), the American Society of Pediatric Hematology/Oncology, the American Academy of Pediatrics, the American Society of Clinical Oncology, the American College of Surgeon's Commission on Cancer, and the NCI in its requirements for approval for comprehensive cancer centers.
	• COG members and other institutions treating children with cancer should ensure that a comprehensive, multidisciplinary system of follow-up care is in place to serve the needs of patients and their families discharged from their care.
	• State comprehensive cancer control plans being developed and implemented with CDC support should include provisions to ensure appropriate follow-up care for cancer survivors and their families.
	• Grant programs of HRSA (e.g., Special Projects of Regional and National Significance [SPRANS]) should support demonstration programs to test alternative delivery systems (e.g., telemedicine, outreach programs) to ensure that the needs of different populations are met (e.g., rural residents or those living far from specialized late-effects clinics, ethnic and minority groups). Needed also are evaluations to determine which models of care confer benefits in terms of preventing or ameliorating late effects and improving quality of life, and which models survivors and their families prefer.
	Recommendation 3 Improve awareness of late effects and their implications to long-term health among childhood cancer survivors and their families.
	• Clinicians providing pediatric cancer care should provide survivors and their families written information regarding the specific nature of their cancer and its treatment, the risks of late effects, and a plan (and, when appropriate, referrals) for follow-up. Discussions of late effects should begin with diagnosis.
	• Public and private sponsors of health education (e.g., NCI, ACS) should launch informational campaigns and provide support to survivorship groups that have effective outreach programs.
Achieving the Promise: Transforming Mental Health Care in America (New Freedom Commission on Mental Health, 2003)	**Recommendation 5.2** Advance evidence-based practices using dissemination and demonstration projects and create a public-private partnership to guide their implementation.

TABLE C-2 Continued

Report	Recommendations
	Quality Measurement
Ensuring Quality Cancer Care (IOM, 1999)	**Recommendation 3** Measure and monitor the quality of care using a core set of quality measures. Measures should: • span the continuum of cancer care and be developed through a coordinated public-private effort; • be used to hold providers, including health care systems, health plans, and physicians accountable for providing and improving quality care; • be applied to care provided through the Medicare and Medicaid programs as a requirement of participation in these programs; and • be disseminated widely and communicated to purchasers, providers, consumer organizations, individuals with care, policy makers, and health services researchers, in a form that is relevant and useful for health care decision-making.
Enhancing Data Systems to Improve the Quality of Cancer Care (IOM, 2000)	**Recommendation 1** Develop a core set of cancer care quality measures. a. The secretary of DHHS should designate a committee made up of representatives of public institutions (e.g., The DHHS Quality of Cancer Care Committee, state cancer registries, academic institutions) and private groups (e.g., consumer organizations, professional associations, purchasers, health insurers and plans) to: 1) identify a single set of quality measures that span the full spectrum of an individual's care and are based on the best available evidence; 2) advise other national groups (e.g., National Committee for Quality Insurance, Joint Commission on Accreditation of Healthcare Organizations, National Quality Forum) to adopt the recommended core set of measures. . . . b. Research sponsors (e.g., AHRQ, NCI, HCFA, VA) should invest in studies to identify evidence-based quality indicators across the continuum of cancer care. . . . d. Efforts to identify quality of cancer care measures should be coordinated with ongoing national efforts regarding quality of care.
From Cancer Patient to Cancer Survivor: Lost in Transition (IOM and NRC, 2006)	**Recommendation 4** Quality of survivorship care measures should be developed through public/private partnerships and quality assurance programs implemented by health systems to monitor and improve the care that all survivors receive.

continued

TABLE C-2 Continued

Report	Recommendations
Childhood Cancer Survivorship (IOM, 2003)	**Recommendation 1** Develop evidence-based clinical practice guidelines for the care of survivors of childhood cancer. The NCI should convene an expert group of consumers, providers, and researchers to review available clinical practice guidelines and agree upon an evidence-based standard for current practice. For areas where bodies of evidence have not been rigorously evaluated, AHRQ Evidence Practice Centers should be charged to review the evidence. When evidence upon which to make recommendation is not available, the expert group should identify areas in need of research.

Research and Demonstrations

Report	Recommendations
Ensuring Quality Cancer Care (IOM, 1999)	**Recommendation 8** Public and private sponsors of cancer care research should support national studies of recently diagnosed individuals with cancer, using information sources with sufficient detail to assess patterns of cancer care and factors associated with the receipt of good care. . . . **Recommendation 10** Studies are needed to find out why specific segments of the population (e.g., members of certain racial or ethnic groups, older patients) do not receive appropriate cancer care. These studies should measure provider and individual knowledge, attitudes, and beliefs, as well as other potential barriers to access to care.
Enhancing Data Systems to Improve the Quality of Cancer Care (IOM, 2000)	**Recommendation 1** b. Research sponsors (e.g., AHRQ, NCI, HCFA,VA) should invest in studies to identify evidence-based quality indicators across the continuum of cancer care. **Recommendation 9** Federal research agencies (e.g., NCI, AHRQ, HCFA, VA) should fund demonstration projects to assess the application of quality monitoring programs within health care systems and the impact of data-driven changes in the delivery of services on the quality of health care. Findings from the demonstrations should be disseminated widely to consumers, payers, purchasers, and cancer care providers.

TABLE C-2 Continued

Report	Recommendations
Bridging Disciplines in the Brain, Behavioral, and Clinical Sciences (IOM, 2000)	**Recommendation 1** Federal and private research sponsors should seek to identify areas that can be most effectively investigated with interdisciplinary approaches. **Recommendation 2** Funding agencies and universities should remove the barriers to interdisciplinary research and training . . . by • Requiring commitments from university administration to qualify for funding for interdisciplinary efforts. These should include supportive promotion policies, allocation of appropriate overhead, and allocation of shared facilities. • Facilitate interactions among investigators in different disciplines by funding shared and core facilities. • Encouraging legislation to expand loan repayment programs to include investigators outside NIH who are engaged in funded interdisciplinary and translational research. • Supporting peer review that facilitates interdisciplinary efforts. • Continuing and expanding partnerships among funding agencies to provide the broadest base for interdisciplinary efforts. • Indicating in funding announcements that training is an integral component on the interdisciplinary research project. Universities should: • Allocate appropriate credit for interdisciplinary efforts . . . including fair allocation of research overhead costs to the home departments of all investigators and a fair credit for faculty contributions. • Review and revise appointment, promotion, and tenure policies to ensure that they do not impede interdisciplinary research and teaching. • Facilitate interaction among investigators through support for shared facilities. • Encourage development, maintenance, and evolution of interdisciplinary institutes, centers, and programs for appropriate problems.
Improving Palliative Care for Cancer (IOM and NRC, 2001)	**Recommendation 2** The NCI should add the requirement of research in palliative care and symptom control for recognition as a "comprehensive cancer center." The Health Care Financing Administration should fund demonstration projects for service delivery and reimbursement that integrate palliative care and potentially life-prolonging treatments throughout the course of disease.

continued

TABLE C-2 Continued

Report	Recommendations
Childhood Cancer Survivorship (IOM, 2003)	**Recommendation 7** Public and private research organizations (e.g., NCI, National Institute of Nursing Research, ACS) should increase support for research to prevent or ameliorate the long-term consequences of childhood cancer. Priority areas of research include assessing the prevalence and etiology of late effects; testing methods that may reduce late effects during treatment; developing interventions to prevent or reduce late effects after treatment; and furthering improvements in quality of care to ameliorate the consequences of late effects on individuals and families. • Research is needed on the long-term social, economic, and quality of life implications of cancer on survivors and their families. . . .
Achieving the Promise: Transforming Mental Health Care in America (New Freedom Commission on Mental Health, 2003)	**Recommendation 5.1** Accelerate research to promote recovery and resilience, and ultimately to cure and prevent mental illness.

TABLE C-2 Continued

Report	Recommendations

Workforce Education and Training

Bridging Disciplines in the Brain, Behavioral, and Clinical Sciences (IOM, 2000)

Recommendation 3 Scientific education at early career stages should be sufficiently broad to produce graduates who can understand essential components of other disciplines while receiving a solid grounding in one or more fields. Criteria for NIH-supported research training should include both breadth and depth of education. Funding mechanisms to support interdisciplinary training in appropriate fields should provide additional incentives to the universities and the trainees along the following lines:

- Through the NIH Medical Scientist Training Program, encourage participating universities to support MD/PhD programs in the social and behavioral, as well as biomedical, sciences. Although existing program language permits such graduate study, training in social and behavioral sciences (e.g., anthropology, economics, psychology, and sociology) is undertaken infrequently. NIH can highlight the need for such graduates and encourage grantees to recruit them.
- Promote translational research, an important aspect of interdisciplinary training by (1) providing clinical experience in PhD programs. This can range from support for single courses that expose students to human pathophysiology to training programs that require both basic research and clinical experience. (2) Supporting PhD programs and postdoctoral mentored career development awards for physicians, nurses, dentists, social workers, and other clinicians.
- Create partnerships with the private sector to develop and support interdisciplinary training. Many of today's students will enter private industry to do translational research. Others will go on to careers in teaching, publishing, science policy, science administration, or law. Interdisciplinary perspectives are as important to success in these careers as they are in research.
- Expand the T32 training grant awards to cover the full direct costs of implementation. This change will provide the resources necessary to support the greater expenses encountered in an interdisciplinary training program.

Recommendation 4 Funding agencies should establish a grant supplement program to foster interdisciplinary training and research. This would be administratively modeled after the supplements that exist for minorities, people with disabilities, and for people reentering research after a hiatus. Investigators with research grants who have interdisciplinary training opportunities should be able to obtain supplemental funds for qualified candidates through a relatively short application with expedited review. Successful pilot efforts will provide data to support further applications for career development and research.

continued

TABLE C-2 Continued

Report	Recommendations
	Recommendation 5 Funding opportunities for interdisciplinary training should be provided for scientists at all stages of their careers.

- Implement career development programs that encourage junior faculty to engage in interdisciplinary research. Junior faculty need to be successful in the early phases of their research, so they are less likely than senior faculty to pursue interdisciplinary research.
- Support midcareer investigators in developing expertise needed for interdisciplinary research. These programs should include sabbaticals, career development awards, and university-based, formal courses for faculty development to enhance interdisciplinary and/or translational research.
- Continue funding for workshops, symposia, and meetings to bring together diverse fields to focus on a particular scientific question. In such an environment, cross training of the investigators and encouragement of collaboration would develop naturally.
- Support consortia and multi-institutional programs that provide integration of research efforts from multiple disciplines.

Childhood Cancer Survivorship: Improving Care and Quality of Life (IOM and NRC, 2003)

Recommendation 4 Improve professional education and training regarding the late effects of childhood cancer and their management for both specialty and primary care providers.

- Professional societies should act to improve primary care providers' awareness through professional journals, meetings, and continuing education opportunities.
- Primary care training programs should include information about the late effects of cancer in their curriculum.
- The NCI should provide easy-to-find information on late effects of childhood cancer on its website (e.g., through the Physician Data Query [PDQ]), which provides up-to-date information on cancer prevention, treatment, and supportive care.
- Oncology training programs should organize coursework, clinical practicums, and continuing education programs on late effects of cancer treatment for nurses, social workers, and other providers.
- Oncology professional organizations should, if they have not already, organize committees or subcommittees dedicated to issues related to late effects.
- Oncology Board examinations should include questions related to late effects of cancer treatment.
- Interdisciplinary professional meetings that focus on the management of late effects should be supported to raise awareness of late effects among providers who may encounter childhood cancer survivors in their practices (cardiologists, neurologists, fertility specialists, psychologists).

TABLE C-2 Continued

Report	Recommendations
Achieving the Promise: Transforming Mental Health Care in America (New Freedom Commission on Mental Health, 2003)	**Recommendation 5.3** Improve and expand the workforce providing evidence-based mental health services and supports.

Palliative Care

Report	Recommendations
Improving Palliative Care for Cancer (IOM and NRC, 2001)	**Recommendation 1** The NCI should designate certain cancer centers, as well as some community cancer centers, as centers of excellence in symptom control and palliative care for both adults and children. The centers will deliver the best available care, as well as carrying out research, training, and treatment aimed at developing portable model programs that can be adopted by other cancer centers and hospitals. Activities should include but not be limited to the following: • formal testing and evaluation of new and existing practice guidelines for palliative and end-of-life care; • pilot testing "quality indicators" for assessing end-of-life care at the level of the patient and the institution; • incorporating the best palliative care into NCI-sponsored clinical trials; • innovating in the delivery of palliative and end-of-life care, including collaboration with local hospice organizations; • disseminating information about how to improve end-of-life care to other cancer centers and hospitals through a variety of media; • uncovering the determinants of disparities in access to care by minority populations that should be served by the center, and developing specific programs and initiatives to increase access; these might include educational activities for health care providers and the community, setting up outreach programs, etc.; . . . • providing in-service training for local hospice staff in new palliative care techniques. **Recommendation 5** Organizations that provide information about cancer treatment (NCI, the American Cancer Society, and other patient-oriented organizations [e.g., disease-specific groups], health insurers, and pharmaceutical companies) should revise their inventories of patient-oriented material, as appropriate, to provide comprehensive, accurate information about palliative care throughout the course of disease. Patients would also be helped by having reliable information on survival by type and stage of cancer easily accessible. Attention should be paid to cultural relevance and special populations (e.g., children).

continued

TABLE C-2 Continued

Report	Recommendations

Reimbursement

Improving Palliative Care for Cancer (IOM and NRC, 2001)	**Recommendation 4** Private insurers should provide adequate compensation for end-of-life care. The special circumstances of dying children—particularly the need for extended communication with children and parents, as well as health care team conferences—should be taken into account in setting reimbursement levels and in actually paying claims for these services when providers bill for them.

Research

Achieving the Promise: Transforming Mental Health Care in America (New Freedom Commission on Mental Health, 2003)	**Recommendation 5.4** Develop the knowledge base in four understudied areas: mental health disparities, long-term effect of medications, trauma, and acute care.

Public Health

From Cancer Patient to Cancer Survivor: Lost in Transition (IOM and NRC, 2006)	**Recommendation 6** Congress should support the CDC, other collaborating institutions, and the states in developing comprehensive cancer control plans that include consideration of survivorship care, and promoting the implementation, evaluation, and refinement of existing state cancer control plans.

Other

Crossing the Quality Chasm (IOM and NRC, 2001)	**Recommendation 1** All health care organizations, professional groups, and private and public purchasers should adopt as their explicit purpose to continually reduce the burden of illness, injury, and disability, and to improve the health and functioning of the people of the United States.
	Recommendation 2 All health care organizations, professional groups, and private and public purchasers should pursue six major aims; specifically, health care should be safe, effective, patient-centered, timely, efficient, and equitable.

TABLE C-2 Continued

Report	Recommendations
	Recommendation 4 Private and public purchasers, health care organizations, clinicians, and patients should work together to redesign health care processes in accordance with the following rules:

1. *Care based on continuous healing relationships.* Patients should receive care whenever they need it and in many forms, not just face-to-face visits. This rule implies that the health care system should be responsive at all times (24 hours a day, every day) and that access to care should be provided over the Internet, by telephone, and by other means in addition to face-to-face visits.

2. *Customization based on patient needs and values.* The system of care should be designed to meet the most common type of needs, but have the capability to respond to individual patient choices and preferences.

3. *The patient as the source of control.* Patients should be given the necessary information and the opportunity to exercise the degree of control they choose over health care decisions that affect them. The health system should be able to accommodate differences in patient preferences and encourage shared decision making.

4. *Shared knowledge and the free flow of information.* Patients should have unfettered access to their own medical information and to clinical knowledge. Clinicians and patients should communicate effectively and share information.

5. *Evidence-based decision making.* Patients should receive care based on the best available scientific knowledge. Care should not vary illogically from clinician to clinician or from place to place.

6. *Safety as a system property.* Patients should be safe from injury caused by the care system. Reducing risk and ensuring safety require greater attention to systems that help prevent and mitigate errors.

7. *The need for transparency.* The health care system should make information available to patients and their families that allows them to make informed decisions when selecting a health plan, hospital, or clinical practice, or when choosing among alternative treatments. This should include information describing the system's performance on safety, evidence-based practice, and patient satisfaction.

8. *Anticipation of needs.* The health system should anticipate patient needs rather than simply reacting to events.

9. *Continuous decrease in waste.* The health system should not waste resources or patient time.

10. *Cooperation among clinicians.* Clinicians and institutions should actively collaborate and communicate to ensure an appropriate exchange of information and coordination of care.

Recommendation 11 The Health Care Financing Administration and the Agency for Healthcare Research and Quality, with input from private payers, health care organizations, and clinicians, should develop a research agenda to identify, pilot test, and evaluate various options for better aligning current payment methods with quality improvement goals.

continued

TABLE C-2 Continued

Report	Recommendations
Childhood Cancer Survivorship: Improving Care and Quality of Life (IOM and NRC, 2003)	**Recommendation 5** HRSA's Maternal and Child Health Bureau and its partners should be fully supported in implementing the Healthy People 2010 goals for Children with Special Health Care Needs. These efforts include a national communication strategy, efforts at capacity building, setting standards, and establishing accountability. Meeting these goals will benefit survivors of childhood cancer and other children with special health care needs.
Achieving the Promise: Transforming Mental Health Care in America (New Freedom Commission on Mental Health, 2003)	**Recommendation 2.2** Involve consumers and families fully in orienting the mental health systems toward recovery. **Recommendation 4.2** Improve and expand school mental health programs.

REFERENCES

IOM (Institute of Medicine). 1999. *Ensuring quality cancer care.* Edited by M. Hewitt and J. V. Simone. Washington, DC: National Academy Press.

IOM. 2000. *Bridging disciplines in the brain, behavioral, and clinical sciences.* Edited by T. C. Pellmar and L. Eisenberg. Washington, DC: National Academy Press.

IOM. 2006. *Improving the quality of health care for mental and substance-use conditions.* Washington, DC: The National Academies Press.

IOM and NRC (National Research Council). 2000. *Enhancing data systems to improve the quality of cancer care.* Washington, DC: National Academy Press.

IOM and NRC. 2001. *Interpreting the volume-outcome relationship in the context of cancer care.* Washington, DC: National Academy Press.

IOM and NRC. 2001. *Improving palliative care for cancer.* Edited by K. M. Foley and H. Gelband. Washington, DC: National Academy Press.

IOM and NRC. 2001. *Crossing the quality chasm: A new health system for the 21st century.* Washington, DC: National Academy Press.

IOM and NRC. 2003. *Childhood cancer survivorship. Improving care and quality of life.* Edited by M. Hewitt, S. L. Weiner, and J. V. Simone. Washington, DC: The National Academies Press.

IOM and NRC. 2004. *Meeting psychosocial needs of women with breast cancer.* Edited by M. Hewitt, R. Herdman, and J. C. Holland. Washington, DC: The National Academies Press.

IOM and NRC. 2006. *From cancer patient to cancer survivor: Lost in transition.* Edited by M. Hewitt, S. Greenfield, and E. Stovall. Washington, DC: The National Academies Press.

National Breast Cancer Centre and National Cancer Control Initiative. 2003. *Clinical practice guidelines for the psychosocial care of adults with cancer.* http://www.nhmrc.gov.au/publications/synopses/_files/cp90.pdf.

NCCN (National Comprehensive Cancer Network). 2006. *Distress management—version 1.2007*. http://www.nccn.org/professionals/physician_gls/PDF/distress.pdf (accessed September 14, 2007).

New Freedom Commission on Mental Health. 2003. *Achieving the promise: Transforming mental health care in America. Final Report*. DHHS Publication No. SMA-03-3832. Rockville, MD: Department of Health and Human Services.

Pirl, W. F. 2004. Evidence report on the occurrence, assessment, and treatment of depression in cancer patients. *Journal of the National Cancer Institute Monographs* 32:32–39.

President's Cancer Panel. 2004. *Living beyond cancer: Finding a new balance*. President's Cancer Panel 2003–2004 annual report. Bethesda, MD: National Cancer Institute, National Institutes of Health, U.S. Department of Health and Human Services.

Index